Praise for *Reflective Practice,* Second Edition

"How we think about our practice and how we actually practice begin with how and what we teach. This beautifully written book explores in detail the essentials of mindful, caring, and intelligent nursing practice that is not only deeply satisfying to the patient but also enriching to the practitioner. Reflective nursing practice is a lifelong developmental quest. This book is *the* guide."

–*Pamela Klauer Triolo, PhD, RN, FAAN*
Novelist, Ghostwriter, Production Editor
Former Chief Nursing Executive, Senior Vice President, and Associate Dean
University of Pittsburgh Medical Center, Houston Methodist, and
University of Nebraska Medical Center

"Florence Nightingale once noted that in our nursing, unless we are making progress every year, every month, every week, we are going back. To make that progress, nurses must master the ability to assess and transform their own practice in a world in which knowledge and evidence are continuously expanding. In this second edition of *Reflective Practice*, Sara Horton-Deutsch and Gwen Sherwood spotlight the critical skill of reflection, a never-ending process that helps nurses critically question their assumptions, knowledge, and prior experiences in a manner that paves the way for progress through new knowledge creation, expanded self-awareness, and improved practice."

–*Beth Ulrich, EdD, RN, FACHE, FAAN*
Professor, University of Texas Health Science Center at Houston School of Nursing
Editor, Nephrology Nursing Journal

"This remarkable second edition needs to be in every clinician's repertoire of learnings. In a task-based, checklist-focused practice environment, having the skills, knowledge, and capacity to reflect, be intentional, and translate reflective practices in education and care delivery will assure the kind of care we all want to deliver. A must-read!"

–*Karen Drenkard, PhD, RN, NEA-BC, FAAN*
SVP/Chief Nurse and Chief Clinical Officer
O'Neil Center at GetWellNetwork

"After 46 years of nursing practice, I find it refreshing to be reminded and renewed by a deeper understanding of the value and meaning of caring. Sara Horton-Deutsch and Gwen Sherwood have done a masterful job of pulling together the many transformative elements of reflective practice and effectively integrating those elements with day-to-day practicalities associated with assuring high quality and safe patient care. Centering the work of the wide variety of chapter authors is the integrating theme that focuses on creating a culture of inquiry, reflective skills, self-awareness, and commitment to advance and improve the care of others. Capping concept exploration in each chapter is a concluding chapter exercise that provides an opportunity to 'breathe into' mindful presence and reflective praxis. What a dynamic and important book this is—an essential read for all who care for others."

–Tim Porter-O'Grady, DM, EdD, APRN, FAAN, FACCWS
Senior Partner, TPOG Associates Inc.
Professor of Practice and Leadership Scholar, The Ohio State University College of Nursing
Professor of Practice, Arizona State University College of Nursing and Health Innovation
Clinical Wound Specialist, Atlanta, Georgia

"The text awakens reader presence in subtle and powerful ways. Prepare to be enlightened."

–Laura Cox Dzurec, PhD, PMHCNS-BC, ANEF, FAAN
Dean and Professor
Widener University School of Nursing

"Building on the solid foundation of their first edition, Sara Horton-Deutsch and Gwen Sherwood have created an even more powerful tool for educators of all levels and types of students. Adding the insights of new authors, along with new frameworks and vignettes, they have given us a foundational resource for contemporary education. What struck me most, however, is that this edition also has great relevance to those of us interested in deepening our professional practice, regardless of our role. So many of the exercises and applications challenged my thinking and prompted me to try different approaches, such as guided reflection, coaching, active listening, using space, and employing Visual Thinking Strategies. Helping others learn, while expanding our own capacities for innovation and authenticity, offers something for all nurses."

–Joanne Disch, PhD, RN, FAAN
Professor ad Honorem, University of Minnesota School of Nursing
Board Chair, Chamberlain College of Nursing
Past President, American Academy of Nursing and American Association of Critical-Care Nurses

"Reading this book is a powerful experience that imparts a message of how to turn vison into action in professional practice. Each chapter provides examples of how to incorporate reflective practice techniques—from the use of journals to shared discourse, to critical analysis in conversation, to self-awareness, and to progress in acquiring true leadership capacity. This book informs nursing faculty in how to transform program curriculum for undergraduate and graduate students, building out the concepts of mindfulness, Caring Science, interdisciplinary practice, QSEN, and social justice. The authors encourage self-reflection as pivotal to the process of empowering interprofessional collaboration for health and healing and wholeness in a global society. This is a book for educators and students in the academic setting as well as for healthcare professionals in clinical practice who are dedicated to fostering transition to practice for new nurses and mentoring compassionate expert leadership while promoting best clinical outcomes for all patients."

–*Kathleen Shannon Dorcy, PhD, RN*
Director, Clinical/Nursing Research, Education and Practice, Seattle Cancer Care Alliance
Staff Scientist, Fred Hutchinson Cancer Research Center
Senior Lecturer, University of Washington Tacoma

"The urgency of teaching, learning, and using reflective practice continues to grow as social and healthcare ecosystems become more complex and uncertain. This book contains specific applications of reflective thinking and learning that translate easily into multiple learning environments and situations, including simulation and interprofessional education. The authors have done an outstanding job of coalescing information from multiple sources and frameworks into an inspiring and useful guide for elevating practice through reflection."

–*Teri Pipe, PhD, RN*
Chief Well-Being Officer
Dean and Professor, College of Nursing and Health Innovation, Arizona State University

"This book is a guide for nurses at every step along a journey of growth and transformation. It is for that person who courageously chooses the unique caring role of nursing. It challenges traditional ways of teaching, learning, and practicing the art and science of nursing and offers healing and hope for delivery of safe, quality care within the backdrop of rapidly changing technology."

–*Beverly Malone, PhD, RN, FAAN*
Chief Executive Officer, National League for Nursing

"The second edition of *Reflective Practice* takes readers into new dimensions to expand and deepen meanings of reflective practice, offering us a more grounded understanding for living out reflective practice. This understanding includes translating the knowledge and process into our personal and professional lifeworld. The book makes new connections between Caring Science philosophy and congruence with reflective practice—guiding educators, administrators, and practitioners alike into new space for revisiting the relevance and foundation of reflective practice. This edition invites any level of student or scholar-educator to engage in and learn more about teaching-learning, moving from political to personal, integrating full emotional self toward reflectively informed moral actions in our daily life—a lasting gift."

–Jean Watson, PhD, RN, AHN-BC, FAAN
Founder/Director, Watson Caring Science Institute
Distinguished Professor and Dean Emerita, University of Colorado Denver

"With our gift of reflection and the ability to dive deeply within ourselves and our practice, we can continually disrupt our thinking and improve. As leaders, educators, and front-line clinicians, we owe it to our patients and our peers to continually improve our outcomes by practicing by choice, not chance—that comes only with reflective practice. This book is an excellent scientific and experiential guide to the art and science of reflective practice."

–Karlene M. Kerfoot, PhD, RN, FAAN
Chief Nursing Officer
Workforce Management Solutions
Healthcare IT, GE Healthcare

Reflective Practice
SECOND EDITION
Transforming Education and Improving Outcomes

Sara Horton-Deutsch, PhD, RN, FAAN, ANEF
Gwen D. Sherwood, PhD, RN, FAAN, ANEF

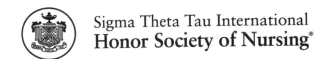

Sigma Theta Tau International
Honor Society of Nursing®

The Honor Society of Nursing, Sigma Theta Tau International (STTI) is a nonprofit organization whose mission is advancing world health and celebrating nursing excellence in scholarship, leadership, and service. Founded in 1922, STTI has more than 135,000 active members in over 90 countries and territories. Members include practicing nurses, instructors, researchers, policymakers, entrepreneurs, and others. STTI's 520 chapters are located at more than 700 institutions of higher education throughout Armenia, Australia, Botswana, Brazil, Canada, Colombia, England, Ghana, Hong Kong, Japan, Jordan, Kenya, Lebanon, Malawi, Mexico, the Netherlands, Pakistan, Philippines, Portugal, Singapore, South Africa, South Korea, Swaziland, Sweden, Taiwan, Tanzania, Thailand, the United States, and Wales. Learn more at www.nursingsociety.org.

Sigma Theta Tau International
550 West North Street
Indianapolis, IN, USA 46202

To order additional books, buy in bulk, or order for corporate use, contact Nursing Knowledge International at 888. NKI.4YOU (888.654.4968/US and Canada) or +1.317.634.8171 (outside US and Canada).

To request a review copy for course adoption, email solutions@nursingknowledge.org or call 888.NKI.4YOU (888.654.4968/US and Canada) or +1.317.634.8171 (outside US and Canada).

To request author information, or for speaker or other media requests, contact Marketing, Honor Society of Nursing, Sigma Theta Tau International at 888.634.7575 (US and Canada) or +1.317.634.8171 (outside US and Canada).

ISBN: 9781945157134
EPUB ISBN: 9781945157141
PDF ISBN: 9781945157158
MOBI ISBN: 9781945157165

Library of Congress Cataloging-in-Publication Data

Names: Sherwood, Gwen, author. | Horton-Deutsch, Sara, author. | Sigma Theta Tau International, issuing body.

Title: Reflective practice : transforming education and improving outcomes / Sara Horton-Deutsch, Gwen Sherwood.

Description: Second edition. | Indianapolis, IN : Sigma Theta Tau International, [2017] | Sherwood's name appears first on the previous edition. | Includes bibliographical references.

Identifiers: LCCN 2017018228 (print) | LCCN 2017018976 (ebook) | ISBN 9781945157141 (Epub) | ISBN 9781945157158 (Pdf) | ISBN 9781945157165 (Mobi) | ISBN 9781945157134 (print : alk. paper)

Subjects: | MESH: Nursing | Creativity | Education, Nursing | Nursing Process | Philosophy, Nursing | Thinking

Classification: LCC RT82 (ebook) | LCC RT82 (print) | NLM WY 16.1 | DDC 610.73--dc23

LC record available at https://lccn.loc.gov/2017018228

First Printing, 2017

Publisher: Dustin Sullivan
Acquisitions Editor: Emily Hatch
Editorial Coordinator: Paula Jeffers
Cover Designer: Rebecca Batchelor
Interior Design/Page Layout: Katy Bodenmiller

Principal Book Editor: Carla Hall
Development and Project Editor: Kezia Endsley
Copy Editor: Erin Geile
Proofreader: Todd Lothery
Indexer: Cheryl Lenser

Dedication

We dedicate this book to our fellow educators and learners who continuously strive for wisdom and personal meaning through reflective and mindful practices that encourage openness, authenticity, compassion, and care for self and others.

Acknowledgments

This book owes its existence to the wisdom and contributions of reflective practitioners and educators, past and present, who daily set an example for those around them, and to the current generation of learners that inspires us to bring presence and reflectivity to practice. We are the sum of our experiences, and this book honors those who have offered us the encouragement, the space, and the confidence to improve our work through reflection—family, friends, teachers, mentors, and coaches.

We also wish to acknowledge and thank those at Sigma Theta Tau International for their creative ideas and commitment to this project as they patiently guided us—Dustin Sullivan, Emily Hatch, Carla Hall, and Paula Jeffers. Thanks also to Katy Bodenmiller for her elegant interior book design and to the sales and marketing teams for all their support, now and in the future, in making this book successful.

About the Authors
Sara Horton-Deutsch

Sara Horton-Deutsch, PhD, RN, FAAN, ANEF, is a Caritas Coach, professor, and the Jean Watson Caring Science Endowed Chair at the University of Colorado College of Nursing. She serves as the director of the University of Colorado College of Nursing Watson Caring Science center with the mission of advancing the art and science of human caring knowledge, ethics, and clinical practice in the fields of nursing and health sciences. The center fosters research, teaching, and practice of human caring through an interprofessional PhD program track and continuing education training programs integrating new knowledge from humanities, arts, cross-cultural spiritual disciplines, and emerging scientific disciplines. In 2015, she also was appointed as an assistant director in the Center for Bioethics and Humanities at the University of Colorado- Denver, which brings together colleagues from across the campus, university, state, and nation to support competent, compassionate, and respectful healthcare through teaching, research, clinical service, and community engagement.

Her work in reflective practice has been published in two co-edited books with Dr. Sherwood: *Reflective Practice: Transforming Education and Improving Outcomes* (2012) and *Reflective Organizations: On the Front Lines of QSEN & Reflective Practice Implementation* (2015). The second was recently recognized as an *AJN* Book of the Year. Clinical nurses and academic programs around the world use the scholarly contributions found in these books to support deep learning—learning that leads to intentional, effective, and thoughtful action. It was through the iterative process of reflection that Horton-Deutsch deepened her own work in reflective practice, resulting in the integration of Caring Science. Like reflective practice, Caring Science calls healthcare professions to action—actions that honor all living things—to health, healing, and wholeness.

Horton-Deutsch has been an active participant in the Quality and Safety Education for Nurses (QSEN) initiative, contributing to the publication of web-based teaching modules on mindfulness, narrative and reflective pedagogies, and cultural equity and inclusion. In 2012, she co-edited a special issue of the *Archives of Psychiatric Nursing*, applying the QSEN competencies to mental health nursing education.

She continues to influence the scholarship and teaching-learning mind-set of nurse educators around the world through her scholarly publications; international, national, and regional presentations; leadership in Caring Science; and service to the profession. Horton-Deutsch currently serves as a leadership mentor in the Nurse Faculty Leadership Academy through Sigma Theta Tau International.

Gwen D. Sherwood

Gwen D. Sherwood, PhD, RN, FAAN, ANEF, has a distinguished record in advancing nursing education locally and globally. She is professor and Associate Dean for Practice and Global Initiatives at the University of North Carolina (UNC) at Chapel Hill's School of Nursing. An expert in teamwork and interprofessional education, her work focuses on transforming healthcare environments by expanding relational capacity of healthcare providers. Her work examining patient satisfaction with pain management outcomes, the spiritual dimensions of care, and teamwork as a variable in patient safety spans education and practice.

Sherwood has been in the vanguard of educators integrating quality and safety in health professions education. She was co-investigator for the award-winning Robert Wood Johnson Foundation–funded Quality and Safety Education for Nurses (QSEN) project to transform education and practice to prepare nurses to work in and lead quality and safety in redesigned healthcare systems. The QSEN Steering Team received the Honor Society of Nursing, Sigma Theta Tau International Nursing Media Award, and its website (www.qsen.org) received the Information Technology Award.

Sherwood was co-investigator for the UNC-Chapel Hill and Duke University Interprofessional Patient Safety Education Collaborative to measure the effectiveness of teaching modalities for interdisciplinary teamwork training for nursing and medical students. She worked with patient safety leaders at the University of Illinois at Chicago School of Medicine who established the Telluride Science Research Institute Roundtable on Redesigning Health Professions Education to improve patient safety, now the Academy for Emerging Leaders in Patient Safety, and was adjunct faculty in the Master of Science in Patient Safety Leadership program.

Her professional service includes the Research Committee of the National Patient Safety Foundation, the Technical Expert Panel of TeamSTEPPS, the QSEN Advisory Board, and past president of the International Association for Human Caring. She is currently faculty for the STTI/Elsevier Nurse Faculty Leadership Academy and advisor for the Technical Expert Panel for the Patient Centered Care AHRQ Task Order at MedStar Health.

Sherwood's distinguished service to the Honor Society of Nursing, Sigma Theta Tau International includes distinguished lecturer, Virginia Henderson fellow, chair of the global task force for the Scholarship of Reflective Practice position paper, and vice president of the board of directors. She chaired the Research Scholarship Advisory Council and speaks frequently for chapters around the world. Her hospital research team received the 2001 Regional Research Utilization Award for implementing relationship-centered care.

Her work bridges U.S. and global organizations to expand nursing undergraduate and graduate education capacity to serve developing regions. Formerly Executive Associate Dean at the University of Texas Health Science Center at Houston's School of Nursing, she bridged academia and practice through a joint appointment as co-director of the Center for Professional Excellence at The Methodist Hospital. She led numerous educational outreach programs in developing areas both on the Texas-Mexico border and around the world. A global ambassador for nursing, she has worked with nurse educators in Kazakhstan, Sakhalin, Macau, Thailand, Taiwan, and Kenya, and helped lead the nursing education renaissance in China. Widely published, she is co-editor of three other books, *International Textbook of Reflective Practice in Nursing*, *Quality and Safety in Nursing: A Competency Approach to Improve Outcomes* (*AJN* Book of the Year), and *Reflective Organizations: On the Front Lines of QSEN & Reflective Practice Implementation* (second place *AJN* Book of the Year). Among many honors, she was awarded Outstanding Alumnus at Georgia Baptist College of Nursing and the University of Texas at Austin, the Special Award for International Interprofessional Education from the Prince Mahidol Conference, and Outstanding Educator Texas Nursing Association District 9.

About the Contributors

Kathryn R. Alden, EdD, MSN, RN, IBCLC, is a clinical associate professor at the University of North Carolina at Chapel Hill School of Nursing, where she serves as course coordinator for maternal/newborn nursing and as the lead academic counselor for undergraduate students. During her 30 years as a nursing educator, Alden has received numerous awards from her students for teaching excellence. She is co-editor for a leading maternity and women's health textbook, *Maternity and Women's Health Care* (10th ed.), and associate editor for *Maternity Nursing* (8th ed.). Alden was an early adopter of simulation and has been instrumental in the integration of human patient simulation into the nursing program at UNC. She has authored obstetrical simulations for Elsevier's Simulation Learning System as well as several chapters on the use of simulation in nursing education and other topics. Her research focuses on promoting academic success and retention in undergraduate nursing students. Alden is a certified lactation consultant who teaches prenatal breastfeeding classes to expectant parents and provides continuing education on breastfeeding to nurses and other lactation consultants.

Gail Armstrong, PhD, DNP, RN, ACNS-BC, CNE, is an associate professor at the University of Colorado in the College of Nursing where she has been on faculty since 2000. Gail's work in reflective practice stems from her previous work in literature and illness narratives. Gail's work in quality and safety began and continues in the national initiative, Quality and Safety Education for Nurses (QSEN). Currently Gail is on faculty with the Institute for Healthcare Quality, Safety and Efficiency Certificate Training Program on the Anschutz Medical Campus. This 12-month training program trains interprofessional clinical teams in the areas of systems leadership, process improvement, and patient safety. Gail's current scholarship focuses on the updating of quality and safety curricula in nursing education, updated concepts of safety, and interprofessional collaboration on healthcare teams.

Kathleen Beck-Coon, MD, is a certified MBSR teacher and currently dedicates her efforts in mindfulness-related teaching and research. Her research interests through the Indiana University Schools of Nursing and Medicine are mindfulness-based interventions in cancer survivors, end-of-life communication, educational pedagogy, and evaluating how mindfulness-based modalities open healing for both caregivers and those they serve. She is director of mindfulness at the center, involved with CompleteLife at the IU Simon Cancer Center, and has been teaching Mindfulness-Based Stress Reduction and Interpersonal Mindfulness Practice at Indianapolis hospitals and universities for 13 years.

Chantal Cara, PhD, RN, is currently a full professor on the Faculty of Nursing, Université de Montréal in Québec, Canada. She earned her PhD from the University of Colorado School of Nursing, under the directorship of Dr. Jean Watson. For almost 30 years, Cara has been actively involved in the understanding of the philosophy of caring in nursing, more specifically in clinical rehabilitation, education, management, and research. She is a researcher at the Centre for Interdisciplinary Research in Rehabilitation (CRIR) of Greater Montreal as well as the Quebec Network on Nursing Intervention Research for humanistic nursing practices, Quebec, Canada. Recently, she was awarded the honorific title *Distinguished Caring Science Scholar* by the Watson Caring Science Institute, Colorado, USA.

Andy Davies, PhD, MEd, has been a nursing educator for 2 decades in hospitals and universities in Australia, Saudi Arabia, and Qatar. He is a keen advocate of using transphilosophical lenses to reexamine and appreciate the many ways of knowing, being, and caring. His extensive health and health education experience has deeply influenced his understanding and pedagogical application of yoga and meditation teaching. His broad yoga and meditation teaching experience has nurtured how he perceives nursing, nursing education, and nursing care models of delivery. He has co-authored two educational research books with Palgrave Pivot—*Contemporary Capacity-Building in Educational Contexts* and *Educational Learning and Development: Building and Enhancing Capacity*. He has co-edited two educational research books: with Cambridge Scholars—*Publishing Metaphors for, in and of Education Research*, and with Sense Publishers—*Echoes: Ethics and Issues of Voice in Education Research*. He is interested in the many intersections of Caring Science, yoga, meditation teaching, and nursing education.

Kristina Thomas Dreifuerst, PhD, RN, CNE, ANEF, is an associate professor at Marquette University College of Nursing in Milwaukee, Wisconsin. Her research is at the forefront of disciplinary efforts to develop, use, and test innovative teaching methods to improve students' clinical reasoning skills. Her work also investigates how teachers can best be prepared to use evidence-based methods, including simulation and debriefing, to enhance clinical teaching. She is best known for *Debriefing for Meaningful Learning* or DML, an evidence-based and theory-based debriefing method she developed which has been adopted by schools of nursing and interdisciplinary schools in health sciences across the US, Canada, Australia, China, and the United Kingdom. DML is being successfully used in clinical and simulation settings as well across the curriculum in all teaching and learning environments. Dreifuerst is the recipient of numerous national and international awards recognizing the contribution of her research to the field.

Barbara L. Drew, PhD, RN, PMHCNS, is an associate professor and coordinator of the Psychiatric Mental Health (PMH) Nurse Practitioner concentration at the College of Nursing, Kent State University and teaches PMH nursing. Barbara is past president of the American Psychiatric Nurses Association (APNA). She also received recognition from APNA as the Psychiatric Nurse of the Year in 2011. Her research interests are suicide prevention, self-management of mood disorder symptoms by adolescents and young adults, the use of self-care strategies to promote mental health, as well as PMH nursing workforce issues.

Carol F. Durham, EdD, MSN, RN, ANEF, FAAN, is a professor and director of the Education-Innovation-Simulation Learning Environment at the University of North Carolina at Chapel Hill School of Nursing. She is a visionary educator and consultant with expertise in practice-based education for all levels of nursing. As a member of the RWJF's Quality and Safety Education for Nurses (QSEN) project, Carol has developed simulation-based educational experiences that reflect cutting-edge pedagogy. Durham has made significant and sustained contributions in interprofessional education and is a leader in preparing faculty to integrate quality and safety into their curriculum and their teaching in the preparation of the next generation of reflective healthcare providers. She uses innovative strategies such as Friday Night at the ER to demonstrate the system of care in which health professionals influence outcomes, and to uncover bias and behaviors that affect quality in patient care.

Jamie Evancio, MEd, BN, RN, is a Caritas Coach and nursing instructor with Assiniboine Community College (ACC) in Winnipeg, Canada. She started her career working in trauma surgery at Health Sciences Centre, Winnipeg and moved to home care for the Victorian Order of Nurses. After moving to Alberta, Jamie lectured in community health at University of Alberta (returning RN program) and worked in an urban public health clinic. Jamie has also held positions working with school-aged community clients and with high-priority parenting teens in Vancouver, British Columbia. Before moving to ACC, Jamie taught for several years in the BN program at University of Manitoba. Jamie holds a master of education degree from U of M specializing in the area of post-secondary education. She has an interest in experiential learning and in helping students to enrich their practice through Caring Science. When not working with students, Jamie can be found with her family, enjoying the gifts of nature.

Jasmine Graw, MSN, RN, CPNP, is a certified pediatric nurse practitioner and PhD candidate with a focus area in children's health and asthma at the University of Texas Health Science Center at San Antonio. Currently, she is providing clinical experience to students in the Childbearing Family Course in the hospital and community setting by incorporating service learning and caring in the nursing curriculum. She helps students merge the knowledge of providing acute and preventative nursing care to improve the quality of nursing care provided. In addition to teaching, she is also researching ways to improve nursing care and practice through a systems theory and social justice perspective for the childbearing family in her PhD program.

Cheryl Woods Giscombe, PhD, RN, PNMNP-BC, is the Melissa and Harry LeVine Family Distinguished Associate Professor of Quality of Life, Health Promotion and Wellness at the UNC Chapel Hill School of Nursing; she has a secondary appointment in the UNC Department of Social Medicine and serves as faculty for the Harvard Macy Institute for Health Professions Educators. Her research focuses on reducing biopsychosocial stress-related health disparities and the benefits of mindfulness meditation. She is also the leader of a wellness initiative for nursing professionals, coordinator for the UNC Psychiatric Nurse Practitioner Program, and the co-director of the Mindfulness and Self-Compassion for Caring Professions course, which enrolls nursing and medical students. She has received numerous honors including designation as a "Leader in the Field" by the American Psychological Association and a Brilliant New Scholar by the Council for the Advancement of Nursing Science. She publishes broadly in nursing, psychology, and interdisciplinary journals.

Marie Hayden-Miles, PhD, RN, CNE, is the former dean of the Theresa Patnode Santmann School of Health Sciences at Farmingdale State College of New York. She has been working with narrative pedagogy for many years and has presented on this topic at regional, national, and international conferences. Hayden-Miles previously served as site director for the Narrative Pedagogy Project at Farmingdale State College. This project brings together faculty from all over the world to explore how to reform courses and curricula in an effort to improve educators.

Pamela Ironside, PhD, RN, FAAN, ANEF, recently retired from Indiana University where she served as a professor and Director of the Center for Research in Nursing Education. Over the past 2 decades, her research investigated the ways new pedagogies influence the practices of thinking in nursing classrooms and clinical courses and the ways students' interactions with faculty and preceptors during clinical experiences foster thinking and learning. She was a member of the National Advisory Council for Evaluating Innovations in Nursing and co-director of the National Nursing Education Research Network project, both funded by the Robert Wood Johnson Foundation. She is the recipient of the Excellence in Nursing Education Research Award from the National League for Nursing, the Scholarship of Teaching and Learning Excellence Award from the American Association of Colleges of Nursing, and the Chancellor's Award for Excellence in Teaching at Indiana University–Purdue University Indianapolis.

Kristen Lombard, PhD, RN, PMHCNS-BC, is a CHCM consultant and co-leader of the *Re-Igniting the Spirit of Caring* service line. She has specialized in psychiatric-mental health nursing, gerontological nursing, Relationship-Based Care, and holistic and integrative care over her 35-year career. She developed her skills in transformational leadership in consultant, clinical nurse specialist, director, nurse manager, clinician, and program developer roles in hospital, long-term care, and home care settings; private practice; and ASN/BSN/MSN education. She has expertise in teaching about Relationship-Based Care, the therapeutic relationship, circle practice, and mindfulness and integrative practices. She is an advanced practitioner of meditation and circle practice, a Certified Healing Touch practitioner, a Therapeutic Touch practitioner, and a Reiki Master. She is author or co-author of many scholarly articles and book chapters, including "The Circle Way to Authentic Leadership" and "Relationship-Based Care and Meaningful Recognition: A Formula for Success in Long Term and Sub-acute Care."

Keith McCandless, MMHS, is the co-author of *The Surprising Power of Liberating Structures—Simple Rules to Unleash a Culture of Innovation.* In a diverse array of public and private organizations, Keith helps people take on complex challenges and innovation efforts. He has guided the launch of health and business innovation initiatives in Latin America, Europe, Canada, and the US. Keith specializes in unleashing everyone to work at the top of their collective intelligence and imagination. He calls himself a *structured improvisationalist.* Born in Cincinnati, Ohio, he holds a masters in management of human services from Brandeis University in Boston and a BA from Evergreen State College in Olympia, Washington. He lives in Seattle with his wife and Deacon, a whippet with talent to amuse.

Angela McNelis, PhD, RN, FAAN, ANEF, CNE, is at the forefront of national efforts to transform clinical nursing education so that new nurse graduates, from entry to advanced levels, are better prepared to provide high-quality and safe patient care. She has systematically established a body of work that now informs new models of clinical teaching and best practices that are currently improving nursing education. Through sustained funding, her scholarship and research has focused on: exploring and developing models to improve clinical and didactic education in undergraduate and graduate programs; increasing the number and diversity of advanced practice psychiatric mental health nursing students and graduates; improving the practice skills of advanced practice nurses and social workers to screen and intervene with clients who have substance use disorders; increasing the prevalence and rigor of interprofessional education; and exploring and developing programs and curricula to increase the number of well-prepared faculty in schools of nursing nationally.

Meg Moorman, PhD, RN, WHNP-BC, is a clinical assistant professor at Indiana University School of Nursing and coordinator of the MSN in Nursing Education program. Her research is based on the use of Visual Thinking Strategies and art in nursing education. She has presented her work at both the national and international levels. She teaches undergraduate and graduate students in the BSN and MSN in Nursing Education programs on the Indianapolis campus. She has been a women's health nurse practitioner for 20 years and an RN for 30 years with a focus on women's health and obstetrics.

Michael Moran, DHA, ACC, LFACHE, is an educator and executive coach who specializes in leadership development in healthcare. Michael has an advanced certification as a personal and executive coach through the College of Executive Coaches and is certified to administer and interpret the EQi-2.0 assessment of emotional intelligence, a highly respected and sophisticated tool for evaluating 15 different skills that make up our emotional intelligence. As an educator, Michael helps learners develop skills to learn from their experiences, identify and overcome barriers, and make choices that support their long-term goals. His teaching approach utilizes evidence-based coaching tools such as emotional intelligence, motivational and adult learning theory, Appreciative Inquiry, and positive psychology. Michael has over 30 years of executive experience in acute care hospitals. He holds master's degrees in counseling and health administration and recently completed a doctorate degree in health administration. His doctoral dissertation focused on managerial coaching in the workplace.

Pamela O'Haver Day, APRN, PMHCNS-BC, is a full-time practitioner at Indiana University Health Physicians Behavioral Health, an interdisciplinary psychiatric group practice. She utilizes mindfulness approaches with traditional psychopharmacological and psychotherapeutic interventions in the care of individuals and families.

Daniel J. Pesut, PhD, RN, FAAN, is the director of the Katharine J. Densford International Center for Nursing Leadership at the University of Minnesota School of Nursing, and professor of nursing, Population Health and Systems Co-operative Unit. He holds the Katherine R. and C. Walton Lillehei Nursing Leadership Chair. Pesut served on the board of directors of the Honor Society of Nursing, Sigma Theta Tau International for 8 years and as president of the Honor Society of Nursing (2003–2005). He is a fellow in the American Academy of Nursing and a board-certified clinical nurse specialist in adult psychiatric mental health nursing, as well as a Certified Hudson Institute coach. He is an award-winning master teacher. He is a popular author and speaks frequently on a number of topics including creative and futures thinking, clinical reasoning, leadership development, and interprofessional health professions education.

Rhonda Schwindt, DNP, RN, PMHNP/CNS-BC, is an assistant professor with the George Washington University School of Nursing and director of the Psychiatric/Mental Health Nurse Practitioner program. Schwindt is an ANCC certified psychiatric/mental health clinical nurse specialist and nurse practitioner with extensive experience as a nurse educator. Prior to joining the faculty at George Washington University, Schwindt taught at the Indiana University School of Nursing, Indianapolis. Her research focus is on reducing the disproportionate impact of tobacco use among high-risk populations. Schwindt has developed innovative online educational models to teach healthcare professionals an interprofessional, collaborative approach to care for persons with mental illness and co-occurring substance use disorders and has presented her work at national and international conferences.

Sharon L. Sims, PhD, RN, FAANP, is a professor emerita in the Indiana University School of Nursing. She was a nurse educator for 30 years prior to retirement in 2013. In collaboration with Dr. Melinda Swenson, she developed a narrative-centered curriculum for family nurse practitioners at IU. They have published extensively on this topic. Also with Swenson, she developed and implemented the Self-Evaluation~Peer Evaluation process. She is a fellow in the American Academy of Nurse Practitioners. Sims is also a pediatric nurse practitioner and currently works in a large pediatric practice in Indianapolis. She has also worked with Keith McCandless and has used Liberating Structures in a variety of settings.

Laura Sisk, DNP, RN, is an assistant professor at the University of Texas Health Science Center at San Antonio in the School of Nursing. She serves as the course coordinator for the Care of the Childbearing Family Clinical Course and co-clinical coordinator for the Family Nursing Course. She has extensive experience in maternal child nursing with expertise in obstetric and neonatal nursing. Laura implemented a Student-Led Pregnancy and Parenting Program for Teen Mothers. As the lead faculty on this project, she used her love for community and maternal child nursing as the inspiration for this program. Additionally, she integrated the Service Learning Education Model—along with the art of reflection and human caring—into this project, contributing to the program's success and impact on social justice and health promotion. She recently obtained her doctorate of nursing practice (DNP) degree, in which she focused on nursing education and leadership with a focus on integrating service-learning into nursing education.

Melinda M. Swenson, PhD, RN, FNP, FAANP, was a teacher of nurse practitioners and PhD nurses at Indiana University for 32 years, before her retirement in 2012. She continues clinical practice in college health and volunteer clinic settings. Along with Sharon Sims, she developed the narrative-centered curriculum at Indiana University, used in the Family Nurse Practitioner MSN program for nearly 20 years. This approach to teaching and learning focuses on clinical stories, on listening to the narratives of patients and clinicians, and on the family as the unit of care. She learned about Appreciative Inquiry and Liberating Structures from Keith McCandless and used these strategies in work with faculty and staff at IU, as well as in workshops and national presentations.

Dawn Vanderhoef, PhD, DNP, PMHNP-BC, FAANP, is board certified as a psychiatric mental health nurse practitioner (PMHNP) with over 16 years' experience as an APRN. Her current practice and research interests include working with persons diagnosed with a severe mental illness (SMI), cardiometabolic side effects from antipsychotic medication, and integrated care models. In addition to her role as the PMHNP Academic Director at Vanderbilt University School of Nursing, she has an active practice working at VUMC in the outpatient psychosis clinic. She is an active member of the American Psychiatric Nurses Association (APNA), National Organization of Nurse Practitioner Faculties (NONPF), Neuroscience Education Institute (NEI), and American

Academy of Nurse Practitioners (AANP) and was inducted as a fellow in 2016. Her passions include clinical education and preparing practice-ready PMHNPs. Her work has been recognized by a variety of organizations, most recently by APNA as the recipient of the Award in Education 2015.

Robin R. Walter, PhD, RN, CNE, is an assistant professor in the Doctoral Nursing program of the College of Nursing and Health Sciences at Barry University. She is a nurse educator with expertise in health and public policy, committed to developing nurses as leaders in policy advocacy and as social justice allies. Her research on health disparities is anchored in understanding and exposing how unearned social privilege influences policy at state, national, and global levels. Her work advocates for system change to promote population health and well-being for marginalized, stigmatized, and at-risk groups locally, nationally, and worldwide. She has received grant funding to implement a statewide leadership development program preparing nurse leaders in Florida with a range of skills related to influencing health and public policy. She completed her undergraduate nursing education at Towson University, her graduate education in nursing and health policy at the University of Maryland, and her PhD in nursing at Barry University.

Table of Contents

Foreword

Nursing practice is both a science and an art informed by many disciplines, requiring both emotional and scientific knowledge and skill sets. Whilst patient care has become extensive and far-reaching, with increasingly complex technological interventions, the act of caring has always been a human endeavor.

The provocative and thoughtful chapters in the second edition of this text remind us that, in these deeply interactive processes of caring, there is an expectation that the person delivering care will be both professional and deeply engaged. Generally, this expectation has been accepted by patients, carers, practitioners, and their employees. However, one might question the degree to which it is human to have such high expectations of those who, at times, feel so undervalued by their employers, politicians, commissioners, and, unfortunately, by their own colleagues.

The second edition of *Reflective Practice: Transforming Education and Improving Outcomes* has an underlying narrative running through the carefully constructed chapters that points to the question of what it is to be a nurse in the current context of deeply perplexing and, at times, bewildering global challenges. But also fundamentally related is the existential question of what it is to be human in these contested times. Compassion, which is described as the emotional state of feeling pity for one who suffers—that is, to feel with—is both revered and maligned in the context of contemporary nursing practices. It is also poorly addressed in nursing curricula.

As Stickley and Freshwater (in press) note, offering human qualities such as compassion to complete strangers is a remarkable phenomenon. The expectation that healthcare professionals do this all the time is worthy of deep reflection during the education and development of practitioners, whether they be novice or expert. The concept of compassion fatigue is well-rehearsed in the literature relating to healthcare professionals. Loss of one's ability to nurture, experiences of physical and emotional weariness, chronic fatigue, and complacency have all been examined in the context of the emotional caregiving required of practitioners and have led to wide-ranging discussions around the impact of compassion fatigue.

As this text points out, albeit indirectly, financial cuts in public services make compassion and consumerism uncomfortable bedfellows. This political and economic environment is not clearly understood in nursing practice, and yet it begs this question: Does society have a right to receive compassion from healthcare professionals when it is not fulfilling its responsibility to provide adequate funding and resources for those very professionals to fulfill the moral obligation to provide compassion? It is imperative that we, like the authors of this text, continue to apply a critical and reflective lens to such questions and concepts as we seek to sustain and maintain the essence of nursing and nursing care—the light that is passed on.

I would like to suggest a call to action as you—academics, educators, researchers, and practitioners who employ and enjoy the beauty of pluralistic kaleidoscopes—read this text. How can we ensure that we continue to apply a critical evaluative and reflective lens to our tendencies toward formulaic and algorithmic thinking around the future of practice, education, and research in nursing? That kind of thinking treats people and professionals as numbers and treats practices as formulas to be metricized.

Reflecting on the work of moral philosopher Charles Taylor, I suggest that we would do well to care deeply for our own values whilst continually (and relentlessly) subjecting them to scrutiny and interrogation. In other words, we should take a reflexive stance that applies a rational, objective, technical lens—as well as an emotional, subjective, professional lens—to the subject for which we have both compassion and a deep passion.

–Dawn Freshwater, PhD, BA(Hons), RN, RNT, FRCN
Vice-Chancellor, University of Western Australia

Reference

Stickley, T., & Freshwater, D. (in press). An introduction to emotional intelligence. Wiley Blackwell.

Introduction

Similarly to when the first edition of this text was published in 2012, we continue to see multiple forces converging to influence nursing education and practice. The eye-opening reports on healthcare quality and safety from the Institute of Medicine (IOM) *Quality Chasm* series revealed serious gaps in patient care outcomes and fueled a debate on changes required in healthcare education. The 2010 IOM report, *The Future of Nursing*, outlined a transformative path for nurses to help lead healthcare quality. These reports remain relevant beside innovations in the sciences and the social contexts of human understanding, advances in technology and treatments, new pharmacology that prolongs lives, and radical and seemingly endless changes in healthcare payment systems that continue to act as forces of change.

The ongoing convergence of these forces makes it clear that to improve healthcare quality, we must be responsible for changing how we prepare those who deliver patient care. Patricia Benner, long a champion for advancing nursing, led a Carnegie report that gave voice to the need for an educational renaissance to transform nursing through innovative approaches to nursing education, to develop the nursing skill set to take advantage of this opportune time and respond to the melding of market forces (Benner, Sutphen, Leonard, & Day, 2010).

Reflective Practice: Transforming Education, Transforming Practice

In the recently published *The Power of Ten: A Conversational Approach to Tackling the Top Ten Priorities in Nursing* (Hassmiller & Mensik, 2016), Chow (pp. 4–8) and Young (pp. 9–14) call for nurse educators to prepare learners to continually refine their practice to integrate new knowledge and technology. In response, the second edition of this book, *Reflective Practice: Transforming Education and Improving Outcomes*, offers educators and learners an expanded path to transform nursing education and practice to help guide healthcare and academic institutions, focusing on new and expanding models and paradigms of quality and safety that incorporate new knowledge, technology, and lifelong learning.

The emotional labor of nursing takes a demanding toll on nurses as they cope with workforce issues, increasingly complex patients, and the impact of human factors. Still, for the vast majority of nursing programs, little is incorporated into nursing education to help nurses with compassion fatigue, the demands of working with multiple providers across multiple settings, and increasingly complex workplace issues that deplete energy and motivation. Nursing is a value-based profession; the motivation to make a difference in the lives of people is a chief reason nurses enter the profession. When work is counter to values, nurses are disenfranchised and become disengaged, and work becomes rote, cynical attitudes become pervasive, and quality of care suffers. To sustain nurses in the profession and improve patient care outcomes requires incorporating innovative pedagogies that change input, reshape educational processes, and consider new ways to assess and evaluate outcomes. For these reasons, Watson's Caring Science model permeates this second edition to provide a lens for practitioners to care for self as they care for others. The 10 Caritas Processes™ (Watson, 2008) are listed in Chapter 1.

Changing the Learning Paradigm

Though advances in science and related fields tempt us to add yet more content based on rational science, believing we need to teach every disease, we can't continue with the same educational processes and expect changes in outcomes. How do learners manage the information overload in trying to integrate this wealth of information into practice applications when most clinical learning schedules comprise 1 or perhaps 2 days per week? Where do we incorporate the self-care practices and thinking time required for integration of rational knowledge with person-centered aspects of care? Do nurse educators have preparation for integrating other forms of knowledge that derive from aesthetics, ethics, personal reflection, and other ways of knowing? How do these converge for making sense of practice and understanding the broad dimensions of humanness relevant to health? This book describes how reflective practice can guide nurses in making sense of their practice and build resiliency to sustain them within their practice. New teaching boxes provide exemplars and instructions to help nurses with the practical application.

How we teach is as critical as what we teach. Lecture alone rarely achieves behavior change. Reflective practice is part of a new paradigm for nursing education that is learner-centered to help develop the person who comes to work as a nurse. Reflection provides a systematic way to integrate knowledge from experience with continued learning from multiple sciences; that is, developing the practical tacit knowledge important in developing clinical judgment. Reflection is a systematic way of thinking about our actions and responses in order to change future actions and responses. It is learning from experience by considering what we know, believe, and value within the context of an event. Reflection helps make sense of events so we can feel more effective, leading to greater satisfaction. It contributes to working according to our sense of mission and purpose and, as such, helps us develop spiritual resources for managing meaning in life. Reflection is a lifelong learning process based on inquiry that helps shape and mold the novice learner and propels practicing nurses toward expert practice.

Deeper learning that incorporates the complex nature of practice is difficult for educators and self-paced learners to master without additional instruction. Reflection is used by almost all nursing educators, yet few have models by which to guide reflective learning experiences. Learners are often asked to "write about your experience in a reflective journal," yet no particular model or framework is provided to the learner to know how to structure the reflective process so that it leads to new awareness and insights that can result in behavior change. Reflection used as a systematic way to "make sense of experience" can be the avenue by which we improve the outcomes of our work. In this sense, reflection becomes a change process by which we can improve practice and the focus of our work.

Healthcare workers want to do their jobs well; they come with a value of contributing to the greater mission of improving health. They need the tools and system support to do their work effectively and to experience the satisfaction of a job well done. In this new edition, we build on how reflection provides the process for asking critical questions that can lead to improvements in quality and safety and health for all. It helps open the possibility of change; questions are the first step in the change process. Promoting a spirit of inquiry helps identify potential gaps in the system where errors might occur. Exercises illustrate how to apply Appreciative Inquiry through reflective models to examine system improvements to promote a culture of quality and safety.

Reflective Practices: Integrating Caring Science With QSEN

Recently adopted quality and safety competencies are threaded throughout the book. The work of the Robert Wood Johnson Foundation project Quality and Safety Education for Nurses (QSEN) is a vehicle for transforming nursing education to integrate a quality and safety framework (Cronenwett et al., 2007; Cronenwett et al., 2009). To further engage learners in reflective practice and aid in tapping into the deeply human aspects of care, we integrate Caring Science as a foundation for how learners connect with self and others—to be more present, authentic, and intentional in their practice. Narrative pedagogy, particularly the use of unfolding case studies, can stimulate learners' imagination and spirit of inquiry—to encourage learners to continually ask questions to appreciate and discover all ways of knowing for the care they deliver, to not only examine standards of care for the most current evidence, but to assess patient needs and preferences for person-centered care and increase their situational awareness of the potential for error. Reflection helps develop leadership capacity, improve responses through emotional intelligence, and develop mindfulness as part of working in interprofessional teams.

This book expands on the original text and further establishes the pedagogy of reflection by providing frameworks with specific applications of reflective thinking and learning in learner-centered environments, implications for reflective educators, and the futuristic complexity science and integral theory. This new edition incorporates complementary paradigms that emphasize the desire to learn, to grow, and to be in community with others, including Caring Science, emotional intelligence, and social justice. *Reflective Organizations: On the Front Lines of QSEN & Reflective Practice Implementation* (2015) is a valuable companion resource from the same editors that delves deeper into application of reflective practice, with exemplars of reflective learning environments in interpersonal education and practice, application in organizational systems, and transforming education in clinical and academic settings.

What's in This Book

The revised edition serves as a timely resource; despite the resurgent interest in pedagogy and in reflective learning experiences based on narrative pedagogies, few resources focus on reflective learning strategies. The book provides a rich resource for nurse educators in both academic and clinical settings, nurses and graduate students interested in developing leadership capacity, and nurses seeking to advance professional development from novice to expert. The book pulls together multiple approaches to reflective pedagogy for self-improvement through exercises that are adaptable to any form of nurses' personal life and professional work. It serves independent learners seeking personal or professional growth and development. It can be used both individually and for group discussions, or with a coach, preceptor, or mentor.

Five parts guide the reader. Part I introduces reflective practice with three chapters. The opening chapter examines the various reflective frameworks and perspectives to create transformational learning opportunities and explores the way nurses integrate experience into their knowledge. Reflection is critical in expanding personal and professional leadership, developing self-awareness, promoting individual accountability, and changing behavior. Through the lens of Caring Science, nurses learn to deepen their reflective ability in and on practice. Chapter 2 integrates the work of the Quality and Safety Education for Nurses (QSEN) project, which seeks to change nurses' professional identity to include quality and safety competencies; the prelicensure and graduate competencies for quality and safety are included in the appendices. Changing education is a first step to achieve the competencies for improving healthcare systems. The quality and safety goals are based on a culture of inquiry, the art of asking questions both to determine the evidence for why actions are implemented but also to consider other ways to complete a task. Application of reflective methods is a model of change agency that can help to uncover gaps in the system for improvement. A new chapter on emotional intelligence completes this part with an introduction to applying reflective practice to a coaching model and self-assessment to enhance emotional intelligence. Educators and learners alike find more relevance and meaning in their personal and professional lives through exploring who we are and what we bring to our being and our practice.

The three chapters in Part II describe how we create opportunities and sacred space for reflection. Mindfulness is considered from multiple perspectives as a cornerstone for reflection. Our presence, our being, is the most powerful teacher and is explored in Chapter 4. *Authentic presence* has been defined as a practice of genuineness, self-knowledge, and the ability to self-reflect; being in the moment; caring communication; and being honest with oneself and others. Mindful educators, discussed in Chapter 5, must themselves develop self-awareness. Mindful educators nurture a learning community in which learners grow academically, socially, and emotionally. Mindful educators master their experiences and emotions to be more skilled, focused, present, confident, and flexible in working with learners. Chapter 6 moves on to develop the mindful learner by offering strategies and exercises to develop mindful attention and self-awareness to hone mental focus that can improve academic and clinical performance. Through this process that emphasizes self-care and compassion, nurses learn to carry these values into their professional practice, becoming reflective practitioners committed to patient-centered care. Each chapter in this part concludes with breathing exercises to support mindful presence and reflective praxis.

The four chapters in Part III examine reflective learning in both didactic and clinical practice. Pedagogies in action are the focus of Chapter 7, and the chapter considers learning through reflection and reflection-on-learning. How to deepen reflective practice through the integration of Caring Science principles and processes is further examined. Reflective and caring frameworks and exemplars are presented for co-creating engaging learning experiences with learners. Chapter 8 illustrates the practice of narrative pedagogy, which uses the patient's experience in an unfolding way to help learners with complex knowledge integration. Chapter 9 describes how reflection is applied to simulation learning using reflection-before-, -in-, -on-, and -beyond-action. Clinical assessment and evaluation match method and objectives, as well as reflection as learning and reflection as assessment, are explored in Chapter 10. Engaging learners in helping create reflective, learner-centered classroom and clinical environments, reflective course evaluation, and Appreciative Inquiry as a reflective change model seeks to instill habits of the mind that reinforce lifelong learning.

Part IV explores ways to deepen the foundations of professional practice through reflection and ways that exemplars help make sense of the emotional labor of nursing, develop practice knowledge, and expand leadership capacity and professional maturity. Chapter 11 presents strategies to develop professional practice. The focus is both on attending to self and on making sense of practice. Reflection helps develop emotional intelligence to monitor feelings, discriminate among emotional reactions, and use the information to guide future responses and actions. Reflection can employ unlimited applications of aesthetics, story, clay, art, photojournalism, dance, and movement. Personal development is the basis of transformative leadership. Reflection provides a mirror to the self by helping us to confront and resolve actual and desired work practices. Chapter 12 focuses on changing the culture of educator evaluation. We explore how reflective evaluation can promote growth, make sense of work, and sustain educators in both academic and clinical settings in developing and preserving roles. An exemplar illustrates how evaluation can be a means of welcoming reflection and sustaining the teaching role. Chapter 13 is about working together, a key to transformation in healthcare. Through the use of Liberating Structures, a reflective methodology derived from complexity theory, we demonstrate how to create new, more effective and reflective ways of working together, whether within nursing teams or interprofessionally.

Part V poses future perspectives on reflective practice and challenges educators and learners to further expand their capacity for deep learning through incorporation of other theories. Educators and learners can use these added theoretical perspectives to further facilitate personal transformation, work with interprofessional healthcare teams, and advocate for the underserved. These perspectives also support the development of leadership capacity and the ability to guide much-needed healthcare transformations. Chapter 14 introduces readers to integral philosophy and theory as a way of knowing that strives for a comprehensive understanding of a situation. As a comprehensive framework, integral theory supports multiple perspectives and enables practitioners to become more aware of their self and patients through analysis, consideration, reflection, and understanding of any situation. Reflecting on the Quality and Safety Competencies through an integral lens provides a path to navigate the complex nature of caring for self and others and opens a way to study quality and safety through integral theory's eight zones of inquiry. Chapter 15 goes a step further in considering how integral theory, action inquiry, and principles of reflection can transform interprofessional practice among the health professions. Developing an integral perspective in combination with methods of action is a skillful means to enhance interprofessional practice. The adoption of integral perspectives and action inquiry methods supports transformational learning and expands capacity for interprofessional reflection, teamwork, and health professions education. In the final chapter, we are encouraged to expand the boundaries of our thinking about reflective practice and how this process carries over into our professional responsibility to address inequities and barriers to healthcare. Globally, nursing and other healthcare professionals are being called to address social justice issues through the Sustainable Development Goals (SDGs). Reflective practice grounds healthcare professionals in the sense of self needed to act in a manner that supports a sustainable world. This chapter illuminates how emancipatory practice directs social justice goals and outcomes through reflection, action, and transformation. This part provides the foundation for expanding leadership capacity through models and frames that support emancipatory practice, a profoundly caring and transformational force to empower all healthcare professions to expand their roles and influence toward health, healing, and wholeness in the world.

–Sara Horton-Deutsch, PhD, RN, FAAN, ANEF
–Gwen D. Sherwood, PhD, RN, FAAN, ANEF

References

Benner, P., Sutphen, M., Leonard, V., & Day, L. (2010). *Educating nurses: A call for radical transformation*. Stanford, CA: Jossey-Bass.

Cronenwett, L., Sherwood, G., Barnsteiner, J., Disch, J., Johnson, J., Mitchell, P., . . . Warren, J. (2007). Quality and safety education for nurses. *Nursing Outlook, 55*(3), 122–131.

Cronenwett, L., Sherwood, G., Pohl, J., Barnsteiner, J., Moore, S., Sullivan, D. T., . . . Warren, J. (2009). Quality and safety education for advanced nursing practice. *Nursing Outlook, 57*(6), 338–348.

Freshwater, D., Horton-Deutsch, S., Sherwood, G., & Taylor, B. (2005). *The scholarship of reflective practice*. Indianapolis, IN: Sigma Theta Tau International. Retrieved from http://www.nursingsociety.org/docs/default-source/position-papers/resource_reflective.pdf?sfvrsn=4

Hassmiller, S. B., & Mensik, J. S. (2017). *The power of ten: A conversational approach to tackling the top ten nursing priorities* (2nd ed.). Indianapolis, IN: Sigma Theta Tau International.

Institute of Medicine (IOM). (2010). *The future of nursing: Leading change, advancing health*. Washington, DC: The National Academies Press.

Sherwood, G., & Horton-Deutsch, S. (2015). *Reflective organizations: On the front lines of QSEN & reflective practice implementation*. Indianapolis, IN: Sigma Theta Tau International.

Watson, J. (2008). *Nursing: The philosophy and science of caring*. Boulder, CO: University Press of Colorado.

Part I

The Transformation of Nursing Education Through Reflective Practice

Chapter 1
Turning Vision Into Action: Reflection to Develop Professional Practice

–*Gwen D. Sherwood, PhD, RN, FAAN, ANEF*
–*Sara Horton-Deutsch, PhD, RN, FAAN, ANEF*

Educators are agents of change. Promoting learning and thinking to achieve both personal and professional development has long been a hallmark of nursing, habits that begin during formative academic programs. The challenges and opportunities of preparing nurses for practice have never been greater. Advances in science and technology, patient-shared decision-making, market-driven healthcare, and the changing nature and setting of nursing practice have changed practice environments. Education and practice are like mirrors; practice changes affect nursing education, and vice versa.

In its *Quality Chasm* series (2001, 2003, 2004), the Institute of Medicine (IOM) issued a call to action. In response to its staggering reports of poor patient outcomes, the IOM called on nurses to transform healthcare, to uphold and transmit core professional values for reducing risk while understanding and managing the full dimensions of evidence-based, quality, patient-centered care. Nurses and all health professionals must be able to deploy a complex array of competencies while maintaining a deep commitment to each patient's best interests; these competencies—patient-centered care, teamwork and collaboration, evidence-based practice, quality improvement, safety, and informatics—were identified by the 2003 IOM report on health professions education. The definitions have been operationalized for nurses through the Quality and Safety Education for Nurses (QSEN) project funded by the Robert Wood Johnson Foundation (Cronenwett et al., 2007; Cronenwett, Sherwood, & Gelmon, 2009). The work completed through the QSEN project identified the role of reflective practice in preparing nurses to catalyze practice improvements in providing safe quality care (Cronenwett et al., 2009).

This chapter will explore a new vision for education to develop transformative learners who cultivate self-awareness and apply a critical reasoning process that both questions actions and reassesses what is known. *Critical reasoning* is a form of learning that raises consciousness and supports all healthcare professionals to more carefully examine and purposefully enact the care they provide. We will explore how reflective practices engage learners to participate in formal and self-directed learning activities, and explain how reflection supports transformative learning. Finally, we describe how a Caring Science framework can be used to further guide and deepen reflective practice and transformative learning in a supportive and caring environment where critical thought is valued and authentic dialogue and debate of ideas are encouraged.

A New Vision for Education

Unprecedented changes in practice are revising professional practice models, thereby changing expectations for new graduates; therefore, traditional nursing education program outcomes may no longer be congruent with market needs, because technical, instrumental knowledge is insufficient to provide safe, quality care (Day & Sherwood, 2017a). Instrumental or empirical knowledge is vital to learn to predict and control the environment—to assess cause-and-effect relationships. Instrumental knowledge by itself, however, does not account for the full range of competencies needed to manage the complexities of twenty-first century practice and intersubjective human interactions and connections. Current practice incorporates other ways of knowing that help practitioners consider the social norms, traditions, and values underlying their work culture and influence decisions in practice (Johns, 1995a, 2016).

Reflective practice is a change strategy used informally by almost all nursing educators, yet few have models by which to guide systematic reflective learning experiences. Frequently, learners are asked to write about their clinical experiences in a reflective journal without a model or framework or writing cue. Cues that frame questions or provide a topic for concentration guide learners in structuring the reflective process so that it can lead to new awareness and insights that can, in turn, lead to behavioral changes. Reflective practice used as a systematic way to "make sense of experience" can be the avenue to promote practice improvements and satisfaction in our work. In this sense, reflective practice becomes a transformative change process by which we can improve practice, refocus our work, and increase meaning and satisfaction from work well done—all of which foster nurse retention.

Benner, Sutphen, Leonard, and Day (2010) examined historical roots of nursing education and explored best education practices among several professions. After interviewing and observing across nursing education sites, they noted the major nursing education paradigm has remained largely unchanged for 4 decades—students have didactic classes, go to clinical learning experiences in small groups with an instructor, care for one or two patients, and participate in post-clinical conferences. Most classrooms focused on the taxonomy of disease or nursing diagnosis; few integrated clinical realities or the patient perspective.

Due to the move of nursing education from hospitals to academic settings, educators began to emphasize abstract and formal knowledge and classifications of knowledge. Pressures to move toward professional prestige and the explosion of healthcare knowledge led to an encyclopedic approach to teaching. Benner et al. (2010) proclaim nursing education should be built on rich and powerful learning that illuminates the human condition as part of the care process.

Learners have to prepare for a practice that straddles the mechanistic medical diagnosis and treatment with patients' lived experience of illness. Educators have the dilemma of finding ways to teach an ever-increasing knowledge base balanced with helping learners know how to use it in practice.

To address these challenges, Benner et al. (2010) propose that nursing education for the twenty-first century should be composed of three apprenticeships: the knowledge base, skilled know-how and clinical reasoning, and ethical comportment. These are integrated rather than separate compartments of learning: Learners develop a moral sense of what it is good to be and good to do in a situation on the basis of evidence-based knowledge; they develop skilled know-how (*competence*) and learn how to act within an ethical framework based on values and beliefs (*human caring literacy*).

Effective, contemporary educators invite and lead learners to develop clinical imagination within a sense of salience and clinical reasoning. The goal is preparing nurses who use evidence-based knowledge and cultivate habits of thinking to deepen their clinical judgment and increase skilled know-how. Teaching is integrative, learner-centered, and focused on the patient as subject; experience melds with various knowledge forms to develop an approach to practice. Experiential learning theory (Kolb, 1984) guides how learners develop situated cognition (knowing), skills (what to do), and ethical comportment (attitudes and values). Educator coaches lead learners in professional identity formation, ignite their imaginations, and engage them in learning from experiences as they move along the professional development continuum.

Acquisition of skills for effective practice is a necessary part of professional development—keeping in mind, however, that professions are distinguished from skills-based work by development of professional artistry (Schön, 1983). The capacity to respond in-action—that is, reflecting-in-action—to deal with complex and sometimes contradictory circumstances constitutes growing toward professional maturity and artistry. Mezirow (1991) believed adults learn not only by developing skills and acquiring new knowledge but also, equally importantly, through critical reflection and transformative learning; adults transform perspective as they reflectively reconstruct experience (Cranton, 1996, 2006).

Creating a radical new vision to transform nursing education that prepares nurses "fit for practice" focuses on developing multiple advanced competencies, clinical judgment skills, and ethical standards with a patient-centered focus, based on integration of the IOM/QSEN competencies. Transformation can only happen with new innovative pedagogical approaches that are strong in situated coaching and experiential learning to develop nurses who have a deep sense of professional identity and commitment to professional values.

Education paradigms are shifting to meet the needs of twenty-first century healthcare needs. Over the past 40 years, educators have scrambled to incorporate unprecedented change in society, knowledge, technology, and healthcare delivery, creating curricula this is often fragmented, overloaded, and content-heavy. Benner et al. (2010) cited paradigm shifts that catalyze radical transformation to integrate learning across settings from classroom, clinical, and simulated lab experiences:

- Replace the focus on decontextualized knowledge with emphasizing teaching for a sense of salience, situated cognition, and action in particular clinical situations.

- Shift from the sharp separation of didactic and clinical teaching to integrative teaching in all settings.

- Reframe the emphasis on critical thinking to emphasizing clinical reasoning and multiple ways of thinking, including critical thinking.

- Move away from an emphasis on socialization and role-taking to emphasizing professional identity formation.

Drago-Severson (2004) identifies two basic forms of learning: informational and transformational. With the exponential explosion of knowledge in nursing's domains, educators have had a natural tendency to overload curriculum with content and to focus on knowledge and skill acquisition—in other words, informational learning became the major developmental goal.

The predominance of lecture by PowerPoint has trained students to diligently take notes that are expected to provide the blueprint for the next exam.

Little discussion or engagement in the deeper understanding of the material (transformational learning) takes place that can help integrate clinical learning experiences with classroom material so learners are challenged to "think like a nurse." How can questions be framed to meld clinical and classroom experiences so that the physiology related to disease categories, the signs and symptoms, the evidence-based interventions, and the outcomes are not just taxonomies to be memorized, but become real, realizing that someone's life will depend on the ability to bring this array of knowledge to bear in a real-world situation? What are pedagogical strategies that engage learners and spark their imaginations to use knowledge as they think and act in ever-changing clinical situations (Day & Sherwood, 2017b)?

Transformational learning is a necessary aspect of practice development. Developing practice derives from critical reflection on the assumptions that often lie under the surface yet guide decisions and actions. Transformation is a process of both personal and professional growth; it is often said that who we are is who we bring to practice. Development inherently moves beyond acquisition of new knowledge and skills to our capacity to question the assumptions, values, and perspectives influencing the decisions we make in practice and our choices in how we treat others.

Practice requires more than simply applying learned knowledge content in practice. Nursing is a high-stakes profession that requires developing multiple types of knowledge, with the capacity to sift through the evidence and make critical decisions in complex situations. Benner et al. (2010) describe how the teacher can lead an ongoing dialogue between information and practice needs, between the particular and the general, that helps build a multiplicity of knowledge applied within one's experiences to develop a sense of salience (i.e., the ability to recognize what is urgent and important in particular clinical situations); we circle back to the importance of nurses knowing how to make critical judgments in the middle of practice dynamics (Tanner, 2006). The typical structured, objective-based nursing education classroom experience delivered via PowerPoint slide is not conducive to understanding the dynamics of practice that lead to personal transformation. Changes in knowledge, skills, and attitudes—competencies—develop when learners are engaged in both informational and transformational learning experiences through which they experientially apply what they know, what they know how to do, and how they align attitudinal adjustments in making critical decisions. The level of inquiry, of engaging in the moment, of asking critical questions, creates a synergy through which nurses actively think and reason in changing situations and act to work for the good of the patient.

TRANSFORMATION

Conversion that comes from a change in behavior, attitudes, and skills for improved performance.

TRANSFORMATIVE LEARNERS

Those who apply critical reasoning by constantly asking questions to reassess what is known—in concert with a well-developed emotional intelligence—to improve their work.

REFLECTING ON . . . WAYS OF KNOWING

How can nurses develop multiple ways of knowing that take into account empirical, aesthetic, legal and ethical, and personal knowledge?

Reflection to Engage Learners in Learning Experiences

Reflective practice helps us access and build on experiential or tacit knowledge as well as other forms of knowledge development (Carper, 1978; Johns, 1995a; Tanner, 2006). Historical debates of whether nursing is an art or a science are outdated in reality (Freshwater, 2008). The processes of reflection help practitioners move between seemingly polar opposites, helping articulate and make evident all ways of knowing. This in turn contributes to the full understanding of nursing.

The views of reflection and its use in practical contexts have been evolving since Dewey (1933) defined it as the active, persistent, and careful consideration of beliefs supported by knowledge and the resulting conclusions. The goal was learning

TACIT KNOWLEDGE

Knowledge that is subconsciously understood or implied and difficult to articulate objectively but may be shared through interactive conversation or narrative. It is the integration of knowledge with experience for new understanding and operating related to specific situations in practice.

how to recognize which beliefs are based on tested evidence. Schön (1983) described a different perspective; instead of a rational view of reflection, Schön included the intuitive and open. Learners consider the tacit norms that underlie decisions, the theories that guide practice, and their feelings that lead to reframing the problem. Through reflection, they explore a detailed view of a situation, opening to multiple dimensions. The process of rational thinking delays action until the situation is understood, a goal for action is determined, alternatives are considered, and a plan is developed (Cranton, 1996). However, this view of thinking did not account for the affective domain; thus Cranton expanded the definition to include feelings and beliefs through the reflective process, *transformative learning* in which the learner changes behavior, attitudes, and skills for a new way of thinking and acting.

Johns (1995b, 2000, 2016) applied reflection to practice, developing a classic definition of reflective practice as one's ability to access, make sense of, and learn through experiences in one's work toward a more desirable, effective, and satisfying work experience. This definition takes into account the conflict or cognitive dissonance that arises in practice between the ideal and the actual. People often say one thing as their beliefs but proceed to do something else, thus creating a contradiction between attitudes and actions. This might also manifest as the dissonance between theories of practice and actual practice, such as forgoing evidence-based practice by taking shortcuts that introduce risk.

Freshwater (2008) and Taylor (2000) describe reflection as a focused way of thinking about practice, whatever that practice or work is. Taylor includes any type of attentive consideration such as thinking, contemplation, or meditation that helps make sense of cognitive acts and leads to contextually appropriate changes. In this way, reflection potentiates change. Freshwater further distinguished critical reflection as thinking not just about current practice, but also questioning the underlying political, ethical, historical, and cultural traditions.

Goulet, Larue, and Alderson (2016) completed a concept analysis of reflective practice based on 42 articles cited in the Cumulative Index to Nursing and Allied Health Literature (CINAHL) database. Reflective practice is inquiry-based, asking questions that examine theory-practice gaps, foster professional development, and undergird human caring. It can also guide knowledge development, explore social change, and make sense of emotions and contradictions in practice. Reflection represents both the constructed experience and how we deconstruct it in order to reconstruct it. By asking questions about what they are doing, why, and how it can be improved, practitioners deconstruct and reconstruct experience or situations to be able to realign future actions. Reflective practice helps novice nurses as they transition from carefully constructed academic learning to the clinical dynamics that welcome them as new graduates in practice (Hatlevik, 2012; Spector, Barnsteiner, & Ulrich, 2017).

The act of reflection enables us to question the assumptions on which we base our work or interact within social contexts, allowing us to reconstruct what we think about how we work. The underlying philosophy of reflection is an individual process of learning that reflects individual experience and meaning. Cranton (1996) challenges the idea of individual reflection, believing that interacting or critical reflection with others is what helps the learner raise questions that identify assumptions to explore a change in perspective. In fact, when one person engages in reflection with another, both are learning; through this type of dialogue we can say "educators learn with their students" (Cranton, 1996, p. 78), which is explored more in Chapter 10.

The questioning aspects of reflection help develop habits of the mind for constantly asking questions and building an environment that nurtures ideas.

REFLECTION

Reflection-before-Action: Thinking through a particular situation in advance.

Reflection-in-Action: Thinking in the moment of action, using self-awareness to manage the moment with both instrumental and tacit knowledge.

Reflection-on-Action: A retrospective process of the thinking that occurs after an incident to make sense of it and using process outcomes to influence future actions.

Overreliance on technical rationality in practice ignores the context of an actual practice situation. Do practitioners make decisions on technical knowledge, or are decisions based more on experience? Critical reflection examines the assumptions underlying content, processes, or premises that guide actions and decisions in practice. Critical reflection links transformative learning theory with adult learning characteristics (emotional maturity, awareness, empathy, and control) to embolden nurses in caring for the full dimension of humanness (Kear, 2013).

Reflection has been linked to the essential nursing skill of developing self-awareness as part of emotional intelligence (Freshwater, 2002; Horton-Deutsch & Sherwood, 2008; Sherwood & Horton-Deutsch, 2008) and is explored in more depth in Chapter 10. A study by Paget (2001) identified how practitioners view the impact of reflective practice on clinical outcomes and how perspectives were transformed. Kear (2013) validated the impact of integrating reflective practice into the nursing curriculum to help learners transform into competent, balanced professionals. Reflective practice helps develop caring intervention and was a necessary component in how learners understood nursing and caring.

Reflection-on-action is a retrospective process; it's the thinking that occurs after an incident. The goal is to make sense of what happened and process the outcomes to rethink future actions. *Reflection-in-action* relates to the intuitive art of thinking in the moment or, as we say, thinking on one's feet (Freshwater, 2008). *Reflection-before-action* is thinking through a particular situation before making decisions or taking action (Burton, 2000). The process of planning, acting, and debriefing—that is, reflecting-before, -in, or -on-action—does not mean reflective practice is a linear process, nor does it mean it occurs on a continuum, but it may occur in cycles of interpretation as one analyzes what happened.

There are arguments to have clearer reflective practice processes, yet the very nature of reflection does not lend itself to the prescriptive approach some practitioners might desire (Ruth-Sahd, 2003). However, evidence demonstrates that learning how to systematically examine assumptions, extract key ideas from experience, and transform those ideas back into the next experience can be facilitated through a variety of reflective learning activities. Jacobs (2016) shares her personal teaching experience, in which she realized the importance of providing structure to student reflections to be able to process practice improvements. Dewey (1933) asserts that reflection is developed through the capacity for open-mindedness, wholeheartedness, and responsibility. As such, employing a variety of reflective approaches to facilitate learning supports adult development, transformational learning, and personal and professional growth (Bulman & Schutz, 2004; Burns & Bulman, 2000).

Reflection to Engage Learners in Practice Development

"Deep learning can only be made known as it comes to the surface. Reflection enables that process."

Educators are change agents propelling learners forward, not "keepers of the status quo." Educators foster the growth and development of learners by serving as role models and mentors for practice through their own spirit of inquiry. Educators with a vision for continuous learning share a mutual commitment with the learner to constantly ask reflective questions that help integrate knowledge and experience, which develops a sense of salience as learners learn to make choices (Benner et al., 2010). Reflective practice helps create a world that more faithfully reflects our personal and professional values and beliefs, so the ideal and real-world practice are congruent (Taylor, Freshwater, Sherwood, & Esterhuizen, 2008).

Practice—however it is defined—is by its very nature not linear, but unfolds with multiple dimensions. Learners need guidance in knowing how to apply the knowledge, skills, and attitudes from formal, didactic learning; application provides informal learning that helps them go deeper into understanding what they know to apply in the real world. All professional situations have the potential for learning. "Reflection enables a continuum of learning and development in which the practitioner grows in and through their practice" (Freshwater, 2008, p. 9). Reflection is a means of formalizing informal learning and development through practice and can be a component of the professional development or learning portfolio (referred to in Chapter 10). Reflection gives more intention to practice to more effectively impact patient outcomes by refining and defining safe quality care, moving the learner toward expert practice (Benner, 1984).

Learners need flexible and dynamic frameworks to guide their development as they move from content to application (practice). Therefore, applying what one knows in making clinical decisions does not necessarily unfold in a linear pattern—more likely, it occurs in back-and-forth deepening reflection as learners continually develop knowing in situations. Deep learning can only be made known as it comes to the surface. Deep learning is more than content acquisition; classroom and clinical learning based on Kolb's (1984) experiential learning theory positions learners to be able to apply content in an inquisitive way to learn how to make clinical choices, and thus gain a sense of salience. Reflection enables that process through the ability to construct, deconstruct, and reconstruct an experience.

Learners need to understand the process of reflection to be able to consciously think deeply about their choices. One early model developed by Atkins and Murphy (1993) from a literature synthesis explains three phases:

- **Noticing:** Aware of inner discomfort about feelings or thoughts about something of importance

- **Reflection:** Critical analysis of the particulars of a situation, past experience, or understanding; remaining open to new information and perspectives; deep immersion in the situation

- **Action/intervening:** Developing a new perspective from a range of options, deciding whether and how to take action; perspective transformation; cognitive, affective, and behavioral changes that result in action

Another model widely adopted in nursing is the Clinical Judgment Model developed by Tanner (2006). The four stages help explain how learners develop the skills to construct or deconstruct an experience, by moving back and forth in a fluid and circular pattern and gaining insights through the reflective process (see a more detailed explanation in Chapter 11):

- Noticing, to gain perceptual grasp of the situation as it unfolded

- Interpreting, to develop sufficient understanding to act

- Responding, to develop a plan of action appropriate to the situation

- Reflecting, to be aware of the patient's responses while caring for them, and assessing outcomes

In this discussion, we are moving back and forth between the role of the educator and the learner; both are significant in reflection for transformative learning. A more complete examination of the role of the educator is explored in Chapter 5 and elsewhere in this book. Understanding the role of situated coaching or clinical supervision is vital. Reflection is an individual activity—and we need to respect the privacy of learners' thoughts—but it is through dialogue, written or verbal, that learners develop the skill to critically appraise their own work and receive feedback from another in a way that is informative for professional development. The dialogue with the educator or coach can illuminate facets of the situation and bring them to the surface to build onto the evidence base of practice.

Then, reflective practice becomes a companion as well as a precursor to improving practice by helping to assess whether practice behavior is congruent with best practices or espoused values and beliefs. Benner (1984) and Benner and Wrubel (1989) demonstrate that reflection is a vital process in building competence along the novice-to-expert trajectory. Through reflection, nurses develop autonomy through self-monitoring and accountability toward professional maturity. Reflective learning as part of a professional development portfolio or course assignment can be part of assessment and evaluation by using rubrics or other dialogue in giving feedback, as discussed further in Chapter 10. Miller (2014) provides an example of how a requirement to include reflective practice writings in her professional development portfolio helped change her perspectives to see her practice in a new way, leading to action.

Reflective practice has been described as a deepening of the learning process to see other perspectives in a situation, which can be applied in almost all situations. Truglio-Londrigan (2013a, 2013b) applied a reflective practice model to decision-making as part of learning to work with others to reach consensus. Reflective practice can be used for individual development but also applied with systems thinking. The national QSEN Pilot Learning Project underscored the essential role of reflective practice in creating practice changes to deliver safe, quality care (Cronenwett et al., 2009). Exemplars of reflective practice applications in academic and clinical settings are further explored in Sherwood & Horton-Deutsch's (2015) *Reflective Organizations: On the Front Lines of QSEN & Reflective Practice Implementation*.

Freshwater (2008) describes three levels of reflection that demonstrate the ever-deepening of learning as one develops the skills of reflective practice with the ingrained habits of asking questions about practice that move one to decision-making and action. Reflective practice may begin with developing awareness of what happens in practice to be able to bring hidden aspects of a situation to the surface. Deepening reflection, nurses then may develop skills in sharing their reflections with others to critically self-question one's actions and responses. The three levels can help guide learning assignments or professional portfolio development. The three levels can guide development of an evaluation rubric, particularly as shown in Table 1.1:

- **Descriptive reflection:** Practice becomes conscious. Clinicians engage in reflection-on-action. Mentors encourage nurses to develop descriptive reflection through reflective journals and to share critical incidents through narratives.

- **Dialogic reflection:** Practice becomes deliberative. Clinicians develop dialogic reflection through formal clinical supervision or through discourse with peers, coaches, supervisors, or other experts to gain feedback on how they are thinking.

- **Critical reflection:** Engage in self-questioning by applying critical reasoning to reframe how one acts, thinks, or knows. Engaging in continuous improvement of practice leads to innovations that transform practice.

Table 1.1 outlines these levels of reflection and stages of development.

TABLE 1.1 Levels of Reflection (Freshwater, 2008)

LEVEL OF REFLECTION	MODEL OF REFLECTION	STAGE OF DEVELOPMENT
Descriptive	Reflective journals, reporting incidents, reflection-on-action	Practice becomes conscious
Dialogic	Discourse with peers in various arenas, including clinical supervision	Practice becomes deliberative
Critical	Able to provide reasoning for actions by engaging in critical conversation about practice with self and others	Transformative practice, practice improvement, move to innovation

Clarifying the purpose of reflection creates a more deliberative learning experience. Reflective models foster dialogue between knowing and doing. Reflecting on beliefs, values, and norms leads to more conscious, deliberative, and intentional interventions. Reflective questioning of the validity of previous learning can lead to regeneration of knowledge and to melding experience with knowledge and can help avoid complacency and reliance on routine in everyday practice.

Guided by beliefs, values, and norms to more conscious, deliberate, and intentional practice, educators and learners are ethically challenged to address new questions:

- How do we integrate facts with meanings?

- How do we demonstrate that the personal and professional are integral to one another?

- How do we create, develop, and engage in reflective, caring practice?

Reflection: The Key to Transformative Learning

Self-directed learning is the foundation for transformative learning. Mezirow (1991) developed the theory of transformative learning that permeates adult education. *Transformative learning* is a reflective process in which the nurse or learner recognizes a disorienting dilemma and applies critical reflection to reach a changed meaning perspective. This form of learning builds the foundation for adult development to advance growth and development, moving from one stage to the other. Real change and growth in our practice are ongoing processes of examining and questioning our assumptions, values, and perspectives. Critical reflection, whether written or verbal, is the central process toward transformative learning.

To illustrate the paradigm shifts, Day & Sherwood (2017a) describe the new classroom as patient-centered, in which learning is situated in clinical contexts. Learning is interactive, beyond content acquisition, and in dialogue with educator coaches. Learners reveal how they are thinking and how they are processing knowledge to apply to practice, and thus educator coaches facilitate practice development.

Contextualized learning should spark clinical imagination to continually question the status quo, seek new approaches, and integrate new evidence—that is, prepare learners "fit for practice."

Critical reflection is key to transformative learning that can lead to changes in practice. Not all reflection leads to transformation; we can question things without changing anything. Transformative reflection is a change process; transformation involves or leads to a change in perspective or way of doing or acting. It is a way of solving problems that arise in practice. Mezirow (1991) described content, process, and premise reflection as three distinctions about how reflection leads to transformative learning:

- **Content reflection:** Focuses on the description of the problem or situation of interest

- **Process reflection:** Focuses on thinking about the strategies used to solve the problem rather than the content of the problem only

- **Premise reflection:** Leads to questioning assumptions, values, and beliefs underlying the situation

We use deeply embedded assumptions to interpret the world around us. Assumptions carry a connotation of "taken for granted," something that might not be challenged without engaging in critical reflection. Learners can be asked to explore these to articulate assumptions about their developing practice and record the basis for the assumption in a reflective journal. They can engage in written dialogues with the educator, a preceptor, a coach, or a professional peer. Assumptions can then be questioned for their validity through deeper dialogue, which can lead to consideration of alternatives. This might happen in a variety of learning settings, such as classroom, clinical, or simulation, and can include presentations and discussion, readings, brainstorming, debates, role-play, simulations, scenarios or unfolding case studies, narratives or story, or aesthetic imaginations. Many of these are explored in a white paper titled *The Scholarship of Reflective Practice*, developed by the Sigma Theta Tau International Task Force on Reflective Practice and posted at http://www.nursingsociety.org/docs/default-source/position-papers/resource_reflective.pdf?sfvrsn=4 (Freshwater, Horton-Deutsch, Sherwood, & Taylor, 2005).

By introducing alternatives through reflective analysis, learners can begin to visualize and reconstruct their views of how to act in a situation. Educators not only help learners question their assumptions but also help lead them to develop new approaches. Thus, we see the duality of learning that happens in the reflective dialogue between learners and educators, requiring an open approach to themselves as mindful teachers, as explored further in Chapter 5. Most educator development is based on the process of instrumental learning, and few are prepared in the reflective or transformative processes.

Educators help to create the context, organization, and culture of the learning environment and also engage in dialogue with learners to understand the context, organization, and culture of the practice setting. Including teaching and learning of the reflective process in educational programs allows educators to utilize various tools and strategies to facilitate the growth of reflective learners at all levels (Epp, 2008). Educator development, however, is a major consideration in developing reflective learning, so educators have the skills and their own self-awareness to help learners engage in self-managing their individual growth and development. By coaching and leading learners to continually ask questions, educators help foster a spirit of inquiry that forms the basis for developing a lifelong learning philosophy that comes from the process of critical reflection. Equally important in helping learners along the learning continuum is for educators to continue as change agents as learners grow toward professional maturity, as learners move beyond their own individual influence and develop influence for change in the organization and in the community culture (Cranton, 1996).

> ### REFLECTING ON . . . TRANSFORMATIVE LEARNING
>
> *If we view learning and development for adult learners as a process of questioning our beliefs about and perspectives on our practice, what changes do we need to make to move from educator-controlled environments toward learner-centered environments?*

The Intersection of Reflective Practice, Transformative Learning, and Caring Science

As we have emphasized throughout this chapter, reflective practice is about tapping into things deeply human: our own as well as others' experience, knowledge, understanding, and wisdom. Transformative learning emphasizes the process of change in understanding ourselves as well as revision of beliefs and behaviors. It also emphasizes how the words we use and how we use them carry much power to influence others (Bache, 2001). Similarly, Watson's Philosophy and Science of Caring (2008) emphasizes self-knowledge, self-discovery, and shared human experiences, combined with the study of human emotions and relations that reflect our shared humanity. Combined, these concepts provide a foundation for and guidance on how nurses and other healthcare professionals can more deeply reflect on their own practice, including their language (Watson, 2016), and how they use it to connect with self and others. Ultimately, reflective practice and Caring Science serve as a guide for transforming one's way of thinking, acting, and leading in a way that nurtures and sustains professional practice.

Integrating Caring Science into reflective practice further supports transformational learning by integrating art and science. Together, art and science reveal what is beyond the visible world, to "see" that which is deeper, glimpsing into the human spirit. Art helps us to bear witness to joy, pain, suffering, love, and struggle of our own human soul. "When one is engaged in human caring and healing, one cannot ignore the element of aesthetics and beauty and the spiritual domain of life's journey" (Watson, 2008, p. 21). A Caring Science perspective focuses on educating learners for a values-based practice that is morally guided to create reflective practitioners. This comes from pedagogies directed toward transformative teaching and learning that integrates a moral and scientific model for considering caring as an ethic ontology, an epistemic and praxis endeavor (Watson, 2008).

At the core of Caring Science is the transpersonal caring relationship. This form of care occurs when, through caring, one connects with and embraces the spirit of the other. This happens through authentic, full attention, in the present moment, and conveys concern for the inner life and personal meaning of another human being (Sitzman & Watson, 2014). The degree a learner is able to fully connect with another's body-mind-spirit depends on his or her cultivation of conscious loving and caring intentions as he/she enters the space of the other. When the meeting recognizes and focuses on the uniqueness of the self and other, it is life-giving and -receiving. This form of coming together supports the emergence of new possibilities for healing, wholeness, and health.

Transpersonal caring is cultivated through Caring Science or caritas literacy and results in authentic caring moments with another. *Caritas* means to cherish, appreciate, and give special loving attention through compassion and generosity of spirit. It involves being literate in ways relating to critical reflection of what it means to be human: our ability to deepen our understanding of cultural, ethic, and human social views (Horton-Deutsch, 2016; Watson, 2016). Caritas literacy emphasizes an understanding of being and becoming. It involves being morally informed with the capacity—beyond task-conscious learning—toward an evolved, heart-centered consciousness of learning that recognizes the connection of all human beings to affirm and sustain humanity (Cowling, Smith, & Watson, 2008).

Watson (2008) has developed and refined 10 Caritas Processes™ to guide nurses and other healthcare professionals to cultivate transpersonal caring and reflection that support an in-depth exploration of humanity and what it means to be human. Applying the 10 Caritas Processes nurtures self-knowledge, self-discovery, and shared human experiences that are life-giving and receiving. These processes serve to model the way for others, support authentic dialogue, and affirm and confirm others by holding them in high ethical regard.

CARING SCIENCE AND THE 10 CARITAS PROCESSES

According to Watson (2008), Caring Science is defined as follows: Caring Science is an evolving philosophical-ethical-epistemic field of study, grounded in the discipline of nursing and informed by related fields. Caring is considered as one central feature within the metaparadigm of nursing knowledge and practice. Caring Science is informed by an ethical-moral spiritual stance that encompasses a humanitarian, human science orientation to human caring processes, phenomena, and experiences. It is located within a worldview that is non-dualistic, rational, and unified, wherein there is connectedness to ALL; the universal field of Infinity: Cosmic LOVE. Caring Science within this worldview intersects with the arts and humanities and related fields of study and practice (pp. 18–19).

Caritas Processes bring love and caring together to form a deep transpersonal caring focusing on how to Be while doing the work of nursing. The 10 Caritas Processes include (Watson, 2007):

1. *Embrace altruistic values and practice loving kindness with self and others.*
2. *Instill faith and hope and honor others.*
3. *Be sensitive to self and others by nurturing individual beliefs and practices.*
4. *Develop helping-trusting-caring relationships.*

5. *Promote and accept positive and negative feelings as you authentically listen to another's story.*

6. *Use creative scientific problem-solving methods for caring decision-making.*

7. *Share teaching and learning that addresses the individual needs and comprehension styles.*

8. *Create a healing environment for the physical and spiritual self, which respects human dignity.*

9. *Assist with basic physical, emotional, and spiritual human needs.*

10. *Be open to mystery and allow miracles to enter.*

Final Reflections

Reflection is sometimes referred to as critical thinking with the addition of the multiple ways of knowing that account for the affective domain. Reflection is a systematic way of thinking about our actions and responses that contributes to a transformed perspective, or the reframing of a given situation or problem, and it determines future actions and responses. It is learning from experience by considering what we know, believe, and value within the context of a particular situation in our work. Reflection contributes to working according to our sense of mission and purpose, and as such helps develop spiritual resources for managing life. Reflection helps us make sense of events, develop leadership capacity, improve responses through emotional intelligence, develop mindfulness to engage in work activities, and thus improve quality and safety for patients. Caring Science deepens reflective practice by connecting reflection with caring and love as the basis for practice in a way that supports healing, health, and wholeness of self and others.

References

Atkins, S., & Murphy, K. (1993). Reflection: A review of the literature. *Journal of Advanced Nursing, 18*(8), 1188–1192.

Bache, C. (2001). *Transformative learning.* Sausalito, CA: Noetic Sciences Institute.

Benner, P. (1984). *From novice to expert: Uncovering the knowledge embedded in clinical practice*. Boston, MA: Addison-Wesley.

Benner, P., Sutphen, M., Leonard, V., & Day, L. (2010). *Educating nurses: A call for radical transformation*. San Francisco, CA: Jossey-Bass.

Benner, P., & Wrubel, J. (1989). *The primacy of caring: Stress and coping in health and illness*. Saddle River, NJ: Prentice-Hall.

Bulman, C., & Schutz, S. (2004). *Reflective practice in nursing* (3rd ed.). London, UK: Blackwell Publishing.

Burns, S., & Bulman, C. (2000). *Reflective practice in nursing: The growth of the professional practitioner* (2nd ed.). Oxford, UK: Blackwell Science.

Burton, A. (2000). Reflection: Nursing's practice and education panacea? *Journal of Advanced Nursing, 31*(5), 1009–1017.

Carper, B. A. (1978). Fundamental patterns of knowing in nursing. *Advances in Nursing Science, 1*(1), 13–23.

Cowling, W. R., Smith, M., & Watson, J. (2008). The power of wholeness, consciousness, and caring. A dialogue on nursing science, art, and healing. *Advances in Nursing Science, 31*(1), E41–E51.

Cranton, P. (1996). *Professional development as transformative learning: New perspectives for teachers of adults*. San Francisco, CA: Jossey-Bass.

Cranton, P. (2006). *Understanding and promoting transformative learning: A guide for educators of adults*. San Francisco, CA: Jossey-Bass.

Cronenwett, L., Sherwood, G., Barnsteiner, J., Disch, J., Johnson, J., Mitchell, P., . . . Warren, J. (2007). Quality and safety education for nurses. *Nursing Outlook, 55*(3), 122–131.

Cronenwett, L., Sherwood, G., & Gelmon, S. B. (2009). Improving quality and safety education: The QSEN learning collaborative. *Nursing Outlook, 57*(6), 304–313.

Day, L., & Sherwood, G. (2017a). Transforming education to transform practice: Using unfolding case studies to integrate quality and safety in subject centered classrooms. In G. Sherwood & J. Barnsteiner (Eds.), *Quality and safety in nursing: A competency approach to improving outcomes* (2nd ed.) (pp. 199–220). Hoboken, NJ: Wiley-Blackwell.

Day, L., & Sherwood, G. (2017b). Quality and safety in clinical learning environments. In G. Sherwood & J. Barnsteiner (Eds.), *Quality and safety in nursing: A competency approach to improving outcomes* (2nd ed.) (pp. 253–263). Hoboken, NJ: Wiley-Blackwell.

Dewey, J. (1933). *How we think: A restatement of the relation of reflective thinking to the educative process*. Boston, MA: D. C. Heath.

Drago-Severson, E. (2004). *Becoming adult learners: Principles and practices for effective development*. New York, NY: Teachers College Press.

Epp, S. (2008). The value of reflective journaling in undergraduate nursing education: A literature review. *International Journal of Nursing Studies, 45*(9), 1379–1388.

Freshwater, D. (Ed.). (2002). *Therapeutic nursing: Improving patient care through reflection*. London, UK: Sage Publications.

Freshwater, D. (2008). Reflective practice: The state of the art. In D. Freshwater, B. Taylor, & G. Sherwood (Eds.), *International textbook of reflective practice in nursing* (pp. 1–18). Oxford, UK: Blackwell Publishing.

Freshwater, D., Horton-Deutsch, S., Sherwood, G., & Taylor, B. (2005). The scholarship of reflective practice (position paper). Indianapolis, IN: Sigma Theta Tau International. Retrieved from http://www.nursingsociety.org/docs/default-source/position-papers/resource_reflective.pdf?sfvrsn=4

Goulet, M. H., Larue, C., & Alderson, M. (2016). Reflective practice: A comparative dimensional analysis in nursing and education studies. *Nursing Forum, 51*(2), 139–150.

Hatlevik, I. K. R. (2012). The theory-practice relationship: Reflective skills and theoretical knowledge as key factors in bridging the gap between theory and practice in initial nursing education. *Journal of Advanced Nursing, 68*(4), 868–877.

Horton-Deutsch, S. (2016). Thinking, acting and leading through Caring Science literacy. In S. Lee, P. Palmieri, & J. Watson (Eds.), *Global advances in human caring literacy* (pp. 59–70). New York, NY: Springer.

Horton-Deutsch, S., & Sherwood, G. (2008). Reflection: An educational strategy to develop emotionally-competent nurse leaders. *Journal of Nursing Management, 16*(8), 946–954.

Institute of Medicine (IOM). (2001). *Crossing the quality chasm: A new health system for the 21st century*. Washington, DC: National Academies Press.

Institute of Medicine (IOM). (2003). *Health professions education: A bridge to quality.* Washington, DC: National Academies Press.

Institute of Medicine (IOM). (2004). *Keeping patients safe: Transforming the work environment of nurses.* Washington, DC: National Academies Press.

Jacobs, S. (2016). Reflective learning, reflective practice. *Nursing, 46*(5), 62–64.

Johns, C. (1995a). Framing learning through reflection within Carper's fundamental ways of knowing in nursing. *Journal of Advanced Nursing, 22*(2), 226–234.

Johns, C. (2000). *Becoming a reflective practitioner.* London, UK: Blackwell Science.

Johns, C. (2016). *Mindful leadership. A guide for the health care professions.* London, UK: Palgrave Macmillan.

Johns, D. (1995b). The value of reflective practice for nursing. *Journal of Clinical Nursing, 4,* 23–30.

Kear, T. (2013). Transformative learning during nursing education: A model of interconnectivity. *Nurse Education Today, 33* (2013), 1083–1087.

Kolb, D. A. (1984). *Experiential learning: Experience as the source of learning and development.* Englewood Cliffs, NJ: Prentice-Hall.

Mezirow, J. (1991). *Transformative dimensions of adult learning.* San Francisco, CA: Jossey-Bass.

Miller, L. (2014). Reflective practice for appraisal and revalidation in general practice: Towards new learning and improved patient safety? *Education for Primary Care, 25*(2), 119–121.

Paget, T. (2001). Reflective practice and clinical outcomes: Practitioners' views on how reflective practice has influenced their clinical practice. *Journal of Clinical Nursing, 10*(2), 204–214.

Ruth-Sahd, L. A. (2003). Reflective practice: A critical analysis of data-based studies and implications for nursing education. *Journal of Nursing Education, 42*(11), 488–497.

Schön, D. A. (1983). *The reflective practitioner.* San Francisco, CA: Harper Collins.

Sherwood, G., & Horton-Deutsch, S. (2008). Reflective practice: The route to nursing leadership. In D. Freshwater, B. Taylor, & G. Sherwood (Eds.), *International textbook of reflective practice in nursing* (pp. 157–176). Oxford, UK: Blackwell Publishing.

Sherwood, G., & Horton-Deutsch, S. (Eds.). (2015). *Reflective organizations: On the front lines of QSEN & reflective practice implementation.* Indianapolis, IN: Sigma Theta Tau International.

Sitzman, K., & Watson, J. (2014). *Caring Science, mindful practice.* New York, NY: Springer Publishing Company.

Spector, N., Ulrich, B., & Barnsteiner, J. (2017). Improving quality and safety with transition to practice. In G. Sherwood & J. Barnsteiner (Eds.), *Quality and safety in nursing: A competency approach to improving outcomes* (2nd ed.) (pp. 281–300). Hoboken, NJ: Wiley-Blackwell.

Tanner, C. (2006). Thinking like a nurse: A research-based model of clinical judgment in nursing. *Journal of Nursing Education, 45*(6), 204–211.

Taylor, B. J. (2000). *Reflective practice: A guide for nurses and midwives.* Buckingham, UK: Open University Press.

Taylor, B., Freshwater, D., Sherwood, G., & Esterhuizen, P. (2008). International perspectives in reflective practice: Global knowledge reservoirs. In D. Freshwater, B. Taylor, & G. Sherwood (Eds.), *International textbook of reflective practice in nursing* (pp. 71–96). Oxford, UK: Blackwell Publishing.

Truglio-Londrigan, M. (2013a). Shared decision making through reflective practice: Part I. *MedSurg Nursing, 25*(4), 260–264.

Truglio-Londrigan, M. (2013b). Shared decision making through reflective practice: Part II. *MedSurg Nursing, 25*(5), 341–346.

Watson, J. (2008). *Nursing: The philosophy and science of caring* (Rev. ed.). Boulder, CO: University of Colorado Press.

Watson, J. (2016). Human caring literacy. In S. Lee, P. Palmieri, & J. Watson (Eds.), *Global advances in human caring literacy* (pp. 3–20). New York, NY: Springer Publishing Company.

Chapter 2

Reflection and Mindful Practice: A Means to Quality and Safety

–Gail Armstrong, PhD, DNP, RN, ACNS-BC, CNE
–Gwen D. Sherwood, PhD, RN, FAAN, ANEF
–With Learning Activity by Gail Armstrong

Quality and safety are major drivers in patient outcomes, and critical data supports the need for healthcare system improvements. Though many factors contribute to healthcare quality and safety, the 2003 Institute of Medicine (IOM) report cited major gaps in health professions education related to quality and safety (IOM, 2003). Largely led by the national Quality and Safety Education for Nurses (QSEN) project (Cronenwett et al., 2007; Cronenwett, Sherwood, & Gelmon, 2009) funded by the Robert Wood Johnson Foundation, many nursing education programs have reconceptualized their curricula by integrating quality and safety competencies; redesigning pedagogical approaches for learners to achieve the knowledge, skills, and attitudes defining the quality and safety competencies; and rethinking clinical learning experiences. The demand to improve quality and safety, and thus patient outcomes, raises a corresponding demand for educators prepared to achieve the call for transformation cited in the 2003 IOM.

New graduate nurses often struggle to know how to integrate quality and safety into their daily work roles and responsibilities. According to one study, 39% of new nurses think they are "poorly" or "very poorly" prepared, or had "never heard of" quality improvement (Kovner, Brewer, Yingrengreung, & Fairchild, 2010). Changing mind-sets for quality and safety is more than introducing content. How do nurse educators help learners (both in academic settings and in transition to practice programs) to incorporate competencies in quality and safety as part of their daily work? Nursing theorist Patricia Benner calls for innovation in how nurses are taught to think (Benner, Sutphen, Leonard, & Day, 2010). Applying a standard model of engagement in practice can guide nurses in their development to consider what they know, make interpretations, and determine thoughtful action; engagement and reflexivity bring the presence of mind to recognize potential gaps in care and thereby improve outcomes. Tanner (2006) developed a multistep model of clinical judgment—including reflection-on-action and reflection-in-action—which helps learners process information to make decisions about their work and develop clinical reasoning to "think like a nurse." It is nurses' critical thinking and analyses that provide the foundation for a practice that's ready for the twenty-first century (Benner et al., 2010).

As clinical agencies and nursing programs provide development experiences to expand new graduate nurses' professional value systems to include quality and safety, strong evidence suggests that reflective inquiry facilitates meaningful exploration of nurses' own roles and sense of professional responsibility (Freshwater, 2008; Johns, 1994, 1995; Spector, Ulrich, & Barnsteiner, 2017). New graduate nurses are increasingly exposed to foundational content in practice quality standards and national safety initiatives but lack focus on systems approaches. That is, early nursing education often focuses on the tasks involved in providing patient care with episodic exposure to systems approaches to care. Nursing students do not always understand that safe systems of care and safe provision of care are different facets of the same phenomenon. Quality and safety are not only systems phenomena; clinicians continually make important decisions at the individual practice level that influence quality and safety outcomes. Eventually, clinicians must wrestle with the call for increased quality and safety in their individual practice. This chapter will illustrate how reflective practice can be an effective learning strategy to help bridge the chasm that sits between quality and safety at the systems level and the consideration of quality and safety in an individual nurse's practice. We will explore the unique kind of learning immersed in quality and safety that serves as a deeper educational experience through an exemplar teaching strategy.

REFLECTIVE INQUIRY

The process of using reflection to ask questions, challenge assumptions, and investigate one's practice.

Reflective Practice and Emotional Intelligence

"By increasing emotional intelligence, nurses raise their awareness so they can make better choices in the future. This process enhances nurses' abilities to have emotional intelligence inform their practice."

The call for radical transformation to improve quality and safety in patient-care delivery requires nurses to reach beyond their intellect to their emotional intelligence. Quality and safety are value-laden concepts that should undergird a nurse's professional stance, whether as a clinician, an educator, or a learner. Doing good work, doing the right thing, and being a good team member are core values in nursing and confirm the will nurses have to improve quality and safety. To improve outcomes requires both a mind-set—i.e., the will—and the skills to use a set of tools—i.e., the ideas and execution.

EMOTIONAL INTELLIGENCE

The ability to monitor feelings and emotions, to discriminate among them, and then use that information to guide thinking and actions.

Teaching nurses about reflective practice is an effective approach to developing *emotional intelligence* (EI) (Foster, McCloughen, Delgado, Kefalas, & Harkness, 2015; Shanta & Gargiulo, 2014). Goleman (1998) describes EI as the ability to monitor feelings and emotions, to discriminate among them, and then use that information to guide your thinking and actions. Emotional intelligence involves recognizing your own feelings as well as those of others and employing this insight in managing yourself and your relationships. Broken down into four realms, EI comprises self-awareness, self-management, social awareness, and relationship management (Goleman, Boyatzis, & McKee, 2002). By increasing EI, nurses raise their awareness, so they can make better choices in the future. This process enhances nurses' ability to have EI inform their practice. Emotional intelligence is the trademark of effective leaders, and this capacity contributes to developing clinical maturity. Reflection helps fit the puzzle together to make sense of experience and knowledge, so that nurses can improve performance and move toward professional maturity. More recently, information science has utilized specific theories related to "sense-making" (Rhodes, McDonald, Campbell, Daker-White, & Sanders, 2016). The process of sense-making provides a theoretical framework by which individuals work to address the "cognitive gap" experienced when attempting to make sense of observed data (Dervin, 1998). The reflective process, when informed by elements of EI, is an effective method for neophyte nursing students to begin a sense-making process to understand their practice and increase awareness of patient safety and quality.

Quality and Safety: Moving from the Political to the Personal

New graduate nurses have a value system that inherently recognizes that safe practice and quality improvement are "right action" and important processes, but their introduction to the mechanics of quality and safety may be at the systems level, employing resources found on the QSEN website (www.qsen.org). New clinicians can experience a sense of cognitive dissonance in their practice when they face an incongruity between standards they have learned and what they observe in practice. Learners often experience inner conflict as they begin to consider compromises in quality and safety and the effect of compromised care at the patient level. In observing a lapse in safety, learners can better appreciate the consequence for a specific patient. For example, in witnessing a medication error, the learner now begins to reflect on the possibility of potential harm to Mr. Smith in Room 204. Quality and safety become transformed from a concern of the quality assurance department to an important facet of an individual clinician's bedside practice, melding how the system problem is enacted at the individual level. The individual concern highlights and informs the larger system issue, helping inspire participation in system repairs to prevent future adverse events.

Models of Reflective Practice That Influence Practice

CREATIVE TENSION
The experience where uncertainty or conflict ultimately leads to improved ideas or outcomes.

Johns (1999) extensively explored the rich potential in a clinician's sense of contradiction. In essence, reflective practice is the process of exposing contradictions in practice, and it demands nurses confront themselves and the conditions of practice that limit the achievement of "good" work in which one "does the right thing." In exposing contradictions, nurses use a reflective process first to understand their definition of ideal practice, then examine the multiplicity of factors within the clinical interaction that either hindered or enhanced their ability to achieve ideal practice, and then consider alternative actions for the future (Johns, 1998, 1999). Johns offers the potential of "creative tension" in the uncomfortable experience of contradiction (2009), wherein improvement of practice is a natural outcome of this creative tension.

As discussed in Chapter 1, Freshwater (2008) describes three models of reflective practice as *descriptive, dialogic,* and *critical,* and they build on each other. Descriptive practice helps one develop consciousness of one's actions with a focus on reflection-on-action through journaling or critical incident reporting. Dialogic reflection is deliberate and it includes talking with peers or clinical supervision. Critical reflection, perhaps the most difficult, brings changes in practice; practitioners are able to provide reasoning for actions by engaging in critical conversation about practice with self and others.

Creative Tension Related to Quality and Safety

A natural overlap exists between quality and safety and reflective practice in the concept of *contradiction.* Reflective practice provides an ongoing process for learners to consider their responses to practice contradictions they see in addressing quality and safety. As learners are educated about emerging standards in quality and safety, they imagine evidence-based standards, well-organized patient care delivery systems, and ideal circumstances within the environment. Sometimes, disillusionment arises as novice learners see the profound divide between the ideal values they were taught about the healthcare system and the flawed care delivery systems they encounter in practice.

Learners struggle with the limits of their own abilities, yet feel a unique gravity as they observe contradictions in quality and safety standards that transcend other realities they witnessed during prelicensure education. The contradictions they see in how patients are safeguarded amid lapses in quality demand attention because of the potential for patient harm. Nurses carry a continuing concern that they might harm a patient. Any safety incident becomes an opportunity for applying a reflective practice framework to analyze imperfect systems and the response within their own nursing practice. By exposing contradictory circumstances around how healthcare systems should protect patient safety even with existing gaps in the system, nurses are forced to examine their commitment to quality and safety in their own practice and their ultimate desire to improve healthcare systems.

Providing guidance to learners within these uncomfortable realities is vital because of the natural tendency to limit experiences of feeling uncomfortable. Despite their discomfort, helping learners sit in the contradiction is the heart of the fertile reflective process. The essence of learning through reflection is for practitioners to draw out contradiction between what they intend to achieve within any situation and the way they actually practice. Contradiction creates a sense of internal conflict, an uneasy sense deep within the practitioner, which learners naturally want to avoid. In teaching a reflective approach to practice, we help nurses learn that contradictions exist because, for whatever reason, practitioners are unable to act congruently with their beliefs (Johns, 1999). When nurses are introduced to reflective practice early in their practice, they gradually develop an awareness of practice contradictions (Miller, 2014). Reflective practice enables them to learn to act on this discomfort by reflecting to understand the incongruities and eventually to develop skills to understand these experiences in a way that allows them to practice in tune with their values.

The Time and Space to Reflect

Nurses are bombarded by stimuli. Reflective practice provides temporal distance from an experience. Within this time and space, learners can intentionally review an experience in the context of their emerging professional values. Without encouragement to consciously reflect on discrete experiences, overwhelmed neophytes potentially bypass rich learning. Inviting learners to engage in reflection and mindful practice gives them vital avenues to make sense of their emerging practice. With space, learners can deconstruct an incident observed in practice and begin to harvest insights. Reflective practice means thinking about practice, your relationships with others, and the way you feel about performing certain tasks. In a sense, reflective practice means becoming more self-aware of your own practice (Burnard, 2002).

DASHBOARDS

In an electronic health record, a dashboard is a user interface that presents quality information in a succinct, easy way for the user to read and reference.

An Exemplar for Teaching Quality and Safety Using Reflective Practice

Learners find an easy pairing between reflective practice and quality and safety in ways that are often surprising. The following exemplar outlines a learning strategy to create space for learners to engage in reflection and develop mindful practice. Because of the integration of the quality and safety competencies defined in the QSEN project (www.qsen.org; Cronenwett et al., 2007; Cronenwett et al., 2009) into nursing education essentials, all nurses should be exposed to learning opportunities in their educational program to understand quality and safety science (Sherwood & Barnsteiner, 2017). From this, learners should know about national safety initiatives such as the National Patient Safety Goals, the 5 Million Lives Campaign, and the National Quality Forum's Safe Practices for Better Healthcare (Barnsteiner, 2017). Accreditation standards (American Association of Colleges of Nursing [AACN], 2008; National League for Nursing [NLN], 2010) include quality-improvement strategies such as the use of dashboards and benchmarks for comparison of quality data. The learning strategy described here is an example of *reflection-on-action*, a retrospective reflection that helps make sense of an experience, thus influencing future practice (Schön, 1987).

Initially, nurse educators provide content and background about reflective practice. Reflective practice content gives learners a schemata and language for future assignments. The strategy helps learners develop a foundation in reflective practice using Johns's (1998) conceptualization, through which they are introduced to the idea of tacit knowledge. *Tacit knowledge* can be described as embedded knowledge. A review of the literature on tacit knowledge (McAdam, Mason, & McCrory, 2007) defines tacit knowledge as "knowledge in practice developed from direct experience and action; highly pragmatic and situation specific; subconsciously understood and applied; difficult to articulate; usually shared through interactive conversation and shared experience" (p. 46). In nursing, Benner (1984) examined the clinical development of nurses and identified access to tacit knowledge as a hallmark of expert clinicians. The expert nurse is able to understand the multiplicity of factors at play within a situation. Benner clarifies, however, that nurses must develop access to their tacit knowledge, and this occurs over time—both through reflective learning and experience. As novices, early learners do not believe that they have any embedded knowledge. It is helpful to give new nurses a foundation in the different ways of knowing to demonstrate that expertise is more than extensive content knowledge. When novice learners see expert clinicians grasp the multiplicity of factors at play within a clinical situation, learners have language and a framework for understanding and articulating such expertise. As learners progress in their clinical development, the process of reflection provides access to tacit knowledge gained in practice (Benner, Kyriakidis, & Stannard, 2011).

"Reflection papers" are one way to guide students to apply the process of reflective practice, whether in an academic setting or with new graduates in a transition-to-practice program. One- or two-page reflection papers completed on a weekly basis are an effective way to demonstrate that all experiences become part of the learning process; the practice of regular writing helps tap all the ways of knowing and helps students recognize how they are building a knowledge base on which to base future actions. These papers become requisite parts of the learners' course of study—perhaps part of a portfolio—and focus on what the learners are experiencing in the provision of care. Learners receive written responses to each paper, offering support and coaching to continue to explore questions and encouraging learners to listen to their emerging inner voices. Helping learners become cognizant of their inner voices, despite the inevitable subjectivity, opens the door for increased awareness and consciousness (Johns, 2009) of their experiences. The weekly reflection and feedback become a one-on-one written dialogue between the educator and each learner. Learners gradually come to trust the space provided and settle into the process. This foundation in the language of reflective practice provides a framework through which they can articulate and understand the "uneasiness" and distress common for novice clinicians. Learners have a natural tendency to reflect on experiences that compromise quality and safety; these experiences, if unprocessed, can lead to a sense of uneasiness about their practice.

As an initial assignment, learners are asked to write a reflection paper that outlines the three top values that they believe will shape their practice standards. This writing creates the foundation for contradictions they might encounter in their experiences of providing care. Safety is often identified as a core value for practice, and this focus facilitates the development of mindfulness about risks to patient safety. Learners' values conceptualization becomes a prime source of dialogue in their weekly reflection papers. Table 2.1 outlines the subsequent open-ended prompts for weekly reflection papers that create a consistent, safe space for learners to examine emerging practice questions. All learners have questions about experiences, and their weekly writing invites them into a space of inquiry, thereby facilitating self-awareness, practice awareness, and ultimately a foundation in mindfulness, which is discussed more fully in Chapter 6.

TABLE 2.1 Writing Prompts for Weekly Reflection Papers (By Gail Armstrong)

1. Tell me about your top three priorities for your nursing practice. What are the barriers you are encountering to these priorities?
2. How does what you are currently seeing at the bedside challenge what you have learned about quality and safety?
3. Describe a clinical experience that affirmed your decision to enter nursing.
4. What was a notable experience from your time at the bedside today? Why do you think it was important for you?

5. Have you noticed similarities among those individuals whom you consider to be positive role models? Negative role models?

6. When today were you unsure of what to do? How did you feel? What steps did you take to be able to make an informed decision?

7. What do you value most about the work you do (or can do)?

8. What do you value most about the contributions you make?

9. What are the core values and best practices that define your work?

10. What are the three things that you commit to in order to improve patient safety?

Guiding learners in the reflective process rather than allowing a more random process is valuable. Guided reflection is a distinct process for reliving your experiences. A variety of models describe, deconstruct, and employ reflective practice in nursing education (Ruth-Sahd, 2003). When educators guide learners in the process of reflective practice, they can ensure more consistency in the guided reflection and less circling on the learner's part, so the learner can get to the point more clearly. If educators observe a learner "spinning" in the process, meaning he or she just circles without coming to a conclusion, they can pose a potent question to move the learner along. Learners often feel able to explore their own reflections in more depth when they receive feedback, encouragement, and support from a clinician familiar with reflective practice. Additionally, guided reflective practice is a progressive process in which learners are encouraged to stay with a question until its natural conclusion.

Learning Through Reflection: Common Themes in Reflection Papers

Through the process of reflection, learners often arrive at a deeper understanding of patient-centered care. One learner who had written about her love of the "technicality of the machines" in nursing wrote one of her last reflection papers on a patient for whom she cared who had been hospitalized with burns to his hands:

> I was assisting the burn nurse with changing the bandages and dressings and the removal of the staples that had been placed to adhere the artificial surface to his own flesh. It looked as though it was healing fairly well. At first I was intrigued with the process that I was watching, and then I looked at the face of the patient. It was plain that this was the first time he had seen the extent of his injuries since he was admitted. He was horrified.
>
> This experience was rich in caring moments for me as a nurse...It was an awakening for me to put the human context to the clinical conditions that I have only read about in books or simulated in lab. This was not a limb with a second and third degree burns to be debrided and bandaged. This was a person with a family to support and a crew of men who looked to him for their livelihood. This was a man used to being in charge of his environment and able to create things with the work of his hands. Now his life will be changed forever.

The striking part of this reflection paper was the learner's dramatic shift away from objectifying her patient as a diagnosis to humanizing her patient as an individual person with a rich human context and life. Freshwater would classify this reflection as a *critical reflection*. You can hear the learner's own surprise in this shift. Even her use of the phrase "caring moments" was indicative of a transformation for this young clinician: Her previous reflection papers had focused solely on the technical aspects of care for her patients.

When a learner observes an explicit compromise in patient safety, the experience can be confusing and upsetting. The example that follows outlines a learner's observation of an extreme compromise in patient safety around the insertion of a Foley catheter and her multilayered response to the experience.

I had quite the striking experience at the bedside this week. One that I believe I won't ever forget. In my EBP class this week, we were discussing implementation of EBP, and these discussions have informed some of my questions. As much as we wish it wasn't still happening, many of our preceptors on the floor show us learners "the right way" to do a task, and then "the way they do it." When a nurse is showing me something "her way" and I know from class or lab that it is not the right way, it can have a tendency to make me very emotional for the patient. For example, this week I inserted a Foley catheter and of course took my time to do it the correct way that we were shown in our lab, all the while talking to the patient. Then later I went into a room with my preceptor who was inserting a Foley. She put the same Foley completely in and out (all the way to the Y bifurcation) three times. She did this regardless of the fact that it had the woman's menses on it, never once talking to the patient to let her know what was happening (in fact she was on the phone the whole time).

I was in shock by these actions. I had never felt so far from our fundamentals lab. I kept thinking about the extreme risk for infection my nurse had created. I have been wondering why nurses do things the wrong way, when they obviously know the right way. Is it a time constraint thing? Or did my nurse not want to have to charge the patient for three separate Foley catheter trays? Or did she not want to take the time to get off the phone and go down the hall to get another sterile catheter? Would she even feel guilty if she knew her actions had put her patient at risk for infection? As confused as I was by this "role modeling," it has made me think about my own responses to time constraints, inconveniences, and putting patients at risk.

In this exemplar, one can hear and feel this particular learner's sensitivity. Because this student has engaged in how she would improve her practice now and in the future, it is an example of Freshwater's critical reflection, as cited in Chapter 1 (Freshwater, 2008). In previous reflection papers, this learner had written about the "burden" of her sensitivity and how poignantly she felt compassion and empathy. In her subsequent reflection paper, the learner followed with an insightful response to this very upsetting event. The learner articulated that she felt powerless in the learner role as she watched her preceptor compromise patient safety, but she would not be powerless in her own practice. In her follow-up reflection paper, she clearly articulated her commitment to safe practice, evidence-based practice, and doing things "the right way."

Many learners choose to write about the reality-based difficulties of effective teamwork and collaboration in the clinical setting. Not being educated alongside other health professionals, nurse learners are often surprised at the varied models other healthcare disciplines employ in providing patient care.

Doctors and nurses see the same patient through different lenses. Nurses have the opportunity to spend considerably more time with each patient than a doctor does and are able to witness the patient's abilities and hindrances in achieving recovery. It is not a matter of whether the doctor or nurse is right or wrong; it is about working together as a medical team to provide the care that is appropriate for each patient. In optimal patient care, the interventions necessary are seen through each lens and provide the patient with holistic care toward healing. But sometimes the picture of the patient is seen through different lenses and [we] do not agree. This was the case when I took care of a patient whose diagnosis was status-post modified radical neck dissection, left tonsillectomy with parapharyngeal tumor removal. The patient's physician visited him in the hospital, saw how his incision was healing and wrote orders for him to be discharged. From a nursing perspective, this patient was NOT ready to be discharged from the hospital. The patient continued to have difficulty swallowing (he was on a liquid diet) and used oral suction every couple of minutes to help clear his secretions. He had mild nausea that was not well relieved. His pain was not managed well despite receiving morphine slow IVP every 2 hours. And despite teaching, the patient had a knowledge deficit of how to manage the

> care of his two JP drains. The patient lived alone and stated that he
> did not have any family members or friends that would be able to
> assist him at home. As a nurse, part of my role is to be my patient's
> advocate. In observing his struggles, I did not feel comfortable with
> the order to discharge him. I spoke with the RN I was working with,
> and she called the physician to try to paint a picture of what our
> experience had been in caring for this patient all day.

This learner remains nonjudgmental about the physician's different assessment of the patient. She attributes the varying assessments of the patient as different "lenses." This learner is a logical thinker and a critical thinker and demonstrates critical reflection. In her reflection paper, she provided clinical evidence supporting her judgment that the patient was not ready for discharge. This learner also makes explicit the importance she places in the professional value of being the patient's advocate, taking this responsibility very seriously, thinking carefully about the action associated with that value in this particular clinical situation. This learner is to be commended for her insight about the expanded awareness of nurses because of their prolonged exposure to patients and how communication of extra information to the healthcare team is part of what nurses do. She included a description of how her preceptor "paints a picture" for the physician.

Many learners write about an awareness of their own personal and clinical growth. Although they rarely describe it as "tacit" knowledge, learners begin to develop a consciousness for knowing what they know.

> I passed one of my patients that I had taken care of last week in
> the hall. She was back for an outpatient visit and looked great! It's
> amazing how people's personalities need to rest and almost become
> dormant in a time of healing. I think meds also affect a patient's
> personality. Health and peace in people are becoming increasingly
> visible to me. It's almost like noticing a person's outfit or hair color.
> Health and peace can radiate from people; their energy is almost
> striking. I'm amazed that I can now see and appreciate these different
> nuances in patients.

In early clinical rotations, learners can begin to appreciate what they do not understand or know in their practice; however, reflection provides the opportunity for learners to see their own development, however slight it might feel. This learner exemplifies Freshwater's dialogic reflection as fits the criteria cited in Chapter 1.

Later in their development, nursing students cultivate an increased sensibility of their own growth. Reflections from students just prior to graduation demonstrate this evolution:

> I have learned, through the process of my nursing education, how to listen. All my life I have been a great talker. Sitting with my patient last week while the pain medication took effect, I was quiet. My patient was quiet. It was a great moment. I might actually choose to be quiet more often. Also connected to my increased sense of myself is my increasing comfort with not knowing. Patient safety has been emphasized in all of my QSEN work. I ask better questions now. I know my limits. I understand that when I am given the responsibility of caring for people, part of that caring is saying when I don't know something.

This student demonstrates critical reflection; she has clearly developed an increased sense of herself, of her strengths, and of areas that she is still developing. Reflective nurses value the process and outcomes of critically examining practice through engagement and critical reasoning to reconsider practice; thus through critical reflection they are continuously improving their practice.

Learner Responses to Reflection Papers

Few learners realize the value of weekly reflection papers when the assignment is introduced. They might not be accustomed to writing every week and might resist the assignment. However, resistance wanes after learners receive the instructor/educator comments on their first assignment; they quickly recognize the value of the individualized, substantive written response from their "teacher" that launches a continuing one-on-one dialogue throughout the term. Though these examples are from an academic perspective, the same coaching approach can help new graduates in transition to practice or nurses moving along the novice-to-expert continuum (Chapter 3), when they reflect on their new experiences with their preceptor. Similarly, experienced nurses can use the same process, because they are continually "making sense of practice" and incorporating new knowledge. After all, nursing is a lifelong learning process, and reflection is a way to continually update awareness, actions, and responses.

Practicing nurses may use journal writings as part of their development portfolio similar to how students may use course evaluations. In this excerpt from a student evaluation of the course, appreciation for the opportunity to learn reflectively emerges as an important part of the course:

> I appreciate the time the professor took to respond to every assignment I submitted. It was refreshing to see that our papers were read, and to receive individualized feedback. I started looking forward to the comments on my reflection papers. They were supportive, yet encouraged me to stretch in my thinking and in my practice. I developed a familiarity with my inner clinical voice through these papers.

> I wish more professors would use reflection papers. I learned so much about my own thinking through this assignment. It actually felt like valuable work. I feel more aware of my own values as a nurse and how I want to enact those values in my emerging practice.

> I was a pretty big critic of the reflection paper assignment when I first learned about it. Weekly writing, really?? I could not imagine any value to such an overwhelming assignment. But I quickly came to love this weekly outlet. I started hearing "Stephanie the Nurse." I didn't know she existed before this. I think the writing helped me see more clearly which values will guide my practice. There was a lot that I saw in my clinical rotation that upset me, but the weekly writing provided a place to figure out some of that confusion.

Though we have concentrated on learner responses, the constant dialogue between learner and mentor becomes a simultaneous learning experience for the educator. Feeling seen, known, and connected can be beneficial to educators' experience of the teaching process, as well as learners' experience of the learning process (Gillespie, 2005). As educators "hear" back and forth with the learners, they too expand their own capacity as "teachers," as explored in other chapters of the book. Similar conversations may occur between the nurse educator or manager and a nurse in practice as part of professional development.

Final Reflections

Nurses are important members of the healthcare team in helping healthcare systems integrate ongoing improvement in quality and safety. Patient outcomes, quality, and safety are learned both at the systems level and at the personal level to advance professional development. When nurses understand those system improvements in the context of their individual patient, a transformation in mind-set takes place, and quality and safety become an integral part of their daily work. Reflective practice pedagogy, whether in academic or clinical settings, provides important opportunities for nurses to explore their professional and individual commitment to quality and safety in their emerging practice. Written reflective dialogue with teachers, mentors, or other nurses provides systematic learning; this reflecting-on-action is a process of sense-making of experience, thus building tacit knowledge to move toward professional maturity. Insights into improved systems begin in a nurse's own practice; improved systems are often the result of collaboration among professionals who are first committed to improving their own practice.

References

American Association of Colleges of Nursing (AACN). (2008). *The essentials of baccalaureate education for professional nursing practice.* Retrieved from http://www.aacn.nche.edu/education-resources/BaccEssentials08.pdf

Barnsteiner, J. (2017). Safety. In G. Sherwood & J. Barnsteiner (Eds.), *Quality and safety in nursing: A competency approach to improving outcomes* (2nd ed.) (pp. 153–171). Hoboken, NJ: Wiley-Blackwell.

Benner, P. (1984). *From novice to expert: Power and excellence in nursing practice.* Menlo Park, CA: Addison-Wesley Publishing Company.

Benner, P., Kyriakidis, P. H., & Stannard, D. (2011). *Clinical wisdom and interventions in acute and critical care: A thinking-in-action approach* (2nd ed.). New York, NY: Springer Publishing.

Benner, P., Sutphen, M., Leonard, V., & Day, L. (2010). *Educating nurses: A call for radical transformation.* Stanford, CA: Jossey-Bass.

Burnard, P. (2002). *Learning human skills: An experiential and reflective guide for nurses and health care professionals.* Portsmouth, NH: Butterworth Heinemann.

Cronenwett, L., Sherwood, G., Barnsteiner, J., Disch, J., Johnson, J., Mitchell, P., . . . Warren, J. (2007). Quality and safety education for nurses. *Nursing Outlook, 55*(3), 122–131.

Cronenwett, L., Sherwood, G., & Gelmon, S. B. (2009). Improving quality and safety education: The QSEN learning collaborative. *Nursing Outlook, 57*(6), 304–313.

Dervin, B. (1998). Sense making theory and practice: An overview of user interests in knowledge seeking and use. *Journal of Knowledge Management, 2*(2), 36–46.

Foster, K., McCloughen, A., Delgado, C., Kefalas, C., & Harkness, E. (2015). Emotional intelligence education in pre-registration nursing programmes: An integrative review. *Nurse Education Today, 35*(3), 510–517.

Freshwater, D. (2008). Reflective practice: The state of the art. In D. Freshwater, B. Taylor, & G. Sherwood (Eds.), *International textbook of reflective practice in nursing* (pp. 1–18). Oxford, UK: Blackwell Publishing.

Gillespie, M. (2005). Student-teaching connection: A place of possibility. *Journal of Advanced Nursing, 52*(2), 211–219.

Goleman, D. (1998). *Working with emotional intelligence.* New York, NY: Bantam Dell.

Goleman, D., Boyatzis, R., & McKee, A. (2002). *Primal leadership: Realizing the power of emotional intelligence.* Boston, MA: Harvard Business School Publishing.

Institute of Medicine (IOM). (2003). *Health professions education: A bridge to quality.* Washington, DC: National Academies Press.

Johns, C. (1994). Nuances of reflection. *Journal of Clinical Nursing, 3*(2), 71–74.

Johns, C. (1995). Framing learning through reflection within Carper's fundamental ways of knowing in nursing. *Journal of Advanced Nursing, 22*(2), 226–234.

Johns, C. (1998). Caring through a reflective lens: Giving meaning to being a reflective practitioner. *Nursing Inquiry, 5*(1), 18–24.

Johns, C. (1999). Reflection as empowerment? *Nursing Inquiry, 6*(4), 241–249.

Johns, C. (2009). *Becoming a reflective practitioner* (3rd ed.). West Sussex, UK: Wiley-Blackwell.

Kovner, C. T., Brewer, C. S., Yingrengreung, S. N., & Fairchild, S. (2010). New nurses' view of quality improvement education. *Joint Commission Journal on Quality and Patient Safety, 36*(1), 29–35.

Mamykina, L., Smaldone, M., & Bakken, R. (2015). Adopting the sensemaking perspective for chronic disease self-management. *Journal of Biomedical Informatics, August 2015*(56), 406–417. doi:10.1016/j.jbi.2015.06.006

McAdam, R., Mason, B., & McCrory, J. (2007). Exploring the dichotomies within the tacit knowledge literature: Towards a process of tacit knowing in organizations. *Journal of Knowledge Management, 11*(2), 43–59.

Miller, L. (2014). Reflective practice for appraisal and revalidation in general practice: Towards new learning and improved patient safety? *Education for Primary Care, 25*(2), 119–121.

National League for Nursing. (2010). *Outcomes and competencies for graduates of practical/vocational, diploma, associate degree, baccalaureate, masters, doctoral and research doctorate programs in nursing.* New York, NY: National League for Nursing.

Rhodes, P., McDonald, R., Campbell, S., Daker-White, G., & Sanders, C. (2016). Sensemaking and the co-production of safety: A qualitative study of primary medical care patients. *Sociology of Health & Illness, 38*(2), 270–285.

Ruth-Sahd, L. A. (2003). Reflective practice: A critical analysis of data-based studies and implications for nursing education. *Journal of Nursing Education, 42*(11), 488–497.

Schön, D. A. (1987). *Educating the reflective practitioner.* San Francisco, CA: Jossey-Bass.

Shanta, L., & Gargiulo, L. (2014). A study of the influence of nursing education on development of emotional intelligence. *Journal of Professional Nursing, 30*(6), 511–520.

Sherwood, G., & Barnsteiner, J. (Eds.). (2017). *Quality and safety in nursing: A competency approach to improving outcomes* (2nd ed.). Ames, IA: Wiley.

Spector, N., Ulrich, B., & Barnsteiner, J. (2017). New graduate transition into practice: Improving quality and safety. In G. Sherwood & J. Barnsteiner (Eds.), *Quality and safety in nursing: A competency approach to improving outcomes* (2nd ed.) (pp. 281–300). Hoboken, NJ: Wiley-Blackwell.

Tanner, C. A. (2006). Thinking like a nurse: A research based model of clinical judgment in nursing. *Journal of Nursing Education, 45*(6), 204–211.

Chapter 3

Reflection and Mindful Practice: Developing Emotional Intelligence Through Coaching

–*Michael Moran, DHA, ACC, LFACHE*
–*Gwen D. Sherwood, PhD, RN, FAAN, ANEF*

The importance of *emotional intelligence* (EI) for nurses is well documented in the literature (Cadman & Brewer, 2001; Evans & Allen, 2002; Smith, Profetto-McGrath, & Cummings, 2009), with a growing number of research studies examining EI among nursing students. However, there is little discussion about the specific set of skills that contribute to EI and a methodology for helping nurses enhance those skills. Educators across all settings can use coaching strategies with a variety of learners to facilitate reflective practice and foster professional development, whether during nursing school, transition to practice programs, enhancing leadership skills, or career development to move from novice to expert (Ball, 2013; Benson, Martin, Ploeg, & Wessel, 2012; Codier, Kofoed, & Peters, 2015; Foster, McCloughen, Delgado, Kefalas, & Harkness, 2015; Rankin, 2013).

This chapter describes how to use a coaching model and self-assessment information to enhance emotional intelligence skills through reflective practice. Four themes of a coaching model are discussed, beginning with a brief overview of EI and its relationship to practice, followed by a description of self-assessment to reveal the learner's profile of EI skills, a review of the coaching model, and application of reflective practice to evaluate and integrate change. The last section illustrates a coaching conversation, learner examples with expected outcomes, and consideration of integrating emotional intelligence development into educational curricula.

A Coaching Model to Develop Emotional Intelligence

Peterson (1996) defines coaching as "a process of equipping people with the tools, knowledge, and opportunities they need to develop themselves and become more effective" (p. 78). The following scenario of an emotional intelligence coaching conversation illustrates the four interrelated themes of the chapter: emotional intelligence, self-assessment, individual coaching, and reflective practice.

SCENARIO: EMOTIONAL INTELLIGENCE COACHING CONVERSATION

Lacey had just reviewed her emotional intelligence assessment report, and her instructor was facilitating a coaching conversation with her. The conversation began with a discussion about empathy, one of the 15 emotional intelligence skills measured in the self-assessment. As a caregiver, she was not surprised that her empathy score was high, indicating she had no difficulty understanding and being sensitive to the feelings and experiences of others. When asked when it might be helpful to not be overly empathetic, Lacey suggested it was essential that her empathy for suffering patients not interfere with clinical decisions or actions.

Her instructor asked about other situations where it was helpful or harmful to either display empathy or withhold it. Lacey recognized that a lack of empathy could leave patients feeling she was distant and aloof. Conversely, she often worried that, in her current working environment, if she was unable to manage her empathy and always tuned into the pain and suffering of her patients, she would quickly burn out from the emotional strain. The instructor then asked her to describe a specific incident where this strain had occurred. Lacey paused, took a deep breath, and began her story about what had happened a day ago among a patient, a doctor, and herself.

The scenario centers on Lacey's emotional intelligence report, which included detailed descriptions of skills and capabilities that assessed her emotional intelligence. The instructor engaged Lacey in a coaching conversation about the report to guide Lacey to examine her work as a nurse from the viewpoint of emotional intelligence skills. The focus in this conversation is empathy. This examination is intended to lead her to greater self-awareness, more emotional intelligence, and changes in her nursing practice. The coaching process allowed Lacey to see the contextual nature of emotional intelligence skills—how her emotional intelligence skills were linked to specific situations and persons—and consider how modifying her skills accordingly would benefit her professional practice.

Emotional Intelligence

In his landmark book, *Emotional Intelligence*, Daniel Goleman (1995) defined *emotional intelligence* as the ability to monitor feelings and emotions, to discriminate among them, and then use the information to guide thinking and actions. EI is based on five major domains listed in Table 3.1. The more detailed Emotional Competence Framework, which identifies 25 personal and social competencies (Goleman, 1998), can be viewed at http://www.eiconsortium. org/pdf/emotional_competence_framework.pdf. Goleman also referred to these competencies as capabilities or skills, emphasizing the potential for individuals to develop them over time.

TABLE 3.1 Model for Emotional Intelligence (Goleman, 1998)

DOMAIN	DEFINITION
Self-Awareness	Know one's emotions, strengths, weaknesses, drives, values, and goals and recognize their impact on others while using gut feelings to guide decisions.
Self-Regulation	Manage or redirect one's disruptive emotions and impulses and adapt to changing circumstances.
Social Skill	Manage others' emotions to move people in the desired direction.
Empathy	Recognize, understand, and consider other people's feelings, especially when making decisions.
Motivation	Motivate oneself to achieve for the sake of achievement.

The psychologist Reuven Bar-On broadened the emotional intelligence concept to include social intelligence and described it as an array of interrelated emotional and social competencies, skills, and behaviors that determine how well we understand and express ourselves; understand others and relate to them; and cope with daily demands, challenges, and pressures (Bar-On, 2013).

The Bar-On model identifies 15 skills and capabilities, such as self-regard, emotional self-awareness and expression, empathy, assertiveness, and independence that make up an individual's emotional and social intelligence (available at http://www.eiconsortium.org/reprints/bar-on_model_of_emotional-social_intelligence.htm).

Applied to nursing, EI is emotional awareness in relation to self, professional efficiency, and emotional management within the context of the environment (Akerjordet & Severinsson, 2010). EI skills are foundational to effective leadership; leadership is about relationships, working with and through people to create desired results. Transformational leaders motivate engagement, active participation, mindful practice, and presence that lead to change. Transformational leadership is grounded in emotional intelligence skills that develop the capacity to manage self, others, and environmental context. By monitoring one's own and others' emotions, nurses develop the capacity to reflect and use the information to guide thinking and actions.

Throughout this book, EI is cited as an important trait for nurses and other health professionals. In Chapter 2, you read that, by increasing emotional intelligence, nurses raise their awareness so they can make better choices in the future. Chapter 10 also notes that reflection helps develop self-awareness, an essential aspect of emotional intelligence. Educators in both clinical and academic settings can guide nurses and students in developing EI skills that contribute to better work environments, enhance how people work together, and foster patient-centered care—all of which contribute to the quality and safety of patient care (Fitzpatrick, 2016). Application of a coaching model is presented in this chapter to illustrate the strategies used to help learners in any setting develop EI skills.

Self-Assessment for Emotional Intelligence Skills

A variety of assessments measure emotional intelligence (Bar-On, 2006; see http://www.eiconsortium.org/reprints/bar-on_model_of_emotional-social_intelligence.htm). Coaches need to complete EI training, particularly in measurement tools, to be able to effectively work with learners in developing EI skills. Assessments that identify specific skills and measure individual skill levels provide learners with constructs to apply to their experience to further their understanding of EI. Together, a descriptive EI model and the assessment of current skill levels provide learners with a starting point for reflective practice—a language and framework that helps them make sense of what they notice about themselves, their environments, and experiences. Most of these self-assessments are questionnaires that learners complete online. The EI examples in this chapter are taken from work with the Bar-On EQ-i 2.0 Model of Emotional Intelligence (Multi-Health Systems, 2011).

Coaching Conversation

The coaching conversation is conducted by a trained educator who has basic coaching skills, is familiar with a structured coaching process, and understands the emotional intelligence self-assessment tool and the skills it measures. The purpose of a coaching conversation is to enhance the learner's understanding of EI through inquiry and facilitate an action plan for improvement. Through the inquiry process, the coach educator asks the learner to reflect on her own experiences to discover how the EI skills impact her effectiveness and well-being. Following the CAAACS coaching model and using the learner's EI self-assessment results, the coach educator guides the learner through an inquiry and goal-setting process, culminating in reflective learning and action.

Reflective Practice

The reflective practice process is ideal for enhancing emotional intelligence self-awareness and learning from experience. The foundation of reflective practice is a structured and purposeful examination of one's lived experience. A number of processes are described in this book that guide learners through a description of their experience, an inquiry into plausible interpretations, and articulation of informed action plans to reenter the experience in order to learn. Learners use the EI skills and self-assessment to describe and interpret their experiences. The action plan is grounded in a specific lived experience that the learner targets to develop EI skills. The coaching procedure and its guiding questions follow the reflective practice sequence. The following exercise presents selected questions from the coaching process to illustrate the sequence.

COACHING QUESTIONS TO GUIDE REFLECTION ON EI

Description:

- *Describe the results of the self-assessment report.*
- *Describe personal experiences that support the results.*
- *Describe personal experiences that do not support the results.*
- *What observations can I make about specific emotional skills, based on the report results?*

Interpretation:

- *In what instances would enhanced EI skills benefit me?*
- *What are the critical features of this situation?*

- *How would I modulate EI skills in response to circumstances or reactions from others?*
- *What are the specific challenges in managing my emotions in this situation?*

Action Plan:

- *Which EI skill do I want to work on?*
- *How will I work on this emotional skill in this specific situation?*
- *What do I want to be able to do (that I cannot do now)?*
- *How will I evaluate my work on this emotional skill?*

Connecting the Dots: Linking Actions With Results

When learners see that emotional intelligence is composed of specific skills, they see the connection between parts and the whole, between actions and consequences (Shanta & Gargiulo, 2014). Their personal assessment results provide them with feedback about their current skill levels, which they can contrast with their personal experience. The coaching conversation challenges learners (in a nonjudgmental fashion) to reflect on their personal experiences and discover the relevance of various EI skills to their professional practice and their lives. The inquiry process identifies the contexts in which the learners' use of EI skills is helpful or not, inserting the decision-making dynamic into their reflective process. And finally, the coaching conversation addresses the learners' desire to enhance their emotional intelligence with an action plan.

Emotional intelligence is a conceptual framework that lists and categorizes skills that together constitute a model for relationships with self and others. This framework can be used to assess one's emotional intelligence and to serve as a guide for further development—in the form of a self-assessment instrument or questionnaire. When learners complete the self-assessment, the instructor meets with them individually to review the results. Then, using coaching procedures (inquiry and dialogue), the instructor guides each learner through a process of description, interpretation, and identification of an action plan for a specific EI skill, grounded in a specific circumstance of the learner's choice. This process is a guided reflective practice.

REFLECTING ON . . . QUESTIONS TO DEVELOP EMOTIONAL INTELLIGENCE SKILLS

- *Describe: What skills make up my emotional intelligence?*

- *Self-assess: Which of my EI skills are strong? Which ones are underdeveloped?*

- *Contrast: What surprised me about the results? What gaps exist between my assessment results and how I perceive my skill levels?*

- *Identify: In what contexts are my current skill levels helpful or harmful?*

- *Reveal: What EI skills do I need to develop? What EI skills do I need to dial back?*

- *Understand: What do I need to do to build my EI skills? How can I modulate use of certain EI skills in particular circumstances?*

- *Discover: How do my EI skills relate to and impact others?*

- *Experience: What have I learned about my EI skills from trying new behaviors or eliminating others?*

Conducting an Emotional Intelligence Coaching Conversation Using the CAAACS Model

Auerbach (2003) created the CAAACS model to organize the coaching process into six steps:

1. Connection: Establish rapport and gain an understanding of the individual's perspective, thoughts, and feelings.

2. Assessment: Evaluate the individual's current situation, strengths, and areas of development, values, and goals.

3. Articulation: Clarify the individual's goals for coaching.

4. Action: Identify the plan for achieving the goals.

5. Commitment: The coach provides support and accountability.

6. Support: Support the individual to find additional resources to increase the likelihood of success.

As described next, the CAAACS model is easily adapted for helping learners reflect on their emotional intelligence.

The CAAACS model is composed of six coaching steps: Connection, Assessment, Articulation, Action, Commitment, and Support. The EI coach leads individual conversations with learners to review their self assessments and leads reflective practice questions to coach development of their EI skills. Table 3.2 provides an overview of the steps followed by further discussion and explanation.

TABLE 3.2 EI Coaching Conversation Model

COACHING STEPS	REFLECTIVE PRACTICE FOCUS	EMOTIONAL INTELLIGENCE
1: Connection	Reflective Practice: Description	Self-assessment results Establish rapport and create a safe environment for disclosure and discovery
2: Assessment	Reflective Practice: Description Interpretation	Facilitate learners' discovery of their current situation, EI strengths, areas of development, and goals
3: Articulation	Reflective Practice: Action Plan	Clarify the learner's emotional intelligence goals
4: Action	Reflective Practice: Action Plan	Identify the plan for achieving the goals
5: Commitment	Reflective Practice: Action Plan	Provide support and accountability for action and experimentation
6: Support	Reflective Practice: Description Interpretation Action Plan	Provide feedback and help the learners find additional resources to continue the emotional intelligence development process

Step 1: Connection

Establish rapport and create a safe environment for disclosure and discovery.

The connection step of the CAAACS coaching process begins prior to the EI assessment and before learners receive their results. The coach or educator seeks to establish rapport and build trust with the learner from the outset through classroom activities and exercises, one-on-one conferences, assignment feedback, and each learner-instructor interaction. The connection process is more critical during the coaching conversation when learners feel more vulnerable and the conversation is focused on the learner's opportunities for improvement. It is important for the coach/educator to have a solid grasp of coaching skills to enhance confidence and the ability to build trust during the connection phase.

> *Though I always considered myself a strong problem solver, I learned, through the emotional intelligence assessment, this ability quickly dissolves in the presence of strong emotions. Upon reflection, I better understand situations where my problem-solving ability deteriorated because of strong emotions. I learned that becoming more self-aware is vital to addressing emotionally influenced actions and thoughts.*

Step 2: Assessment

Facilitate learners' discovery of their current situation, EI strengths, areas of development, and goals.

The assessment phase of the coaching conversation is a self-discovery process that includes the EI self-assessment results as well as the learners' reflection on how they experience EI in their lives. To introduce the EI concept, describe the individual EI skills as muscles that may be underdeveloped and unavailable when needed or overdeveloped and overused depending on the context. Shankman and Allen (2008) stress the role of context when developing and applying emotional intelligence. It is important to emphasize the relevance of the scores; higher scores are not necessarily better and lower scores may not be negative depending on the context where each skill comes into play.

To begin the reflection process, ask the learners which individual ratings stood out for them as they reviewed their ratings. Follow up with, "What surprised you about that result?" This line of questioning allows the learners to focus the debriefing on what is important to them or what they are curious about.

Learners are often surprised by a higher rating when they don't feel a particular EI skill is a strength. Often, learners focus on lower scores they perceive as weaknesses or gaps in their emotional intelligence. To normalize their results and emphasize the importance of context, ask the learners to describe circumstances when low or high scores may be helpful and when they might get in the way of achieving their goals. Learners attach their own experience to the specific EI skills through the reflective process and identify the circumstances where strong or weak EI skills are either helpful to them or hinder their goals. This reflective process allows learners to see how EI skills could help them be more effective and satisfied, build stronger relationships, and manage their emotions.

The following example illustrates how a learner discovered the contextual nature of emotional intelligence through the reflective self-assessment process.

According to Bar-On, the EI skill *assertiveness* is composed of three components: (1) the ability to express feelings such as anger, warmth, and compassion; (2) the ability to voice opinions, to disagree, and to take a stand; and (3) the ability to stand up for personal rights (Multi-Health Systems, 2011).

Coach/Educator: Can you think of a situation where not being assertive presented problems for you?

> Lately, our team has been discussing shift-scheduling issues. It seems a few nurses always find a way to avoid weekend and holiday shifts. In a recent meeting, we discussed a new approach that would even out weekend and holiday shifts. The conversation was heated and eventually led to a suggestion that we leave things as they are. I didn't speak up when I was clearly annoyed that the strong voices in the room weren't addressing the fairness issue. The scheduling procedure didn't change, and I find myself on the short end of the stick, scheduled to work more than my fair share of weekends and holidays.

Coach/Educator: Can you describe a situation where your low assertiveness score was helpful?

The other day I had to address a scheduling issue with another department. I called the lead [nurse] on duty to describe how the scheduling snafu was affecting our unit. When the lead downplayed my concerns I found myself getting angry and irritated. I didn't express these emotions at the time and, in retrospect, I was glad I didn't. The scheduling problem turned out to be a computer glitch and I found out from my supervisor that the lead I talked with had just lost her husband. I was glad I held back on my feelings and I didn't embarrass the lead or make a fool of myself.

EMOTIONAL INTELLIGENCE AND CONTEXT

Strong emotional intelligence skills can be an asset or a restraining force, depending on the context.

As these examples show, the reflective process and personal change can involve risk for some learners. Emotional intelligence assessments are often threatening because learners hold the misconception that their results will reveal flaws or weaknesses. The coaching conversation is an essential step in the reflective practice process because it reduces the perceived risk of revealing gaps in EI skills. It does this by explicitly addressing the advantages and disadvantages of a particular skill. This allows learners to view the EI feedback more objectively and, as a result, they are much more likely to consider applying the EI framework to their experience. Also, the focus on context reduces risk by normalizing what many learners would consider weaknesses. For instance, when learners focus on low-scoring EI skills, they often discover contexts where their perceived weakness is an asset. By considering the contexts they encounter, learners see EI skills as tools to be applied or withheld to achieve their desired objective.

Step 3: Articulation

Clarify the learner's emotional intelligence goals.

After the learner has the opportunity to discuss how his skill levels affect his life through the inquiry process, he is asked to identify opportunities to enhance his emotional intelligence skills. For some, "enhancement" may involve developing an EI skill that lacks strength. For others, it may involve "dialing back" or relying less on a skill that is too strong or used in inappropriate settings. Learners are then asked how addressing specific EI skills would help them achieve their goals.

Coach/Educator: How could enhancing your assertiveness benefit you?

> This is important to me because I think women are socialized to be less assertive and to adopt more people-pleasing attitudes and behaviors, and I am tired of playing that part. Firstly, it is exhausting and not rewarding to be a people pleaser, because ultimately I cannot please everyone, but in trying, I end up compromising my own interests and needs. I know I am acutely concerned and tuned into other people's discomfort, which has its advantages and disadvantages, especially as a nurse. I do not want to lose my ability to accommodate or empathize; however, I do want to assert myself in situations in which I need something, want something, or need to speak up about something I don't agree with.

In the ensuing discussion, the goal is to ground the development goal in the learners' values and needs.

Step 4: Action

Identify the plan for achieving the goals.

In the action step, learners are asked to develop a written plan to experiment with changes in their EI skills. Reflective practice requires action to complete the learning process—learners benefit when they take their basic understanding of EI gained from the coaching process and apply it to their experiences. Assignments that ask learners to apply EI skills provide an opportunity to test new behaviors and thoughts.

Development Plan Assignment

Coach/Educator: What are the specific behaviors or mental processes to be changed? What will you do differently, with whom, in what circumstances, when will you be carrying out this plan, and what will you be looking for to determine if your changes are having the desired impact?

> In order to ratchet up my assertiveness, my plan is to begin handling things differently with my program director. I find myself slipping into that people-pleasing mode around her rather than speaking up for what I need for my education and career. There is a conference that I really want to attend later this year that I believe will be very important for my career. She has already insinuated that any conference other than the one she wants us to go to would require extensive discussion, including the fact I would need to miss a few days of class in the fall to attend. I know asking her to go will create conflict, but I also know that I need to do this for myself. The early bird registration is almost expired, so I have to ask her in the next two weeks, which is my goal. In speaking with her and others, I can change the use of my words so that I come across as more certain and firm. I can use "I" more and "I think" or "I need" instead of asking for permission or approval of what I think or need.

When learners prepare detailed plans like this one, their subsequent experience will generate specific feedback on their plan. In fact, each experience of using EI skills provides learners with feedback—an opportunity to discover a different outcome more in line with their needs and goals. By repeating the experience, learners gradually transform themselves and develop self-mastery.

Step 5: Commitment

Provide support and accountability for action and experimentation.

Commitment calls for ongoing involvement on the part of the coach/educator. Changing lifelong habits is challenging, and educators can support learners by helping them understand barriers to change. Identifying a plan to enhance EI skills is based on changes in behavior as well as the thoughts learners associate with those behaviors. In many cases, challenging mind-sets and the assumptions that support them is a precondition to trying new behaviors. Learners wanting to be more assertive may develop a plan to act more assertively and test the behavior. Learners who also reflect on the emotions of becoming more assertive may find that their anxiety or fear is holding them back and recognize that those emotions are based on misguided assumptions about the outcome of their assertiveness. Learners may challenge these paralyzing assumptions and apply empowering ones, thus engaging in a context requiring assertiveness, having a more positive or realistic perspective about the risk involved, and experiencing fewer debilitating emotions. You can guide learners through this reflective process by asking them to identify assumptions that may be hindering their ability to try new behaviors or let go of others.

Coach/Educator: What assumptions and associated emotions might get in the way of following through on your plan?

> The assumptions and emotions that underlie my past behavior mostly pertain to being fearful of being different. There is a fear of being "wrong" if I do speak up, take the different route, or create conflict. There is also the working assumption that if I do create this conflict, whoever is involved will see me as difficult or hard to work with and won't like me.

Coach/Educator: What alternative assumptions would help you follow through with your plan?

I can assume that others aren't judging me when I speak up. I can also see them as supportive and invested in my well-being regardless of how they might respond to my request.

To address accountability, learners prepare a reflective paper detailing the outcome of their EI development plans.

Reflective Paper Instructions

Coach/Educator: Prepare a reflective paper summarizing the emotional intelligence skill that you wanted to change, what you did differently, with whom, in what circumstances, how it felt, what the impact was, what you learned from the experience, how this development plan experience has contributed to your emotional intelligence development, and what you will do going forward to continue enhancing your emotional intelligence skills.

My goal was to be more assertive with my director. I asked my director for funding to attend a conference. I was admittedly nervous about asking her and I could feel myself cringing in anticipation of the conflict it might create, but I asked anyway. I told myself that anything I requested that was outside her usual rules and regulations would cause her anxiety but that it did not need to cause me any. I remembered to tell myself that my career interests are paramount to any discomfort I might create for either one of us in asking. I was still not excited about making the request but I did and was told I could probably go. I took that as a victory and felt good about being assertive about my needs. I learned that I often hesitate to be assertive because I make negative assumptions about the outcome. By focusing on my goals and setting aside my negative, paralyzing assumptions, it is easier to assert myself.

I have also tried to be more conscious of my tendency to people please and make note of it as well as what I would have preferred to say or do in those situations. This increased awareness is helping reinforce the behavior, and I plan on continuing this practice. In a recent group project situation, I found myself extremely frustrated with two members who had not been contributing to the work. I did not want to disrupt the peace, call them out on their behavior, or create conflict. I heard my internal mechanisms churning to make accommodations for their lack of participation, trying to downplay it or make excuses for why I did not have time or responsibility to deal with the issue. I recognized that I was worried they would think I was difficult and hard to work with or unlikable if I confronted them. I was able to talk myself into being assertive, however, and I not only confronted them about it (kindly, albeit) but I also complained to the professor about their total lack of contributions. I noticed how uncomfortable this made me and I am still dealing with the fear of being seen as mean or harsh. But I also feel justified in being angry and in calling attention to the problem. I cannot say it feels great to be assertive yet, neither in this situation nor in the one with my director, but I think I will gradually adapt. In terms of my potential, I know it will increase my effectiveness to be able to create and handle conflict when necessary, whether that be asserting my needs or opinion, or standing up for something that needs to change or be said.

The learners' reflections enhance their emotional intelligence self-awareness and reinforce their learning. Their descriptions of successful efforts and disappointments can be opportunities for further discussion and learning with their coach/educator.

Step 6: Support

Provide feedback and help learners find additional resources to continue the emotional intelligence development process.

Learners are given feedback on their reflective paper highlighting the connection between their goals and values and reinforcing their efforts, regardless of how successful. Constructive comments help them connect EI to their professional goals, provide encouragement for continued experimentation, and reinforce the action taken and insights gained.

Ongoing support for learners can take many forms, such as books, articles, videos, and other material specific to the EI skill the learner is addressing. Emotional intelligence can be folded into other courses to reinforce and support the EI focus. On an interpersonal level, continuing to ask learners about their efforts to address their EI skills provides support for their ongoing development. The coaching model provides a structured approach for facilitating learners' conversations about emotional intelligence assessment results.

Developing EI Skills for the Coach/Educator

To effectively integrate an emotional intelligence skill-development strategy into educational learning modules, whether in academic or clinical settings, EI coaches and educators need a sound understanding of an EI model and self-assessment tools and the access for administering and evaluating the assessments. Many EI assessment services require certification to administer and interpret reports. Training programs often provide a limited review of the EI models and assessment tools; it is recommended that coaches and educators have additional study and experience to develop the skill and expertise to effectively use them in an educational setting. Furthermore, to be effective, EI coaches and educators themselves should complete an emotional intelligence assessment and reflect on their own skill levels, the contexts in which they are assets or liabilities, and enhancements that would improve their effectiveness as a coach. Fortunately, testing services usually require a self-assessment and debriefing as part of their certification training programs.

Final Reflections

One of the most challenging aspects for learners interested in developing their emotional intelligence is overcoming the apprehension they have about what an EI assessment will reveal about them. As with many self-assessments, learners tend to focus on the numbers, their rating, and how it compares to the norms of the assessment sample. By itself, assessment anxiety can interrupt the learning process such that learners overemphasize a shortcoming or dismiss results altogether. Coupling a coaching approach with EI self-assessment results can have a powerful impact on learners as they wrestle with who they want to be, what skills they need to be effective and happy, and how they can enhance their emotional intelligence. Who we are is who we bring to practice; developing EI skills is fundamental to improving intra- and inter-professional teamwork, enhancing a positive work environment, and maximizing the quality and safety of patient care.

References

Akerjordet, K., & Severinsson, E. (2010). The state of the science of emotional intelligence related to nursing leadership: An integrative review. *Journal of Nursing Management*, 18, 363–328.

Armstrong, G., & Sherwood, G. (2012). Reflection and mindful practice: A means to quality and safety. In G. Sherwood & S. Horton-Deutsch (Eds.), *Reflective practice: Transforming education and improving outcomes* (pp. 21–40). Indianapolis, IN: Sigma Theta Tau International.

Auerbach, J. E. (2003). *Personal and executive coaching: The complete guide for mental health professionals*. Ventura, CA: Executive College Press.

Ball, L. (2013). Accelerated baccalaureate nursing students' use of emotional intelligence in nursing as "caring for a human being": A mixed methods grounded theory study. *International Journal of Nursing Education Scholarship, 10*(1), 293–300. doi:10.1515/ijnes-2013-0015

Bar-On, R. (2006). The Bar-On model of emotional-social intelligence (ESI). *Psicothema, 18*(Suppl.), 13–25.

Bar-On, R. (2013). A broad definition of emotional-social intelligence according to the Bar-On Model. Retrieved from http://www.reuvenbaron.org/wp/37-2/

Benson, G., Martin, L., Ploeg, J., & Wessel, J. (2012). Longitudinal study of emotional intelligence, leadership, and caring in undergraduate nursing students. *Journal of Nursing Education, 51*(2), 95–101.

Cadman, C., & Brewer, J. (2001). Emotional intelligence: A vital prerequisite for recruitment in nursing. *Journal of Nursing Management, 9*(6), 321–324.

Codier, E., Kofoed, N., & Peters, J. (2015). Graduate-entry non-nursing students: Is emotional intelligence the difference? *Nursing Education Perspectives, 36*(1), 46–47.

Evans, D., & Allen, H. (2002). Emotional intelligence: Its role in training. *Nursing Times, 98*(27), 41–42.

Fitzpatrick, J. (2016). Helping nursing students develop and expand their emotional intelligence. *Nursing Education Perspectives, 37*(3), 124.

Foster, K., McCloughen, A., Delgado, C., Kefalas, C., & Harkness, E. (2015). Emotional intelligence education in pre-registration nursing programmes: An integrative review. *Nurse Education Today, 35*(3), 510–517. doi:10.1016/j.nedt.2014.11.009

Goleman, D. (1995). *Emotional intelligence.* New York, NY: Bantam Books.

Goleman, D. (1998). *Working with emotional intelligence.* New York, NY: Bantam Books.

Multi-Health Systems. (2011). *Emotional Quotient Inventory v. 2.0 (EQ-i 2.0): User's handbook.* Toronto, Canada: Multi-Health Systems.

Peterson, D. B. (1996). Executive coaching at work: The art of one-on-one change. *Consulting Psychology Journal: Practice and Research, 48*(2), 78–86.

Rankin, B. (2013). **Emotional intelligence:** Enhancing values-based practice and compassionate care in **nursing**. *Journal of Advanced Nursing, 69*(12), 2717–2725.

Shankman, M. L., & Allen, S. J. (2008). *Emotionally intelligent leadership: A guide for college students.* San Francisco, CA: Jossey-Bass.

Shanta, L., & Gargiulo, L. (2014). A study of the influence of nursing education on development of emotional intelligence. *Journal of Professional Nursing, 30*(6), 511–520.

Smith, K., Profetto-McGrath, J., & Cummings, G. G. (2009). Emotional intelligence and nursing: An integrative literature review. *International Journal of Nursing Studies, 46*(12), 1624–1636. doi:10.1016/j.ijnurstu.2009.05.024

Part II
Reflection and Mindful Practice

Chapter 4

Creating Space for Reflection: The Importance of Presence in the Teaching-Learning Process

–Kristen Lombard, PhD, RN, PMHCNS-BC
–Sara Horton-Deutsch, PhD, RN, FAAN, ANEF
–With Learning Activity by Andy Davies, PhD, MEd

Introduction

The practice of nursing is fundamentally a framework for learning about love, caring, healing, and humanity. We gather knowledge and wisdom on many levels and seek to blend a way of being with a way of doing (skill/technique). First, however, we must understand our own humanity and develop a relationship with ourselves. The strengthening of our relationship with self has tremendous implications for our ability to stay inspired by our work; remain congruent with our core values; collaborate; and deliver high-quality, safe, and compassionate care. Nursing practice is a reflective journey of personal and professional growth, where learning is continual and always evolving. A key ingredient of a vibrant community of learning is space—noticing its existence, acknowledging it, allowing it, feeling it, appreciating it, and working with it. This chapter explores the notion of space and its relationship to reflective practice: what it is and how we engage with it, or not; what emerges within space; how we become reacquainted with it; and our imperative to offer it, protect it, and claim it.

Reflecting on Space

REFLECTING ON . . . SPACE

- *What is your experience of space?*
- *What do you do with space when you have it?*
- *How do you understand this for yourself?*

Space is an interesting concept to ponder and an experience to bear. In a linear sense, our usual mental model of space is of a physical environment: a building, room, or outdoor space like a park or a plaza. Space can also be something we yearn for when we have hard and pressured workweeks or family lives. We can imagine sitting by the ocean or at the top of a mountain and just being within a wide, open expanse. We look forward to the weekend (space), when we can relax and be at home and perhaps "do nothing" in our own space. In a mental sense, we aspire to openness in thought (space), desiring freedom of expression and endless avenues to accomplish our dreams. Emotionally, we may "need space" when we become overwhelmed or need distance from a situation. We may recognize that we just need to "be" in that space. Spiritually, space may be a state that allows us to access a sense of something greater than ourselves, a greater perspective and meaning, or a place to honor our traditions. Space can represent freedom, hope, release, and support, have a character of its own, clearing out, clarity, home, heaven, or God.

Space is all of that—and more. Heidegger (1973) states that space is the medium through which relationships flow. It can become an interpersonal environment where gathering and ungathering occurs, where we practice being in relationship together. Space can also be a place where we cultivate our relationships with new ways of being, thinking, or feeling. "Holding space" is a term meaning to hold an interpersonally safe container that allows for authenticity or truths to be revealed or unknown possibilities and potential to emerge.

Clinical Reflection

One consultant of relationship-based care facilitates programs that help reconnect caregivers with their passion for the work by holding space for them to deepen their relationships with themselves, their colleagues, and their patients and families. The participants begin to appreciate the space provided for them to reflect, write, draw, imagine, have dialogue, circle practice, and take part in various inter/intra-active group activities. One of the most powerful activities is at the beginning of the program when participants pair off and respond to the question "Who am I?" over and over. A crucial piece is "setting the container" with simple guidelines of protected space, silence by the listener, and confidentiality. The speaker has 2 minutes to verbalize responses to the question. Until thoughts come, there may be silence, which is okay. The listener does not speak or interrupt but merely holds space for the speaker to talk. It is not a conversation. After the 2 minutes are up, the listener repeats back the essence of what he heard. Then they switch with the same guidelines. Round two goes deeper with the same pair. Each speaker shares what inspires them, what they believe in, and what makes them afraid. The listener is silent and then repeats back what she heard.

What were the conditions that made this activity so powerful and insightful? Participants often provided feedback that they felt listened to without judgment, fixing, advice, distraction, or interruption. Shockingly, one 32-year-old nurse stated it was her first experience in her life of feeling completely listened to. There was a play between self-knowing and yet not knowing. They appreciated the time to be able to do such inquiry. As speakers, they felt vulnerable talking about themselves, but it became easier as they went along. They built meaningful relationships with each other and felt closer to their peers in 4 short minutes. As listeners, they often felt anxious, noticing tendencies to want to fill the space, jump in, validate, and tell their own story, instead of remaining silent. They practiced presence and attuning to themselves and each other. They wondered about self and others. They followed what was said. The intentional holding of space made them feel "held" and safe, thus more willing to take risks and share truths about themselves. They began to trust more because of their experience. They also practiced just being. Some said it felt like a relief to not have to talk.

This beautiful reflective activity (Koloroutis, 2016) demonstrates the core therapeutic relationship practices that are foundational to reflective practice and compassionate caring (Koloroutis & Trout, 2012). Participants voiced feeling gratitude for this powerful opportunity to find meaning and new friends by collaborating in this way. They voiced feeling a certain quality of caring and being cared for through the use of listening, silence, and held space.

What Emerges in Space: Potential

Do you remember playing make-believe when you were young? Can you remember when the sky was the limit, no holds were barred, and creativity abounded? Can you remember times when exploration was expected or unexpected, and interesting situations caused you to somehow figure out how to be in those situations and make sense of yourself in the world? There was uncertainty about how the stories in playing would end up, and we delighted and trusted in the evolution of the story. We were masters of improvisation and of imagining all kinds of possibilities. Our worlds became greatly expanded compared to the beginning point.

Becoming reacquainted with space can be like experiences from our youth. The fundamental ingredient is safe space and time. The reflective journey is a similar process: a personal journey of growth toward self-awareness and of comfort with what is (Horton-Deutsch & Sherwood, 2008; Sherwood & Horton-Deutsch, 2015).

Engaging With Space—or Not

Space is not always a comfortable place to be. Our past history and experiences, judgments, and storylines can influence our ability to tolerate space. Ironically, when we create the opportunity for space and expansion, we discover a common habit: feeling the need to fill that empty space by doing, rather than simply being in that space. Our Western and healthcare cultures support this. We have become enculturated to value speed, efficient and quick answers, and measurable productivity and profit. Heidegger (1973) suggests that Westerners are enculturated to fear the unknown, to fear space, and we go out of our way to try to predict outcomes or manipulate control, even in our educational designs. He maintains that any new frontier (space) triggers our worst habits to conquer, fill, measure, or commodify the space. Such control is often seen as strength, whereas letting go of control and trusting are judged to be weaknesses—but are they?

We have become really good at fixating on a problem in order to understand. We value the mental process of logical analysis, or pushing through long agendas rather than creating space for reflection, acknowledging emotions, and accessing many kinds of wisdom. Doing so would engender complaints that we aren't doing anything—but are we? Why is it we have an aversion to slowing down and making space for something to arise organically?

Our professional culture has become one of doing, where tasks have become more honored than the need for human connection, developing relationships with information and people, or making well-considered decisions. Patient surveys and dissatisfied staff are now demanding the latter (Press Ganey, 2016). The question then becomes: How can we get back to the kind of care that is congruent with our core values? How can many of us recover from compassion fatigue and reconnect with our practice? Very simply, by ensuring that the space, time, and means for reflective practice are enculturated into our organizations.

Gadamer (2004), a philosopher of human nature, is concerned that present-day humanity has evolved into societies that are out of balance and fragile. He maintains that we are losing our vital instincts for authenticity, language, and conversation; reflective consciousness; and self-understanding. In this societal disequilibrium, our atrophying vital instincts for connection have affected the health of the individual and, therefore, our larger humanity. Gadamer believes that intentional raising of consciousness, engagement in dialogue, and arriving at new understandings require us to ethically assume responsibility for these

A fear of being vulnerable might contribute to a discomfort with space. The Latin root of the word "vulnerable," vulnus, means wound. It is defined as "being susceptible to physical or emotional injury . . . attack . . . [being] open to censure or criticism" (Vulnerable, 2007, p. 1931). How we respond to our own vulnerability can depend on traditions, social norms, and events in our own lives, where we can tend toward self-protection, staying busy, and nurturing rigid boundaries (Lashley et al., 1994). In contrast, vulnerability can call us to a willingness to be in a space of not knowing and authenticity.

insights. He calls this the path to a healthy society. A way to re-equilibrate back to health and balance is to create space for reconnecting with ourselves and within our nursing practice. We must create space for reflective practice.

What Emerges in Space: Vulnerability

The discussion so far is leading us to explore how space and not knowing (uncertainty) engender individual and collective vulnerability. Lashley, Neal, Slunt, Berman, and Hultgren (1994) suggest that vulnerability is fundamental to the calling of the nurse and the subsequent growth of professional identity. Nurturing "a lived language of vulnerability" (Lashley et al., p. 48) invites the development of new understandings and horizons of experience. It also invites us to find ourselves in the process. Accepting vulnerability is vital in the practice of reflection.

REFLECTING ON . . . VULNERABILITY

- *If space engenders vulnerability, what guidelines do you and your colleagues need to put in place so that everyone feels secure enough to risk authentic communication and reflection in the workplace? In the classroom?*

- *What self-protecting habits do you notice in your colleagues that might be related to protecting their own vulnerability? In what ways are they demonstrated?*

- *What self-protecting habits do you notice in yourself? Are they demonstrated in your workplace? In the classroom? If so, in what ways?*

Our history with space might influence our ability to connect with the present moment. We may feel there is no room for space. Our desire for a spacious future might be short-circuited because of reinforced experiences of a lack of space. Are we doomed to repeat the past and limit our experience of the present and future, or do we have a choice? What perceived and real obstacles are limiting our connection with space?

Clinical Reflection and Activity

Susan finds Maureen to be judgmental, rigid, closed off, and negative. Susan often experiences conflict with Maureen and dreads working with her. She notices that whenever Maureen is around, Susan feels constricted and closed off to communication with Maureen. Susan speaks negatively about Maureen to others; she feels protective of herself and experiences a sense of powerlessness that nothing will ever change. Susan notices how uptight she feels during the entire shift and how that tension feels in her body and how it gets communicated to her colleagues, patients, and families. She also notices that she goes to great lengths to work around Maureen, so that she doesn't have to interact with her. She notices she is more exhausted and pressured than is needed. How could space and reflection possibly address this situation?

This situation addresses several issues at the same time. First is recognizing how the power of our perceptions, judgments, and automatic thoughts can limit our worlds and determine our stress, energy level, and moods, which then can affect our collegiality and patient/family care. Susan has created space to notice various details: specific personality traits of Maureen; her own emotional and physical feelings; how she is protecting herself from feeling vulnerable; how she is different from her authentic self when she is around Maureen; and how that affects her interactions with self and others. Susan is demonstrating mindfulness-awareness and she needs space to figure these things out.

With such mindfulness-awareness, Susan now has a choice with how she will proceed. This is an act of self-care as she manages her energy to be energized or drained. Will she allow the status quo to continue or could she open up to a larger field of view and discover other ways of being? From a patient care standpoint, what is her ethical responsibility in response to this awareness?

"Preconceived notions are the locks on the door to wisdom."–Merry Browne

How can Susan unlock the door to wisdom and how can space help? Further reflection can help her go deeper and create transformation in this situation. Susan already knows what traits Maureen has that challenge her. What if Susan asks herself these questions:

- What are the four qualities that Maureen has that could benefit me?

- Which of Maureen's challenging behaviors might I notice in myself? What parts can I own?

- What is one thing I could imagine doing that could shift this relationship?

In this true story, Susan opened her mind and noted some strengths that Maureen had. Some that she wished she had! Susan also admitted that she was judgmental herself, which projected her toward negativity. She began to understand Maureen differently, with more empathy. She thought that one way she could shift the relationship was to ask Maureen to mentor her in cardiac arrhythmias, an area where Maureen was an expert. The dynamics shifted after Susan gathered the courage to ask Maureen for help. They became friends! Remember that how we learn and grow in nursing can come from many directions!

Many nurses have cited a fear of being vulnerable as a compelling obstacle to allowing space (Lombard, 2011). This fear of vulnerability can play a subtle yet powerful role in healthcare and beyond. Vulnerability researchers identify our culture as one that has lost its tolerance for vulnerability (Brown, 2010). For example, we have been conditioned to avoid and eliminate suffering and have developed destructive behaviors and addictions in order to cope. Additionally, some have played on this fear throughout history as a way to maintain the status quo and social norms (Brown, 2010). More recently, researchers are finding that respect for human vulnerability preserves dignity, and that respect is an important part of building helping-trusting relationships and creating a healing environment (Wiklund, Gustin, &Wagner, 2012). Vulnerability is also a strong tool for survival that creates space for developing new awareness, inviting new levels of sureness and courage to manifest (Brown, 2012; Horton-Deutsch, 2016).

It takes courage to encounter the status quo of what is known and comfortable (or uncomfortable) and go beyond. Making a change can engender fear when we perceive potentially losing acceptance by others or losing status. It also takes courage to work within spacious environments, to broaden our understanding of the world, and to choose to be in the world differently and honestly. It takes daring to be authentic, to encourage that in our teaching (as explored in Chapter 5), or to pause from a focus on content and skill acquisition to sharing our vulnerability with learners, modeling authentic dialogue and the sense-making that comes from creating space (as discussed in Chapter 6). This form of teaching allows for human-to-human connection; it expands our compassion and caring and keeps our common humanity alive (Horton-Deutsch, 2016; Watson, 2008).

What Emerges in Space: Fear

Another thing that can emerge in space is the stimulation of our primitive brain, the amygdala, due to perceived fear. This induces a fight-or-flight reaction, which can influence our ability to allow space; our habitual patterns can pull us back into the comfort of what we already know. Selhub (2010) reminds us that the amygdala is triggered by stressful memories from the past, negative expectations about outcomes, and maladaptive coping and belief systems. Even though a present-moment experience of space might be free of danger or connections with the past, the mind-body connection perceives the trigger as real, hijacks the brain out of the present moment, and initiates a chain of physiological and psychological reactions, as has happened in past negative experiences. The good news is that through learning mindfulness-awareness, this amygdala reaction can be successfully bypassed.

The science of neuroplasticity shows us that individuals can redirect stressful amygdala reactions to higher brain centers like the cerebral cortex. Using these

SELF-CARE

Within a holistic nursing practice, self-care is the intentional cultivation of personal reflection and individualized health-promoting behaviors and activities (Orem, 2001). Self-care develops a deeper understanding of the human healing journey, as well as the resilience to be present to it. Self-care has been shown to improve a nurse's patient care and their experience of their workplace, as well as to strengthen communication skills and their ability to better relate with others (Dossey & Keegan, 2013).

higher brain centers enables us to remain in the here and now, acknowledge what is real and not assumption, stay aware of core values, be better able to act congruently with our values, and be present with authenticity. The use of the breath and positive emotions are two of many ways we can shift a stress reaction. As well, the space or environment held for practicing vulnerability must feel safe. Replacing the negative experiences with positive experiences of connection, emotion, and authenticity can rewire neural pathways.

Awareness and insights about self and other emerge in space. In reflective practice, we are being asked to cultivate a space within ourselves where we become more comfortable examining what is real, being in the present moment and being our authentic selves—aware, connected, and, yes, maybe vulnerable. This sense of comfort with ourselves is an important component of self-care.

We need to acknowledge that vulnerability and suffering are part and parcel of the human experience and, therefore, inescapable. In addition, vulnerability is our strongest ally for survival (Brown, 2010, 2012). According to the literature, vulnerability is strength. It calls us to understand that new awareness and growth are knocking at the door, and it invites a new level of confidence and fearlessness to manifest. So, let's reframe this notion of vulnerability as a necessary ally for growth.

Finally, what emerges in space can be vulnerability, fear, self-protection, stress reactions, awareness and insight, and opportunity for self-care and growth.

Mindfulness-Awareness

"Out beyond ideas of wrongdoing and right doing there is a field. I will meet you there." –Rumi

What would it be like to dwell in a field (or space) free from judgment or storylines, where hearts and minds could meet, be curious, and talk without concern of time, limitations, personal agendas, or fear of feeling shame or small and insignificant? Could such a field be an open expanse of possibilities and unconditional positive regard? Could it be a place where new understanding could occur with simple openness and wakefulness? Is this even possible? We posit that it is, yet it requires the willingness, courage, and discipline to create the conditions necessary for such a space.

Stated simply, mindfulness is paying attention, in the moment, on purpose, and free from judgment (Kabat-Zinn, 2013). We can learn to expand our awareness by cultivating the courage to observe ourselves in order to become more flexible and open with our minds and hearts. Mindfulness grows compassion, as well as the skill of being able to reframe thoughts, perceptions, and judgmental thinking (Baer et al., 2008). Mindfulness-awareness interweaves intentionality, attention, and attitude (Shapiro, Carlson, Astin, & Freedman, 2006). All these qualities are essential in the personal and professional journey of the nurse (Watson, 2012) and contribute to safe care within the complexity of patient care in the twenty-first century (Epstein, Siegel, & Silberman, 2008). Mindfulness-awareness is a way of self-regulating and has been equated with reflection-in-action (Schön, 1987).

However, one's potential cannot be realized until one comes off autopilot and chooses to become fully present to a situation. *Autopilot* is a collection of unconscious habits we engage in without thinking or being aware. It is reacting instead of responding. It is the opposite of mindfulness-awareness. Mindfulness-awareness practice helps us unhook from autopilot and *choose* to be in the moment, on purpose, and without judgment. Noticing when we are on autopilot enables us to then *consciously choose* a path of action or inaction. That said, it takes intention and exertion to notice and change patterns of thought and

AUTOPILOT

The unconscious habitual thoughts and reactions, distraction and behavior where one is not fully present in the moment with one's mind-body-emotions-spirit. Presence cannot occur unless there is a conscious decision to come off of autopilot and engage in the present moment.

behavior. It becomes clearer that internal obstacles seem harder to overcome than external obstacles.

With practice we learn to catch ourselves on autopilot, whether we are driving the car, brushing our teeth, eating a meal, or avoiding a difficult conversation. This awareness brings us to the present moment, where we have the opportunity to fully attend to our experience—thoughts, smells, emotions, and physical sensations; in other words, the embodied experience. What are some ways we can interrupt autopilot to increase awareness of the present moment? In the car, we can purposefully choose a different route, or we can brush our teeth starting on the opposite side than usual. But within our nursing world, how can we turn off autopilot? First, we notice we are not present and then choose to become present and fully experience ourselves and our social context. What are the stories and assumptions we are making up? Is there a possibility that those stories are not true? We can transform our perceptions and overall perspective so we respond rather than react, and move from a tacit to an explicit experience of our own minds and lives.

REFLECTING ON . . . AUTOPILOT BEHAVIORS

- *Are there autopilot behaviors you notice in yourself that prevent you from staying present in your space?*

- *Have you ever been challenged to change a habit? Name the habit. What kind of resolve was necessary to make a shift? What worked and what did not?*

- *Identify one autopilot behavior you have and list one thing you can do to shift into the present moment.*

Space and Intentionality: The Choice to Reflect

Intentionality is needed to come off autopilot. It is a *deliberate decision* to shift into our present moment experience to stay connected with our core values and aspirations as a human being (Parse, 1999; Watson, 2002). The spirit of intentionality in nursing is described by Dossey, Keegan, and Guzzetta (2005) and Rew (2000) as commitment, responsibility, integration, and conscious-focused awareness. Watson (2002) defines intentionality as focused caring-healing consciousness and cites the work of M. Kabat-Zinn and J. Kabat-Zinn (1998), in which intention informs what choices and actions we take.

Research supports how attention and intentional nonjudgment of thoughts and experiences allow us to connect to our lives with greater clarity, objectivity, and compassion. As we shift our relationship with our storylines and open up to new understandings (Shapiro et al., 2006) we can nurture a stronger ability to reflect on values, have clarity about what is needed, and choose congruent actions.

REFLECTING ON . . . INTENTIONALITY

Consider how your autopilot behaviors may be contributing to the status quo (stasis) or, on the other hand, transformation. You can ask: What am I doing? Am I reinforcing my suffering or negativity? What story am I telling myself about that? Is is true? Am I being congruent with my core values? How can I come into the present moment? What different choices can I make in this moment?

Malle, Moses, and Baldwin (2001) distinguish between *having a desire* for a certain outcome and *having a purposeful plan* to accomplish an action. The former remains in the mind and heart, whereas the latter becomes embodied and action-oriented. Making a deliberate decision to pause in the middle of a hectic day is an example of intentionality. Deliberately reconnecting with our breath prior to entering a patient's room or prior to a challenging communication with

PRESENCING

A skill described by nurse theorists as essential to the practice of caring (Newman, 1999; Parse, 1999; Paterson & Zderad, 2007; Rogers, 1990; Watson, 2005, 2008). The term comes from the Latin esse, which means "to be" (Presencing, 2007). To be present is to fully inhabit all aspects of ourselves and use all our senses in order to understand (Paterson & Zderad, 2007) and connect.

a colleague opens a space for self-regulation, as well as expanded awareness of ourselves and the situation. This expanded awareness makes it more likely that you will put forth an intentional and compassionate embodied response (Trungpa, 2008).

Reflective practice requires working with intentionality and getting off autopilot. It is about giving voice, language, and embodiment to our awareness and understanding. It is a "step-by-step unveiling of being [which] comes about" (Gadamer, 1998, p. 50). This process can feel freeing and inspiring!

Space and Authentic Presence

When nurses bring all of themselves into the moment, they are practicing authentic presence—a powerful teacher. It is a practice of being genuine, cultivating self-knowledge, and self-reflecting in real time as we engage in our lives.

Authentic presence requires full attention to the here and now and conveys a concern for the inner life and personal meaning of another (Sitzman & Watson, 2014). In fact, it has been identified as a crucial healing element in the caring process (Paterson & Zderad, 2007; Watson, 1999).

Authentic presence is a claiming of one's space. Gadamer (1996) describes authentic presence as an embodied manifestation of mindfulness. He calls it "wakefulness, being-in-the-world...something which fully occupies a kind of space" (p. 74). Showing up to claim our space or to be seen can be scary. We make choices every day about how much we will reveal of ourselves. The notion of choosing to be authentic might be surprising (Brown, 2010, 2012). Sadly, we see this often in healthcare. We often think that we are being authentic, but if given the space—and if we are honest with ourselves—we can find the opposite to be true. Instead, because of our fear of vulnerability, we might consciously or unconsciously choose not to share our true selves. Reflection brings the unconscious to consciousness. Only with awareness and intention can we begin to notice and then shift negative patterns. Increasingly, nurses are coming to recognize the importance of intentionality in positively transforming professional experiences.

Becoming authentic seems to ignite a *potential* for a powerful experience into an *actual* powerful experience. When nurses are wholly present, there can be a synergy and connection with creative solutions.

Presence has been described as a skill essential to caring in nursing— caring first for ourselves, then for our colleagues, which enhances stronger collaboration, which in turn strengthens our ability to care safely and compassionately for our patients and families. To be fully present is not easy but is a required element for reflection to occur, for our understanding to deepen, and for our relationships to flourish.

An effective path to creating space and authentic presence is the use of the breath. Much evidence exists about the benefits of learning to breathe effectively. Aside from the mental, emotional, and physiological benefits of balance (Benson & Proctor, 2010), paying attention to your breath allows you to come into your body, to interrupt habitual patterns that pull your being from the present moment, and/or to redirect the stress response. There are many techniques of focusing on the breath as a way of becoming present. In the context of yoga, pranayama is used as a means of regulating and harmonizing the flow of *prana* (energy) in the body. A calmer, more focused mind will help you develop a more reflective practice.

PRANIC SQUARE BREATHING

1. *Find a place where you can focus on your breath for 5 minutes without being disturbed.*

2. *Set a gentle, soft alarm for 5 minutes on your watch or mobile phone.*

3. *Commence your inhale for a count of three. This should be comfortable and relaxed; you should feel no anxiety.*

4. *At the end of your inhalation (at the end of the count of three), keep the air in your lungs for a count of three (once again, this should be comfortable and relaxed; you should feel no anxiety). This is a breath inhalation retention.*

5. *At the end of your breath inhalation retention, exhale to a count of three.*

6. *At the end of your exhalation (keeping the same count of three), do not inhale air in your lungs for a count of three (once again, this should be comfortable and relaxed; you should feel no anxiety).*

7. *At the end of the count of three, you repeat the cycle.*

8. *If at any point you feel anxious, decrease your count in all phases of the inhalation/retention/exhalation/retention cycle. Conversely, as you become more adept and comfortable with the pranic square breathing practice, you can lengthen your count times.*

9. *When your alarm sounds, take a moment to honor the opportunity to sit and focus internally.*

Protected Space: Nurturing Communities of Learning

When human beings come together, there is always learning—on many different levels. Continuous change, newness, not knowing, and uncertainty in our daily practice engender vulnerability. We are encouraging you to respond to these experiences in an authentic way. Therefore, if the practice environment/space does not feel safe and healthy, there will be challenges to providing safe, quality, and meaningful care.

Add to that, we learn best within a social context. Healthcare clinicians who practice together form what is known as a *community of learning*. Experts reinforce that successful knowledge-sharing depends on human networks and relies on the personal authenticity, depth, and quality of the community interactions (Allee, 2003; Ives, Torrey, & Gordon, 2000). In order to nurture and sustain a healthy community of learning, we recognize the imperative of a safe learning container that is reflective, cultivates trust, is open to possibilities, and deliberately honors vulnerability (Edmondson, 2004). Everyone in a learning community has a shared responsibility to ensure this happens.

> *"Tell the truth as you know it; always speak for yourself; declare your interdependence."*

There are a few ways to create safe containers for learning and reflective practice. First, create your own unit/department/classroom agreements that support authentic and compassionate interaction and reinforce expectations for all colleagues to behave in those ways. Second, incorporate the use of circle practice into your work environment as a way to practice reflection, authentic presence, and mindfulness in an innovative collaborative approach (Baldwin & Linnea, 2010). In addition, Paris (2008) recommends three principles to guide all interactions with others: (1) tell the truth as you know it; (2) always speak for yourself; and (3) declare your interdependence.

Hence, the development of safe space and trust is critical and is the ground on which successful communities of learning are built. As we engage with new information at every turn, how we make sense of it for ourselves is through interaction and conversation. We become *life-learners,* discovering how safe space and trust are profound lessons about life.

CONTAINER

To Baldwin and Linnea (2010), a container is a safe interpersonal environment that is carefully shepherded to allow for an unfolding of authentic human processes.

LIFE-LEARNER

Life-learner is a play on words that describes an individual who welcomes informal and formal education throughout life, and at the same time learns about life. It is someone with an inquiring mind who is constantly seeking knowledge.

Final Reflections

This chapter has explored the importance of cultivating space as a place for reflection, learning and transformation of individuals, nursing, and healthcare. What would change about our work if we embraced space into our everyday practice? We could feel more connected, intentional, present, aware, and authentic. We could balance our doing with our being. We could just rest! We could learn to offer protected space to others to help them grow or heal. With intention, we could shift from *desiring* a particular outcome to *purposeful and congruent actions* toward an outcome.

We need to ensure that space, time, and means for reflective practice are enculturated into our organizations, leadership, and work environments. The more authentic we can be, the healthier we and our society will be.

How would the creation of internal space change the work environment? These ideas are explored further in Chapters 5 and 6. Mindful and reflective practices provide us with approaches, challenges, and rewards as we reconnect to our authentic nature as nurses and human beings. They allow us to hone our abilities to put words to our experience and to nurture our understanding of self and others. Mindful and reflective practices endow a space in which equilibrium can be established between logical analysis and vital instincts. Most importantly, space and reflective practices connect us with our brave authentic presence, our hearts, and our shared humanity.

References

Allee, V. (2003). *The future of knowledge.* Boston, MA: Butterworth Heinemann.

Baer, R., Smith, G. T., Lykins, E., Button, D., Krietemeyer, J., Sauer, S., & William, J. (2008). Construct validity of the Five Facet Mindfulness Questionnaire in meditating and nonmeditating samples. *Assessment, 15*(3), 329–342.

Baldwin, C., & Linnea, A. (2010). *The circle way: A leader in every chair.* San Francisco, CA: Berrett-Koehler.

Benson, H., & Proctor, W. (2010). *Relaxation revolution: The science and genetics of mind body healing.* New York, NY: Scribner.

Brown, B. (2010). *The gifts of imperfection: Let go of who you think you're supposed to be and embrace who you are: Your guide to a wholehearted life.* Center City, MN: Hazelden.

Brown, B. (2012). *Daring greatly.* New York, NY: Gotham Books.

Dossey, B. M., & Keegan, L. (2013). *Holistic nursing: A handbook for practice* (6th ed.). Burlington, MA: Jones & Bartlett Learning.

Dossey, B. M., Keegan, L., & Guzzetta, C. E. (2005). *Holistic nursing: A handbook for practice* (4th ed.). Boston, MA: Jones & Bartlett Learning.

Edmondson, A. (2004). Psychological safety, trust and learning in organizations: A group-level lens. In R. M. Kramer & K. S. Cook (Eds.), *Trust and distrust in organizations: Dilemmas and approaches* (pp. 239–272). New York, NY: Russel Sage Foundation.

Epstein, R. M., Siegel, D. J., & Silberman, J. (2008). Self-monitoring in clinical practice: A challenge for medical educators. *Journal of Continuing Education in the Health Professions, 28*(1), 5–13.

Gadamer, H-G. (1996). *The enigma of health: The art of healing in a scientific age* (J. Gaiger & N. Walker, Trans.). Stanford, CA: Stanford University Press.

Gadamer, H-G. (1998). *Reason in the age of science* (F. Lawrence, Trans.). Cambridge, MA: The MIT Press.

Gadamer, H-G. (2004). *Truth and method* (2nd ed.) (J. Weinsheimer & D. Marshall, Trans.). New York, NY: Continuum.

Heidegger, M. (1973). Art and space (C. Siebert, Trans.). *Man and World, 6*(1), 3–8.

Horton-Deutsch, S. (2016). Thinking, acting and leading through Caring Science literacy. In S. M. Lee, P. Palmieri, & J. Watson (Eds.), *Global advances in human caring literacy* (pp. 59–70). New York, NY: Springer.

Horton-Deutsch, S., & Sherwood, G. (2008). Reflection: An educational strategy to develop emotionally competent nurse leaders. *Journal of Nursing Management, 16*(8), 946–954.

Ives, W., Torrey, B., & Gordon, C. (2000). Knowledge sharing is a human behavior. In D. Morey, M. Maybury, & B. Thuraisingham (Eds.), *Knowledge management: Classic and contemporary works* (pp. 99–129). Cambridge, MA: The MIT Press.

Kabat-Zinn, J. (2013). *Full catastrophe living: Using the wisdom of your body and mind to face stress, pain, and illness* (Revised). New York, NY: Bantam.

Kabat-Zinn, M., & Kabat-Zinn, J. (1998). *Everyday blessings: The inner work of mindful parenting.* New York, NY: Hyperion.

Koloroutis, M. (2016). *Re-igniting the spirit of caring facilitator manual* (3rd ed.). Minneapolis, MN: Creative Health Care Management.

Koloroutis, M., & Trout, M. (2012). *See me as a person: Creating therapeutic relationships with patients and their families.* Minneapolis, MN: Creative Health Care Management.

Lashley, M. E., Neal, M. T., Slunt, E. T., Berman, L. M., & Hultgren, F. H. (1994). *Being called to care.* Albany, NY: State University of New York (SUNY) Press.

Lombard, K. (2011). *Nurses' experiences of the practice of the PeerSpirit Circle model from a Gadamerian philosophical hermeneutic perspective* (Doctoral dissertation). Indianapolis, IN: Indiana University.

Malle, B. F., Moses, L. J., & Baldwin, D. A. (Eds.). (2001). *Intentions and intentionality: Foundations of social cognition.* Cambridge, MA: The MIT Press.

Newman, M. (1999). *Health as expanded consciousness* (2nd ed.). New York, NY: National League for Nursing.

Orem, D. (2001). *Nursing: Concepts of practice* (6th ed.). St. Louis, MO: Mosby.

Paris, K. A. (2008). *Staying healthy in sick organizations: The Clover Practice.* Charleston, SC: BookSurge.

Parse, R. (1999). *Illuminations: The human becoming theory in practice and research.* Sudbury, MA: Jones & Bartlett Learning.

Paterson, J., & Zderad, L. (2007). *Humanistic nursing.* Retrieved from http://www.gutenberg.org/files/25020/25020-8.txt

Presencing. (2007). *Oxford English dictionary on historical principles* (6th ed.). Oxford, UK: Oxford University Press.

Press Ganey. (2016). Performance redefined: As health care moves from volume to value, the streams of quality are coming together. In *Press Ganey special report: 2016 strategic insights.* South Bend, IN: Press Ganey.

Rew, L. (2000). Intentionality in holistic nursing. *Journal of Holistic Nursing, 18*(2), 91–93.

Rogers, M. E. (1990). Nursing: Science of unitary, irreducible human beings: Update 1990. In E. A. M. Barrett (Ed.), *Visions of Rogers' science-based nursing* (pp. 5–11). New York, NY: National League for Nursing.

Rumi, M. (n.d.). Retrieved from http://www.worldprayers.org/archive/prayers/ meditations/out_beyond_ideas_of_wrong.html

Schön, D. (1987). *Educating the reflective practitioner.* San Francisco, CA: Jossey-Bass.

Selhub, E. (2010). *The love response: Your prescription to turn off fear, anger, and anxiety to achieve vibrant health and transform your life.* New York, NY: Ballantine.

Shapiro, S. L., Carlson, L. E., Astin, J. A., & Freedman, B. (2006). Mechanisms of mindfulness. *Journal of Clinical Psychology, 62*(3), 373–386.

Sherwood, G., & Horton-Deutsch, S. (Eds.). (2015). *Reflective organizations: On the front lines of QSEN & reflective practice implementation.* Indianapolis, IN: Sigma Theta Tau International.

Sitzman, K., & Watson, J. (2014). *Caring Science, mindful practice: Implementing Watson's Human Caring Theory.* New York, NY: Springer.

Trungpa, C. (2008). *True perception: The path of dharma art.* Boston, MA: Shambhala Publications.

Vulnerable. (2007). *Oxford English dictionary on historical principles* (6th ed.). Oxford, UK: Oxford University Press.

Watson, J. (1999). Becoming aware: Knowing yourself to care for others. *Home Healthcare Nurse, 17*(5), 317–322.

Watson, J. (2002). Intentionality and caring-healing consciousness: A practice of transpersonal nursing. *Holistic Nursing Practice, 16*(4), 12–19.

Watson, J. (2005). *Caring Science as sacred science.* Philadelphia, PA: F. A. Davis.

Watson, J. (2008). *Nursing: The philosophy and science of caring* (Rev. ed.). Boulder, CO: University Press of Colorado.

Watson, J. (2012). *Human Caring Science* (2nd ed.). Sudbury, MA: Jones & Bartlett Learning.

Wiklund Gustin, L., & Wagner, L. (2012). The butterfly effect of caring—Clinical nursing teachers' understanding of self-compassion as a source to compassionate care. *Scandinavian Journal of Caring Sciences, 27*(1), 175–183. doi:10.1111/j.1471-6712.2012.01033.x

Chapter 5
The Mindful Educator: Preparing Ourselves to Interact with Learners

–Rhonda Schwindt, DNP, RN, PMHNP/CNS-BC
–Pamela O'Haver Day, APRN, PMHCNS-BC
–Angela McNelis, PhD, RN, FAAN, ANEF, CNE
–With Learning Activity by Andy Davies, PhD, MEd

"Your vision will become clear only when you look into your heart. Who looks outside, dreams. Who looks inside, awakens." –Carl Jung

Introduction

The delivery of caring, compassionate, and patient/client-responsive care requires nurses who are aware of, and attentive to, intra- and interpersonal dynamics and who acknowledge the essential nature of human interactions in healing. Mindful educators recognize the value of an integrated, holistic approach to teaching and

REFLECTIVE LEARNING

Reflective learning involves linking recent experiences to earlier ones to promote a more complex schema. It includes looking for commonalities, differences, and interrelations beyond their superficial elements, with the goal of developing higher-level thinking skills.

learning and purposefully attend to this distinctive human-centered process of caring. The core principles of mindfulness and reflective learning complement traditional approaches of teaching to create an environment in which the mindful educator models the way for reflective learners.

Emerging evidence suggests that mindfulness meditation may cause neuroplastic changes in the brain regions responsible for the regulation of attention (anterior cingulate cortex and striatum), emotion (prefrontal and limbic regions and the striatum), and self-awareness (the insula, medial prefrontal cortex, and posterior cingulate cortex and precuneus) (Tang & Leve, 2016). Because of the association between the ability to self-regulate and mental health, the practice of mindfulness has important implications for educators, practitioners, and patients/clients (Tang, Holzel, & Posner, 2015). Psychological distress is also thought to be associated with a static concept of self, whereas a more fluid, evolving sense of self derived from lived experiences is believed to promote self-acceptance (Tirch, 2010). In *Mindsight: The New Science of Personal Transformation*, Siegel (2010) highlights the human ability to develop ongoing skills in knowing one's mind, as well as sensing the inner world of others. Mindful educators model this capacity through self-awareness, empathy, social skills, and self-mastery. Mindfulness practices offer a promising strategy to enhance self-awareness, promote empathy and self-compassion, and facilitate a sense of well-being (Boellinghaus, Jones, & Hutton, 2014; Tirch, 2010).

"A teacher can help anyone on the path to awareness. The most valuable teacher is not the one with the deepest knowledge of the scriptures or the one most eloquent. It is the one who points you in the direction that enables you to see." –Anonymous

Mindful educators are attentive to cultivating meaningful therapeutic relationships with learners. They accept mindfulness as an essential element in teaching, learning, and caring. A mindful educator suspends judgment and extends thoughtfulness, kindness, and acceptance to all those they encounter (Williams, Mark, & Kabat-Zinn, 2011). In this chapter, we explore the attributes, skills, and processes of mindful educators who facilitate mutually beneficial teaching and learning experiences.

The Essence of Mindfulness

Mindfulness refers to the creation of space and time and the process of being curious, of paying attention in the moment, on purpose, and without judgment (Mars & Oliver, 2016). It is a way of life; a transformational way of being in the world that can be learned and practiced daily (Crane et al., 2012). According to Crane (2015), when we are present with our authentic self we are reminded of our own humanity and the humanity of others. The essence of mindfulness lies in the intention to be authentic, in this case within the context of teaching and caring. Mindfulness is also described as being truly present in moment-to-moment experiences. Mindful educators recognize the intentionality of being fully present and aware as essential to becoming more skillful, confident, and flexible (Schoeberlein, 2009).

MINDFULNESS
Mindfulness involves being completely in touch with and aware of the present moment, as well as taking a nonevaluative and nonjudgmental approach to your own, and others', inner experience.

Being a Mindful Educator

Mindful educators are individuals who are committed to a sustained mindfulness-based approach to teaching, practice, research, and being in the world. They are purposeful about being attuned to their own emotions, thoughts, and behaviors in ways that create a learning environment where learners grow academically, socially, and emotionally (Crane et al., 2012; Williams et al., 2011). Mindful educators recognize that embracing a daily practice strengthens neuronal circuitry responsible for cognitive skills, self-awareness, empathy, social skills, and self-mastery (Siegel, 2010).

> *"Mindfulness begets mindfulness. Unconditional acceptance extended toward oneself promotes unconditional acceptance toward others."*

The mindful teacher integrates formal and informal mindfulness meditation into daily life. Formal mindfulness meditation includes practices such as "sitting with breath" and "mindful walking." Informal practices refer to moment-to-moment, nonjudgmental, and purposeful attention to any daily activity. These are opportunities in daily life to intentionally take time away from "doing something" and allow time for "being with" whatever is presented. Informal mindfulness practice lends itself to frequent and spontaneous practice points (Hanley, Warner, Dehili, Canto, & Garland, 2015). Examples include routine activities of life, such as mindful eating, dishwashing, or journaling. Twenty minutes of formal or informal meditation practiced daily produces positive health benefits including decreased stress (Hindman, Glass, Arnkoff, & Maron, 2015), enhanced self-compassion (Hindman et al., 2015), and improved mood (Hanley et al., 2015).

SITTING WITH BREATH MEDITATION

- *Assume an erect posture while you sit.*
- *Close your eyes if that is comfortable for you.*
- *Breathing your own rhythm of breathing, focus your attention on your abdomen, its expansion on the in-breath and its relaxation on the out-breath.*

- *Follow each in-breath and each out-breath with ease and moment-to-moment attention.*

- *When your mind wanders away from your breath, note where it took you, and then bring your attention right back to your breath.*

–Adapted from Kabat-Zinn (1990)

MINDFUL WALKING MEDITATION

- *Attend to each step as you walk.*

- *Bring your attention to your legs in space as they take each step.*

- *Bring your attention to your feet as they lift away from the ground and as they make contact with the ground at each step.*

- *Bring your attention to the shifting of your body weight as you take each step.*

- *Bring your attention to the shifting in direction of your walking steps.*

- *When your mind wanders away from your attention to walking, gently bring your attention right back to walking.*

–Adapted from Kabat-Zinn (1990)

The attentional aspect of mindfulness promotes the ability to fully experience the richness of the present moment. Mindful educators are aware of the nuances of a learner's presence—their nonverbal expressions and language—during a teacher-learner encounter. Because mindfulness involves purposeful attention coupled with a nonjudgmental stance, practice is reciprocal; it encourages the development of emotional intelligence—a sense of self-acceptance, self-motivation, and self-confidence as well as acceptance toward others (Davis & Hayes, 2011; Walsh & Shapiro, 2006). When a mindful educator models self-acceptance and self-confidence, it encourages learners to be more tolerant of making mistakes and more likely to take necessary risks for self-exposure. This is necessary for learners to benefit from learning opportunities.

This authentic experience enables learners to "name and tame" their emotional reactions, their thoughts, and their behavioral response to academic and clinical issues. Furthermore, this experience can enable educators to manage and learn from their experience, giving them the opportunity to transform a reactionary approach to a more thoughtful, compassionate response. Mindfulness begets mindfulness. Unconditional acceptance extended toward oneself promotes unconditional acceptance toward others. Mindful educators have been shown to demonstrate a universal principle of behavioral psychiatry, called *reciprocal inhibition*, which maintains that individuals are unable to hold contradictory emotions at the same time (American Psychological Association [APA], 2006). Mindful educators who attend to themselves with care and compassion do not simultaneously judge learners harshly.

REFLECTING ON ATTENTIONAL TEACHING: QUESTIONS FOR EDUCATORS

- *Am I being present with my learner? If not, how can I work to be more present?*

- *Am I listening with intention? If not, what can I do to improve my listening skills?*

- *Am I responsive to my learner's nonverbal affect? If not, how can I work to center more awareness and be more consciously observant?*

- *Am I accurately reflecting my learner's reactions? If not, can I spend more time reflecting on my own thoughts and behaviors?*

Burnout is a state of physical, emotional, and mental exhaustion often accompanied by feelings of alienation and reduced performance at work.

Lack of self-care may lead to burnout (Flook, Goldberg, Pinger, Bonus, & Davidson, 2013), and for nurses, this can negatively impact many aspects of their personal and professional lives. Mindful educators, as well as mindful practitioners, are individuals who embrace mindfulness training as a mechanism for self-care. They transfer their practice directly into clinical education and training in hopes of preventing burnout and secondary trauma. Mindful educators recognize that meditation practice reduces stress and increases physical and emotional resilience (Khoury, Sharma, Rush, & Fournier, 2015).

Research in neuropsychiatry demonstrates our ability to intentionally redirect our attention away from more primitive areas of the brain to more complex centers in the neo-frontal cortex. Mindfulness practice encourages neurocircuitry in the neo-frontal cortex. The neo-frontal cortex area of the brain allows individuals to remain aware of core values, reflect on an interaction, and respond with authenticity and behavioral congruence (Siegel, 2010). This is especially relevant in dealing with trauma. Mindfulness practice helps to move beyond a fight-or-flight "reptilian" reaction to a higher-level and skillful human response. Learner anxiety is often locked into a fight-or-flight reactive mode. Mindful educators can help teach learners how to unlock this circuitry.

Mindful teaching can be viewed as the intentional effort to be present with learners and patients/clients, acknowledging the individual as a complex whole with many parts—seen and unseen—which ultimately impacts the educational or clinical encounter and steers decision-making efforts. This intentionality is interpreted by the receiver as genuine respect, attention, and acceptance (Chase, 2009, p. 215; Johns, 2016; Shapiro, Carlson, Astin, & Freedman, 2006). Mindfulness begins with awareness of breathing. Awareness of breathing enables us to interrupt habitual patterns of avoidance and longing that lead the mind away from the present moment to space and time elsewhere. The practice of "sitting with breath" cultivates skill in intentional presence-keeping (Kabat-Zinn, 1990).

REFLECTING ON . . . MINDFUL LISTENING

- *Breathe your normal breath and listen to the sounds around you.*
- *Take note of sounds that are nearby and those that are far away.*
- *Direct your attention to a particular sound and note the pitch, tone, and volume of the sound.*
- *Note any pattern to the sound.*
- *Note any emotion the sound evokes in you.*
- *Note any thoughts you associate with the sound.*
- *Now direct your attention to the overall sound around you.*
- *Reengage with your learner(s). Note this transition. How are the two experiences different? How can you recreate this intentionality in your current work environment?*

Skill in presence-keeping encourages therapeutic relationships between teacher and learner. A reconceptualization of nursing practice as whole and nonlinear recognizes that healthcare concerns are gleaned through deliberate attention to, and knowledge of, a learner's authentic self (Cowling & Repede, 2009). Knowing the wholeness of a person requires a keen observational stance and a purposeful attempt to understand. Mindful educators have a myriad of opportunities to engage and model this attentive stance for learners, who in turn apply it in their professional practice model.

REFLECTING ON . . . CREATING AN ATTENTIVE STANCE

What are some educational approaches for educators to use in creating an attentive stance? Here are two examples:

- *Develop a course on mindfulness practices or thread mindfulness practices throughout your curriculum. For example, guide your learners in a brief mindful breathing exercise before class.*

- *Establish mindfulness practice at your institution. For example, offer to facilitate a brief discussion about the challenges of teaching and lead a brief mindfulness activity.*

The Practice of Mindful Teaching

Educators have numerous opportunities to model the process of mindfulness and demonstrate reflective learning. Educators can model mindfulness strategies as a basis for reflective learning. As a process of internally exploring an issue or concern arising from a lived experience, reflective learning seeks to clarify meaning in terms of self and results in a newer conceptual perspective. Embracing emotion as a moment-by-moment awareness of self is an example of how a mindful educator might engage learners in reflective learning.

Mindful Teaching Leads to Empathy and Compassion

Mindfulness encourages us to attend to, accept, and be present with all experiences, both positive and negative. Over time and with practice, we can turn toward, rather than lean away from, negative emotions, thoughts, or physical sensations. This requires considerable practice and self-acceptance of the human experience. The authentic self attends to the human experience in its entirety. Gradually, mindful individuals develop the skill to allow even unpleasant emotions to arise and pass away by experiencing and witnessing, but not reacting to, the emotion. Mindful educators and learners who safely allow their own emotions to arise and pass away without engaging in a response develop the capacity for empathy and compassion toward others (Shapiro & Izett, 2008). Loving-kindness mindfulness meditations are particularly well-suited to fostering self-nurturing and balance.

REFLECTING ON . . . A LOVING-KINDNESS MEDITATION

1. *Sit with your breath for a few moments.*

2. *On each in-breath, repeat the following phrases:*
   - *May you and I be happy.*
   - *May you and I be peaceful.*
   - *May you and I be well.*
   - *May all beings be happy, peaceful, and well.*

3. *Let go of distress with each out-breath; exhale your stress.*

Empathy and compassion rely on a sense of equanimity that allows educators and learners to be present in the moment (Raab, 2014; Shapiro, Brown, & Biegel, 2007). Because mindfulness practice encourages self-awareness and an understanding of the impermanency of emotions and thoughts, it facilitates acceptance and the ability to examine thoughts and feelings without getting "stuck."

Mindful attention enables educators to deconstruct their own self-denigrating narratives, which block teaching and their ability to engage in more flexible, open dialogue with learners. Educators who take the time and attention for their own growth appreciate the time and space required for learners to construct alternative, healthier beliefs and practices. Mindful educators cultivate learners' skills in self-observation with their patients; they encourage learners to embrace flexibility, develop an openness of head and heart, and begin to recognize biases and distorted thoughts and perceptions (Crane, 2015).

Mindful Teaching Leads to Self-Awareness

Reflection is linked to the cognitive behavioral skill of self-monitoring (Benner, Sutphen, Leonard, & Day, 2010), which is believed to be the overarching goal of mindfulness. Educators who build their own capacity for reflection can effectively engage learners in this essential skill of connecting schematic and thoughtful thinking to achieve successful patient outcomes. Recognition of emotion in self and others encourages the therapeutic relationship between teacher and learner. Mindful educators model attentiveness to despair or distress in a learner and demonstrate caregiving responses. They demonstrate facilitation of a teacher-learner encounter. Mindfulness is closely aligned with reflection-in-action because it involves purposefully paying attention to thoughts, feelings, and judgments.

Encouraging these metacognitive processes helps learners be more aware of themselves in their actions with others. Mindful teaching facilitates increased awareness for learners in their interpersonal and interprofessional interactions. It enables learners to develop insight into how their awareness of self and others shapes their thoughts, emotions, and actions and how this information informs their responses. Individuals must be fully aware of their perceptual experiences and create a sense of balance and tolerance for their conscious experience (O'Haver Day & Horton-Deutsch, 2004). A detached stance enables the mindful educator and learner to respond to—rather than react to—their habituated way of thinking, moving, and behaving. This detached stance is a skill that is cultivated through both formal and informal mindful meditation practices.

Numerous experiential strategies promote mindful teaching and reflective learning. Mindfulness strategies encourage learners to become increasingly aware and attentive to widening experiences of their emotional and physical experience. Learners begin to recognize, name, connect with, and allow for all of their experiences within a process of growth and self-discovery (Forsyth & Eifert, 2016). Educators can use mindful teaching practices, such as *mandalas*, to encourage learners' reflection skills.

USING MANDALAS AND JOURNALING

The mandala is a circular symbol used among many cultures throughout world history as a tool to promote reflection, meditation, and healing. The circle is a symbol of wholeness, connection, and continuity. Circles help individuals focus inward (van der Vennet & Serice, 2012).

1. *Take a few moments to meditate on the breath.*

2. *Using a pre-printed circle about the size of a snack plate, fill in the space with colored pencils or pastels.*

3. *Be present with the movement of creating the mandala, the colors chosen, and the thoughts and feelings that arise during the exercise.*

4. *Remind yourself to take a nonjudgmental stance toward the exercise.*

5. *Allow yourself 15 to 20 minutes to engage in the practice.*

6. *Take a few moments to notice your mandala and any thoughts or feelings you have.*

7. *Spend a few moments journaling your experience or consider discussing this exercise with others who may be present with you.*

8. *Consider how you can integrate this experience into your daily practice and emulate it in your classroom and/or work environment.*

Exemplar of Mindful Teaching

Graduate health-professions students from three disciplines (nursing, social work, and pharmacy) completed an interprofessional simulation experience with a standardized patient. In preparation, the learners attended a collaborative training session that included opportunities to engage in joint decision-making and mutual learning. Immediately following completion of the simulation experience, all learners participated in a faculty-facilitated debriefing session.

Prior to the start of the simulation, one learner shared that she had been feeling anxious and scared for several days and was fearful that her performance would not "measure up" to her peers. She was especially concerned because she did not have any prior experience with simulation and was certain that she "would not know what to do" and as a result "would fail." Being mindful of the importance of compassion and empathetic responses during a teacher/learner encounter, the teacher acknowledged the learner's distress and commended her for openly sharing her feelings. A brief discussion ensued during which her feelings were validated by her peers as they shared their own anxiety about participating in a new experience. The teacher's recognition of emotion in others and her correspondent compassionate response created a safe environment for all learners to reflect upon their feelings and to extend and receive support from each other.

During the debriefing session, the same learner expressed feeling proud of her performance and stated, "I was so scared, but it wasn't that bad . . . and I wasn't the only one freaking out about going into the room. I'm glad I pushed myself to go through with it." The teacher encouraged the learner to reflect upon how her feelings may have affected her interaction with the standardized patient. The learner believed that her anxiety level prevented her from "fully connecting" with the patient. Further reflection from the learner and other members of the group revealed the important role that awareness of self plays during interpersonal interactions.

The teacher's awareness of some of the key components of mindful practice—empathy, acknowledgment, and reflection—facilitated a deeper exploration by all of the learners regarding the relationship between emotions and actions. This mindful approach facilitated the learners' self-awareness and positive self-regard. The teacher chose to respond in a mindful manner, which provided the opportunity for the learners to reflect deeply without internal or external judgment.

CAPACITY-BUILDING COMPASSION, BY ANDY DAVIES, PhD, MEd

How does a mindful educator care and provide caring education? We argue that caring, in this context, arises out of an individual's ability to feel empathy and compassion. For some people this is an inherent skill, but for others it is something that must be learned. A simple and effective means of developing compassion is by placing yourself into another's position (Lama & Cutler, 1998). This allows for a momentary deconstructing of who you are and a reconstructing of yourself as the other person. After observing someone, consider what it is to be them—

their identity, their gender, and their motivations. Imagine being them. In essence, attempt to see the world through their eyes, not your own. Understanding their perception of the world is an effective means of gaining insight. This intentional practice allows the mindful educator to develop compassion and empathy for those they are working with.

1. *Find a place where you can focus on your breath for 5 minutes without being disturbed.*

2. *Set a gentle alarm for 5 minutes on your watch or cellphone.*

3. *Bring to your attention the individual you are intending to build compassion for.*

4. *On an inhale, consider one of their motivations or passions. On an exhale, imagine experiencing this motivation or passion. (You may have to sit for many breaths for the experience to have an impact. Once you have experienced this motivation or passion as if it were your own, move on to another one.)*

5. *Repeat the breath sequence, focusing on facets of the individual that are relevant to your context. These could include gender, race, education level, religious preference, etc.*

6. *When your alarm rings, take a moment to honor the opportunity to sit and focus internally. Observe your understanding of the individual. Can you perceive any shift in your appreciation of the person?*

Final Reflections

In summary, mindful educators strive to create an environment where learners feel safe to engage in deep reflection, explore new ideas, and expand their ways of thinking and being in the world. The fostering of awareness, curiosity, and new discoveries underlies the teaching philosophy of a mindful educator. Mindfulness and reflection are a bridge to develop higher-level cognitive skills (Schön, 1983). Learners who interact with mindful teachers learn to think mindfully, reflectively, and critically. They become more open and inquisitive, developing critical-reasoning skills to avoid premature closure of thinking (Dyche & Epstein, 2011). With a mindful way of being, they are more likely to integrate new knowledge into their clinical practice, experience deeper self-awareness, and develop more respectful relationships.

References

American Psychological Association (APA). (2006). *APA dictionary of psychology.* Washington, DC: APA.

Benner, P., Sutphen, M., Leonard, V., & Day, L. (2010). *Educating nurses: A call for radical transformation.* San Francisco, CA: Jossey-Bass.

Boellinghaus, I., Jones, F. W., & Hutton, J. (2014). The role of mindfulness and loving-kindness meditation in cultivating self-compassion and other-focused concern in health care professionals. *Mindfulness, 5*(10), 129–138. doi:10.1007/s12671-012-0158-6

Chase, S. (2009). Decision making and knowing in nursing: The essentiality of meaning. In R. Locsin & M. Purnell (Eds.), *A contemporary nursing process: The unbearable weight of knowing in nursing* (pp. 251–281). New York, NY: Springer.

Cowling, W. R., & Repede, E. (2009). Consciousness and knowing: The pattern of the whole. In R. Locsin & M. Purnell (Eds.), *A contemporary nursing process: The unbearable weight of knowing in nursing* (pp. 251–281). New York, NY: Springer.

Crane, R. S. (2015). Some reflections on being good, on not being good and on just being. *Mindfulness, 6*(12), 1226–1231.

Crane, R. S., Williams, J., Mark, G., Hastings, R. P., Cooper, L., & Fennell, M. J. V. (2012). Competence in teaching mindfulness-based courses: Concepts, development and assessment. *Mindfulness in Practice, 3*(9), 76–84.

Davis, D. M., & Hayes, J. A. (2011). What are the benefits of mindfulness? A practice review of psychotherapy-related research. *Psychotherapy, 48*(2), 198–208. doi:1037/a0022062

Dyche, L., & Epstein, R. M. (2011). Curiosity and medical education. *Medical Education, 45*(7), 663–668.

Flook, L., Goldberg, S. B., Pinger, L., Bonus, K., & Davidson, R. J. (2013). Mindfulness for teachers: A pilot study to assess stress, burnout, and teaching efficacy. *Mind, Brain, and Education, 7*(3), 182–195.

Forsyth, J. P., & Eifert, G. H. (2016). *The mindfulness and acceptance workbook for anxiety: A guide to breaking free from anxiety, phobias, and worry using acceptance and commitment therapy.* Oakland, CA: New Harbinger Publications.

Hanley, A. W., Warner, A. R., Dehili, V. M., Canto, A. I., & Garland, E. L. (2015). Washing dishes to wash dishes: Brief instruction in an informal mindfulness practice. *Mindfulness, 6*(5), 1095–1103.

Hindman, R. K., Glass, C. R., Arnkoff, D. B., & Maron, D. D. (2015). A comparison of formal and informal mindfulness programs for stress reduction in university students. *Mindfulness, 6*(12), 873–884. doi:10.1007/s12671-014-0331-1

Johns, C. (2016). *Mindful leadership: A guide for the health care professions.* New York, NY: Palgrave Macmillan.

Kabat-Zinn, J. (1990). *Full catastrophe living: Using the wisdom of your body and mind to face stress, pain, and illness.* New York, NY: Bantam Dell.

Khoury, B., Sharma, M., Rush, M. S., & Fournier, C. (2015). Mindfulness-based stress reduction for health individuals: A meta-analysis. *Journal of Psychosomatic Research, 78*(6), 519–528.

Lama, D., & Cutler, H. (1998). *The art of happiness.* New York, NY: Hodder & Stoughton.

Mars, M., & Oliver, M. (2016). Mindfulness is more than a buzzword: Towards a sustainable model of health care. *Journal of the Australian Traditional Medicine Society, 21*(1), 7–10.

O'Haver Day, P., & Horton-Deutsch, S. (2004). Using mindfulness-based therapeutic interventions in psychiatric nursing practice—Part II: Mindfulness-based approaches for all phases of psychotherapy—Clinical study. *Archives of Psychiatric Nursing, 18*(5), 170–177.

Raab, K. (2014). Mindfulness, self-compassion, and empathy among health care professionals: A review of the literature. *Journal of Health Care Chaplaincy, 20*(3), 95–108.

Schoeberlein, D. (2009). *Mindful teaching and teaching mindfulness: A guide for anyone who teaches anything.* Boston, MA: Wisdom Publications.

Schön, D. A. (1983). *The reflective practitioner: How practitioners think in action.* New York, NY: Basic Books.

Shapiro, S. L., Brown, K. W., & Biegel, G. M. (2007). Teaching self-care to caregivers: Effects of mindfulness-based stress reduction on the mental health of therapists in training. *Training and Education in Professional Psychology, 1*(2), 105–115.

Shapiro, S. L., Carlson, L. E., Astin, J. A., & Freedman, B. (2006). Mechanisms of mindfulness. *Journal of Clinical Psychology, 62*(3), 373–386.

Shapiro, S. L., & Izett, C. D. (2008). Meditation: A universal tool for cultivating empathy. In S. F. Hick & T. Bien (Eds.), *Mindfulness and the therapeutic relationship* (pp. 161–175). New York, NY: Guildford Press.

Siegel, D. J. (2010). *Mindsight: The new science of personal transformation.* New York, NY: Bantam.

Tang, Y-Y., Holzel, B. K., & Posner, M. I. (2015). The neuroscience of mindfulness meditation. *Nature Reviews Neuroscience, 16*(4), 213–225. doi:10.1038/nrn3916

Tang, Y-Y., & Leve, L. (2016). A translational neuroscience perspective on mindfulness meditation as a prevention strategy. *Translational Behavioral Medicine, 6*(1), 63–72. doi:10.1007/s13142-015-0360-x

Tirch, D. D. (2010). Mindfulness as a context for the cultivation of compassion. *International Journal of Cognitive Therapy, 3*(2), 113–123. doi:10.1521/ijct.2010.3.2.113

van der Vennet, R., & Serice, S. (2012). Can coloring mandalas reduce anxiety? A replication study. *Art Therapy, 29*(2), 87–92.

Walsh, R., & Shapiro, S. L. (2006). The meeting of meditative disciplines and Western psychology: A mutually enriching dialogue. *American Psychologist, 61*(3), 227–239.

Williams, J., Mark, G., & Kabat-Zinn, J. (2011). Mindfulness: Diverse perspectives on its meaning, origins, and multiple applications at the intersection of science and dharma. *Contemporary Buddhism, 12*(1), 1–18. doi:10.1080/14639947.2011.564811

Chapter 6
Mindful Learners

–Sara Horton-Deutsch, PhD, RN, FAAN, ANEF
–Barbara L. Drew, PhD, RN, PMHCNS
–Kathleen Beck-Coon, MD
–With Learning Activity by Andy Davies, PhD, MEd

The constantly changing, collaborative nature of reflective practice of educators and learners subsumes mindful awareness of one's internal and external milieu. Although the critical benefit of such skills might be obvious, the means to cultivate this innate capacity is often omitted in the educational forum and is frequently relegated to theory. Growing scientific evidence indicates that the moment-to-moment, purposeful, nonjudgmental awareness of mindfulness practice encourages just such neural and functional integration and flexibility (Lutz, Dunne, & Davidson, 2007).

In exploring the neuropsychological underpinnings of mindfulness, Tang, Hölzel, and Posner (2015) identified three key components of mindfulness that might account for its effects: attention control, emotion regulation, and self-awareness. These components interact to enhance self-regulation. Educators who embody and share mindful practice encourage learners in developing this presence and attention, facilitating the engaged, spirited inquiry of active learning that serves to shape their nursing practice.

This chapter explores the use of mindful and reflective practices with learners and offers exercises and methods to help learners pay attention and gain awareness in relation to self and others. By paying attention and honing awareness in the open-hearted nonjudgment of mindfulness, learners improve academic and clinical performance.

Background

Schön, a leading social scientist, recognized that clinical practitioners develop practical knowledge and working intelligence as they make sense of theoretical knowledge in their work. He differentiated between *reflection-on-action* (which happens after clinical practice) and *reflection-in-action* (which happens during the moments of a clinical encounter), in effect, bridging the theory-practice gap and enabling professionals to uncover knowledge in and on action (Schön, 1983).

> *"By being present, learners bring clarity to what they are sensing, feeling, thinking, wanting, and willing to do. Integrating mindfulness into educational pursuits lays the foundation for reflective learning."*

Mindfulness, often equated with reflection-in-action, enhances overall learning by helping learners integrate understanding gained from experience in the present moment. Importantly, it incorporates awareness of the intrapersonal experience of body sensations, emotions, and thoughts as not separate from this metacognitive process. Reflection-in-action is a complex cognitive activity that requires learners to be conscious of what they are doing and how they are doing it in the moment of practice.

Processes for reflecting-in-action are those creative strategies that learners can use in the moment of practice, when learners are "being, thinking, and doing" simultaneously. As learners begin to reflect on personal, professional, and civic dimensions of learning experiences, they increase their ability to be reflective-in-action. This means that learners not only find meaning in their experiences when looking back on them, but also while preparing for them and even in the middle of them. Learners will find that such continuous reflection helps them to be most effective in learning encounters and, indeed, in life.

Mindfulness explicitly recognizes that the reflective process is not limited to cognition alone. People engaging in mindfulness practice perceive reality by liberating attachment to memories of the past and fantasies of the future, bringing the present moment clearly into focus, beginning with grounding in present-moment body sensations. By being present, learners bring clarity to what they are sensing, feeling, thinking, wanting, and willing to do. Integrating mindfulness into educational pursuits lays the foundation for reflective learning. This chapter addresses current pursuits at integrating mindfulness and reflective practices in classroom and clinical settings.

The Need for Introducing Mindful Practices Into Learning

Though health promotion is a core value of nursing, nurses are often "imperfect role models" (Rush, Kee, & Rice, 2005, p. 166) and do not regularly engage in practices of self-awareness and self-care, such as meditation, physical activity, or stress management (Hensel, 2011). This likely holds true for most nursing faculty, as well. As a result, nursing students, with their challenging curricula and other life demands, come to neglect themselves (Ashcraft & Gatto, 2015), mirroring their faculty and practicing nurse mentors.

ATTENTION CONTROL

The capacity to allocate the brain's limited attentional resources (defined as the distinct functional and neuroanatomical subsystems of alerting, orienting, and conflict monitoring) to its intended target.

EMOTION REGULATION

The broad and complex adaptive capacity to respond to biopsychological stimuli in a nonreactive, functional, and situationally appropriate manner. Incorporates the willingness to meet whatever is being experienced.

SELF-AWARENESS

Perception that self is a product of an ongoing mental process rather than a static and unchanging entity (Tang, Hölzel, & Posner, 2015).

Mind-body self-care strategies deliberately introduced to nurse educators and curricula cultivate a more mindful way of being and are associated with less emotional distress, more positive states of mind, and better quality of life (Greeson, 2008). It can begin with caring educator-learner relationships that are hallmarks of successful nursing programs and evolve into an environment that promotes opportunities for the teaching and practice of mind-body self-care by faculty, staff, and students. Caring relationships are the foundation of a caring curriculum and are carried out through modeling, practice, authentic dialogue, and affirmation and confirmation (Noddings, 2013; Hills & Watson, 2011). Nursing programs at Florida Atlantic University and Nevada State University have missions that focus on advancing caring through art, science, and study. Both express their mission through a caring-based approach to teaching and learning nursing.

By contrast, most nursing education programs have historically emphasized ways of doing over ways of being. For nurses to meet the demands of an ever-changing healthcare delivery climate, learners must gain the knowledge, skills, and attitudes to continuously improve healthcare systems in which they work (National Academies of Sciences, Engineering, and Medicine, 2015; QSEN Institute, 2014). This mandate requires using a variety of curricular approaches that extend beyond traditional teaching modalities to methodologies of inquiry, in which students learn from their clinical experiences and are versed in the use of reflection. This also supports the development of lifelong learners who are open, aware, and responsive to change. As such, mindfulness is becoming an important theoretical construct in health promotion education and research (Black, 2010). Teaching students to be present-in-the-now does not preclude learning or performing necessary tasks. Rather, learners who practice increased self-awareness and consciousness reduce the demands of caring as the care provided becomes more accurate, more focused, and generally more fulfilling for both the nurse and the patient (Watson, 2008).

In recent years, a number of colleges and universities have introduced courses that emphasized personal wellness and mindfulness into their curriculum as a way to lay a foundation for learners to develop self-awareness, presence, and intention, as well as an appreciation for the importance of self-care, compassion, and stress reduction. Three different strategies have been described. First, for example, Indiana University School of Nursing offered an elective course entitled Mindfulness-Based Wellness: An Integrative Journey of Health and Well-Being (Beck-Coon, 2010) that introduced mindfulness practice and explored evidence-based applications of mindfulness in healthcare and education.

Second, rather than an elective course, Kent State University embedded a module on mind-body self-care in a first semester course for accelerated nursing students (Drew et al., 2016). The module included 1 hour per week of practices such as yoga, mindful breathing, Reiki, and the use of essential oils. The objectives were to help students manage their stress and approach the care of their clients in a more mindful way.

A third strategy is to infuse academic content with concepts relevant to personal wellness. For example, at Georgetown University School of Nursing, self-reflection related to student mental health and well-being was integrated into the curriculum (Riley & Yearwood, 2012; Yearwood & Riley, 2010).

Introducing reflective practices through formally developed courses that emphasize the concepts outlined in the preceding description lays the foundation for creating mindful learners and practitioners. It is reasonable to believe, though, that learners need to not only be introduced to mindful practice but that the skills should be reinforced with ongoing mindful practices threaded throughout their nursing programs. Additionally, mindful educators create mindful learners by role-modeling and encouraging self-awareness, self-care, and nurturing relationships and by creating the necessary time and space for reflection that supports a personal journey of growth.

Supporting the Development of Self-Awareness and Self-Care

Through the process of mindful and reflective practices, learners become aware of uncomfortable feelings and thoughts. Recognition and awareness of emotional reactions is the first step in reflection (Freshwater, 2008), and openly exploring emotions with a sense of curiosity encourages mutual exploration and discovery. Maintaining a posture of not knowing and being genuinely curious keeps learners open to multiple possibilities. Thus, self-awareness is the first critical component of reflective practice. While further study is needed, moment-to-moment awareness and presence is a vital asset for helping patients and is not about self-absorption, but about paying attention to the self and others (Bein, 2008; Burton, Burgess, Dean, Koutsopoulou, & Hugh-Jones, 2016).

Mindfulness allows bearing witness to one's own pain and responding with the kindness and understanding that allows enhancement of both self-care and caring for all those served by nurses. Furthermore, the insidious nature of stress that directly affects the personal and professional capacity of caregivers, often labeled as *compassion fatigue* (Najjar, Davis, Beck-Coon, & Carney-Doebbeling, 2009), skips over the (self) compassion of so-called "self" care, while mindfulness incorporates self-care as an integral understanding of compassion. Breathing exercises that prompt self-awareness, presented in Chapters 4 and 5, are one strategy for anchoring in mindful presence. In addition, mindfully paying attention while they are completing activities of daily living (such as doing the dishes, walking, driving, and brushing their teeth) can also help learners to develop moment-to-moment presence.

In supporting the goals of Healthy People 2020 (Office of Disease Prevention and Health Promotion, 2016), the American Hospital Association (2011) called for innovative strategies to enable hospital staff to manage stress effectively and improve workplace conditions within all healthcare settings. Professional caregivers—including nurses, physicians, social workers, and all other therapists—struggle with balancing their self-care needs with the demands of the workplace and find it difficult to schedule time for restorative practices that can help manage stress. Mindfulness is a form of self-care, because it involves the use of systematic and routine approaches to promote one's physical, spiritual, and emotional well-being.

Self-care behaviors include appropriate health screenings, physical activity, spiritual growth, proper nutrition, satisfying interpersonal relationships, meaningful work, and stress management. Educators can reinforce these practices with learners and emphasize their importance not only for patients, but also when caring for themselves. Integrating various self-care questions into classroom learning activities is one strategy to consider.

REFLECTING ON . . . SELF-CARE

- *How do I take care of myself?*

- *List the ways I cared for myself yesterday.*

- *How do I know when I am caring for myself?*

- *What are the obstacles to caring for myself?*

- *What are the benefits of caring for myself?*

- *What are the consequences of not caring?*

- *How would I like to improve caring for myself? In other words, what areas need caring?*

Hernandez (2009) proposes a self-care model for nurses based on Watson's Theory of Caring (2008). It is entitled the "Caring Model of Self-Care." Hernandez believes healthcare professionals must cultivate sensitivity to themselves and others through self-reflection, awareness, and spiritual practices of loving-kindness (also part of mindfulness practice). Although Hernandez's model itself is not empirically tested, it holds potential as a succinct visual reminder of the basic tenets for mindful and reflective practice.

REFLECTING ON . . . THE CARING MODEL OF SELF-CARE

C: *Compassion*

A: *Awareness*

R: *Reflection*

I: *Intentionality*

N: *Nonjudgmental Attachment*

G: *Gratitude*

Mindful approaches to health benefit healthcare educators, learners, and patients. Mindfulness training appears to provide a meaningful vehicle for promoting self-care and reduces the impact of work-related stress. Educators who engage learners in mindfulness activities in the classroom support the creation of a culture where self-awareness, self-care, and stress management are viewed as central to providing patient-centered care.

Nurturing Relationships

Compassion, defined as the capacity for empathy and sympathy that desires the resolution of suffering (Bodhi, 1994, p. 39), involves being with the suffering of another with an open heart and often neglects the reality that, as nurses, we often do not know how to be with our own suffering (Beck-Coon, 2010). To be compassionate, the learner must be open to possibilities, be accepting of the responses of others, and be able to adjust to the needs of others. The compassion of mindful reflection acknowledges negative self-talk; instead of getting on the treadmill of self-criticism, it acknowledges suffering, offers loving-kindness to the self, and allows nonjudgmental insights to be known.

Compassionate Reflection

Mindful, compassionate reflection predicts flexibility in tolerating negative emotions (e.g., after receiving ambivalent feedback or in acknowledging our role in negative events without overwhelming guilt and rumination) (Leary, Tate, Adams, Allen, & Hancock, 2007) and enhances students' empathy and well-being in personal and professional relationships (Siegel, 2007a). When educators deliberately practice mindfulness with learners, learners improve in the ability to focus, pay attention, remain open, and improve complex task performance such as responding to the multiple and simultaneous needs of others (Jha, Krompinger, & Baime, 2007; Siegel, 2007b).

Mindfulness, cultivated through intentional attention and nonjudgment, facilitates becoming compassionate with our own lives and the lives of others. It connects us to our common humanity (Neff, 2003). Instead of reactive engagement, wise, kind, responsive, values-based behaviors can then follow. Not only does the practice develop intrapersonal compassion, but interpersonal compassion as well. In essence, those who practice mindfulness lower their risk for burnout, reduce their stress, and have a greater sense of personal accomplishment (Cohen-Katz, Wiley, Capuano, Baker, & Shapiro, 2004, 2005).

Historically, little empirical-based direction has been available to academic programs to help learners cultivate habits of mind necessary for controlling attention and for having an empathetic response. The majority of teaching literature focuses on external and observable responses such as mirroring thoughts or feelings. It is now recognized that inattention to cultivating internal skills can result in decreased self-efficacy and ability to care for others and increased anxiety of the caregiver (Beck-Coon, 2010). Evidence also suggests that cultivation of mindfulness not only wards off burnout and stress, but also helps to develop attention and empathy (Beddoe & Murphy, 2004).

Compassionate Communication

Mindfulness expressed in speaking and listening improves workplace communication (Beddoe & Murphy, 2004). By purposefully paying attention in a nonjudgmental manner, we intentionally pause and maintain a stance of being present, open, and flexible. The act of presencing also releases muscle tension, opinions, and fixed ways of thinking, responding, or acting (Kramer, 2007). This simple act of *noticing* releases the need to control the learning (or clinical) encounter or reactively give advice. Listening open-heartedly, we become more open to outcome and focus on being mindfully responsive. Learners develop patience and understanding and accept that things unfold in their own time. Given that mindfulness is cultivated through experiential learning, engaging students in mindful practices is essential. An introduction of mindful practice to students at Kent State University is described as follows:

> On the first day of the class, students were asked to describe current self-care practices. As one might imagine, students all described physical activities that they practiced, such as running, playing volleyball, and weightlifting. The discussion then transitioned to mental and spiritual self-care. The term mindfulness was introduced, along with a description of documented benefits such as a decreased response to stress, improved focus of attention, increased compassion, and the ability to be truly present in the moment

(Greeson, 2008). All of these are qualities the students would need to provide safe, quality care to patients and to successfully complete an accelerated BSN program (T. Motter, personal communication, 2011).

There is limited emphasis on helping learners develop self-care and compassion in nursing curricula; however, research demonstrates mindfulness facilitates stress management for nurses and prevents burnout (Cohen-Katz et al., 2004; Drew et al., 2016; Shapiro, Astin, Bishop, & Cordova, 2005). Evidence further demonstrates that mindfulness helps decrease depression and anxiety while empathy increases (Greeson, 2008).

Self-Care Curriculum Infusion

The following comments are from Kent State University students during focus groups following a course that included mind-body self-care; they illustrate the positive outcomes experienced (Parsons, Drew, Motter, Bozeman, & Motter, 2015).

I thought it was also helpful because we know that for the rest of our lives now any situation where we are stressed or exhausted or we can't sleep we now have tools that will help us get through that.

I have also been making a conscious effort to mindfully relax at the end of the day when I'm lying in bed. Instead of dwelling on my worries, I am consciously clearing my mind. I always seem to practice deep breathing automatically while clearing my thoughts. This is an instant sleeping aid. Finals are here and I can honestly say that I am not feeling the stress. I think I can attribute this to a more mindful way of approaching my new stressors.

My roommate and I actually do that thing where you put your legs up against the wall together when we're studying. It is like our little break. It is just relaxing to just take a few minutes just to do that.

If you are in clinicals . . . and you have a very stressful situation or stressful patient . . . you could take a step back and just breathe for a minute.

They (faculty) are not just concerned with our education; they are concerned for us. That was nice.

I actually have been practicing (or trying to practice) breath awareness. Without knowing much about it, I have, in times of stress or strong emotions, been trying to focus on the present and just "being" where I am. It is surprisingly calming and I find that it seems to get me out of the chaos more than some of the distractions I try to use. I look forward to learning more and using different techniques.

Yearwood and Riley (2010) explore the impact of pedagogy of curriculum infusion on nursing students' well-being and intent to provide safe and effective care. *Curriculum infusion* is the blending of an issue with course content, and in this study the issue was self-awareness. Student reflections, case analyses, and narrative evaluations were examined in relation to American Association of Colleges of Nursing (AACN) Essentials (2008) and QSEN criteria (Cronenwett et al., 2007). Through this intervention, students experienced the connection between their own agency and quality indicators, prompting more students to express the intention to work more confidently, competently, and holistically with patients (Riley & Yearwood, 2012). Riley and Yearwood (2012) recommend addressing the self more explicitly in the QSEN competencies and through the use of curriculum infusion to promote nursing student well-being.

Creating Space for Reflection in the Classroom

Creating space in classroom and clinical settings for mindful and reflective practices is essential to developing reflective practitioners. Reflective thinking is not what learners do after they acquire content; rather, it is what learners do to acquire content (Shermis, 1992). Content needs to be expanded to include the data of reflection and evidence from any source that bears on the clinical concern. Neurobiology research has established that the brain is wired to change structurally and functionally in response to experience (Cozolino & Sprokay, 2006), and mindfulness is perfectly poised to support this learning. By asking questions and creating assignments that encourage reflection, educators not only facilitate identification of the concern but also all the contextual and relational aspects. For example, during the initial phase of any nursing course or clinical encounter, learners can be introduced to mindful practices. In addition, follow-up questions that are more cognitive and contemplative in nature can be used within a practice to encourage reflection.

REFLECTING ON . . . CREATING MINDFUL LEARNERS THROUGH QUESTIONING

Mindful learners ask themselves:

- *Why am I in this class, program, and profession?*
- *What choices did I have to make to be here?*
- *What do I expect that I can take with me?*
- *What am I willing to invest?*

As nursing courses progress, learners can regularly engage in mindful, reflective writing to reinforce thinking about their own thinking in a way that is consistent with the "attentive attunement" of the hermeneutic process (Smythe, Ironside, Sims, Swenson, & Spence, 2008). For example, an opportunity for 5 minutes of mindfulness meditation followed by a 1-minute reflective writing assignment at the end of each day encourages a nonjudgmental knowing of the unique individual filters that are shaping perception, as well as taking responsibility for personal learning needs and attempting to ensure they are met.

DAILY REFLECTIVE WRITING EXERCISE

Write for 1 minute the most important lessons you learned today. Why were these lessons important and how can they help you? What else do you need to explore to further grow in this area?

When held in the nonjudgmental stance of mindfulness, learners have an opportunity to question and explore the body sensations, thoughts, feelings, and actions of personal and interpersonal experiences in a space that allows wise insights to arise.

Using the Kosha Model (Contributed by Andy Davies, PhD, MEd)

The practices of reflection and mindfulness expand ways of knowing, ways of being, and ways of caring. Educated, thinking, questioning nurses are vital to the discipline of nursing and other healthcare professions seeking to balance conventional science with art, humanities, and spirituality—converging models of mind-body-spirit medicine, often called *alternative* or *integrative* medicine. Avenues to infuse our understanding of the world include trans-philosophical models. One such model is the *Kosha model*.

The Kosha model originated from the Hindu yogic traditions. In the original Sanskrit language, the term *kosha* means layer or sheath. The model considers a human being as an integrated and multidimensional being. This individual is composed of five layers. Each of these layers is considered interdependent and influential. When a stimulus affects one layer, a domino effect occurs in each of the remaining four layers. These five layers are: a physiological layer, an energetic layer, an emotional/mental layer, a wisdom/intellectual discernment layer, and a spiritual layer (see Figure 6.1).

FIGURE 6.1

According to the Kosha model, humans are composed of five layers.

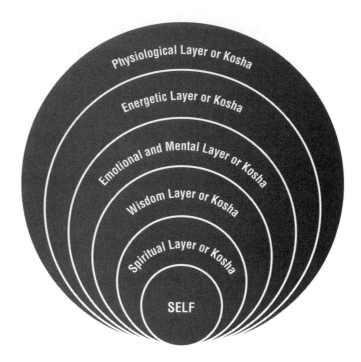

When considering the acts of mindfulness and reflective practice, the benefit of drawing upon a trans-philosophical model to reconsider these notions opens up the possibility of new ways of thinking. The Kosha model perceives the human being as a holistic, interrelated, inter-permeating series of systems. The application of this model opens up new possibilities for nurses when considering reflective practice and being mindful.

When considering the self, the Kosha model allows us to perceive our bodies as five distinct but influential systems. Balance can only be achieved in this system through balance of each of the layers or sheaths. Each layer requires, therefore, sustaining, nurturing actions to facilitate equilibrium. This approach to understanding the individual rejects the either/or understanding of mind or body, heart or soul, brain or brawn. None of the binaries is privileged because each is as integral as the other, mind-body, heart-soul, and brain-brawn. Each is integral to each other. Neglect of one Kosha causes neglect in the others. This influences how we perceive self-awareness.

When we consider the act of self-awareness in this state, we observe not just the body or the mind. We now ponder the five systems that compose the self. Most of us are aware of our first layer—aches, pains, hunger, thirst, and elimination needs—which all represent the obviousness of our physiological sheath. We may be aware of varying energy levels from morning into afternoon and evening, demonstrating our awareness of our energetic layer. But how aware are you of your emotional-mental state? Is it balanced? Is it overextended? How aware are you of your capacity for intellectual discernment? Is your wisdom layer underserved, under-challenged? Or are you prioritizing your intellect over your physical form? Have you nourished your spiritual side recently? Is it crying for connection to community or nature? What might balance this facet of your being? Reevaluating yourself through a new trans-philosophical lens such as the Kosha model affords you the opportunity to reflect upon who you are from a more holistic framework. It also influences how you perceive self-care and self-care behaviors.

When you consider the act of self-care, the Kosha model enables you to consider more nuanced aspects of yourself. Have you fed your body with life-sustaining food? Have you provided your body with enough sleep? Did you overindulge in too much wine or beer during a social night? Every choice influences your collective body. Did you spend too much time lifting weights so now your energy is exhausted? Or have you sat on the couch every night ignoring your walking shoes even though you feel lethargic?

Have you prided yourself on your intellect to the detriment and neglect of your body? Conversely, have you slavishly exercised your body but neglected your intellect? Do you crave companionship incessantly? Or hide from the world in a desire to be alone? Do you listen internally to what is right? Or do you follow the crowd because it is easier? Do you follow your own internal moral compass? Or do you feel distressed because you function against your values? Every choice influences our internal equilibrium. Reflective consideration of our many layers can aid in the development of a self-sustainability and robustness. As we come to understand ourselves through intentional mindfulness, the Kosha model allows us to see others and our communication with others from a different and more nuanced perspective.

Role-modeling, communication, and relationships all require interaction with another individual. When we mindfully consider ourselves from the Kosha model, we can then see others as equally layered and interdependent. Embracing the Kosha model as a means of understanding our human condition aids us in our communication and relationships. It aids us to more skillfully nurture our relationships. Observing for balance or imbalance in others may assist with how and what we say and what we offer.

The Kosha model provides us with a framework by which we may reflectively practice our interactions with others. It offers us an opportunity to see that our balances or imbalances can influence others and that we are all influential and interdependent. Our mindful and reflective consideration of multifaceted selves shows us that we are part of an interdependent collective community and that we desire this spiritual connectivity at the core of our being.

REFLECTING ON . . . YOUR KOSHA LAYERS, BY ANDY DAVIES, PHD, MED

Find a place where you can focus on your breath for 5 minutes without being disturbed and set a gentle alarm for 5 minutes.

- *Consider your physiological layer. Become aware of your body and how it is positioned. Observe comforts and discomforts. Itches and twitches. Gurgle sounds and breath sounds. Reflect upon your treatment of your body. Reflect upon the importance it plays in your life. Do you ignore it? Do you nurture it? Do you take it for granted?*

- *When your alarm sounds, take a moment to honor the opportunity to sit and focus internally. Reflect upon what you have observed and then write these thoughts down.*

- *When you next have 5 minutes, set your alarm and sit in a quiet and comfortable space.*

- *Consider your energetic layer. With your eyes shut, explore internally your body, searching for vibrations and energies flowing through the body. Notice sensations of tiredness or fidgeting. Notice if your body wants to move or twitch. Or if your body wants to go to sleep. Are you kind in your expectations of your body with sleep and rest? Or do you drive your body too hard? If you are tired, what is it you could do to energize your body? Do you ever consider the importance of your body in your life?*

- *When your alarm sounds, take a moment to honor the opportunity to sit and focus internally. Reflect upon what you have observed and then write these thoughts down.*

- *When you next have 5 minutes, set your alarm and sit in a quiet and comfortable space.*

- *Consider your emotional and mental layer. When you are happy, can you feel it in your body? When you are sad, can you feel it in your body? With your eyes closed, feel in your body the places sensations arise when you feel emotional. Are you aware of such places? Do emotions alter how you think? Can your thoughts change your emotions? Do your thoughts and emotions run freely? Or do you control them?*

- *When your alarm sounds, take a moment to honor the opportunity to sit and focus internally. Reflect upon what you have observed and then write these thoughts down.*

- *When you next have 5 minutes, set your alarm and sit in a quiet and comfortable space.*

- *Consider your wisdom or intellectual discernment layer. Do you think you are intelligent? What does intelligence mean to you? Is it important? Do you trust your judgments? Do you feel positive when you give advice? Consider the mental choices you have made today. Were they made with wisdom?*

- *When your alarm sounds, take a moment to honor the opportunity to sit and focus internally. Reflect upon what you have observed and then write these thoughts down.*

- *When you next have 5 minutes, set your alarm and sit in a quiet and comfortable space.*

- *Consider your spiritual layer. Do you value a god? Or do you value an inner connection? Have you ever felt called to do something greater than yourself? Do you see meaning in actions or in community? Do you consider values or mores often? Is being in nature important to you? What is it in you that makes you a good person?*

- *When your alarm sounds, take a moment to honor the opportunity to sit and focus internally. Reflect upon what you have observed and then write these thoughts down.*

The Kosha Layer Reflection

Coming to understand ourselves is a lifetime task and a lifetime journey. We comprise many narratives, and we are composed of many rationalizations. We construct narratives, we arrange vignettes, and we build rationalizations to explain who we are, just as tribal natives constructed narratives and metaphors to explain their world. Our practice of mindfulness and our practice of reflection deconstruct these worlds of narrative, of tasty vignettes and of juicy rationalizations. Mindfulness and reflective practice deconstruct our sense of self, our inner narratives. The adoption of a trans-philosophical model such as the Kosha model enables us to re-perceive ourselves. It enables us to reconsider, to reevaluate, and to reconnect in different ways. It allows us to consider and reflect from a new way of knowing. It permits us to reevaluate how to be in this new world. Most of all, it affords us new opportunities in how we care in the world.

Final Reflections

As educators both embody for learners and engage learners in ongoing mindful and reflective practices through time, learners become skilled at critically considering beliefs and knowledge, raising awareness, and monitoring responses. According to Bolton (2005), the paradox is that reflective practice is required by the educators and by the institution, yet its nature is politically and socially disruptive. Essentially, it opens to question anything taken for granted, and that's the rub. Educators who engage learners in reflective practice must be open to inquiry-based education, creativity, and innovation and must be comfortable with change. Learners must be encouraged to know that it is safe to ask challenging questions, to monitor their reactions to ensure responses were consistent with their intentions, and to openly discuss their mistakes to make better choices in the future.

An additional challenge to supporting the development of mindful learners is the drive for nursing educators to emphasize content delivery rather than allowing time in the classroom and clinical setting for the processes of reflection, learning to be present in the moment, and finding ways to manage stress. Many champions of mindful practices within a faculty group are needed for continuous role-modeling for students and threading of reflective practices throughout the curriculum, or pressure may be exerted to return to more traditional ways of teaching.

A mindful way of being brings present-moment, active engagement that includes the intra- and interpersonal in this real-time learning mode. It taps into discerning wisdom held in kind curiosity rather than the harsh, judgmental style that characterizes much of educational exploration. Engaging learners in mindful and reflective practices, with an emphasis on self-care and compassion, supports the development of nurses who carry these values into their professional practice by enacting patient-centered care and a commitment to lifelong learning.

References

American Association of Colleges of Nursing (AACN). (2008). *The essentials of baccalaureate education for professional nursing practice*. Retrieved from http://www.aacn.nche.edu/Education/bacessn.htm

American Hospital Association. (2011). A call to action: Creating a culture of health. 2010 Long-Range Policy Committee, John W. Bluford III, chair. Retrieved from http://www.aha.org/research/cor/content/creating-a-culture-of-health.pdf

Ashcraft, P. F., & Gatto, S. L. (2015). Care-of-self in undergraduate nursing students: A pilot study. *Nursing Education Perspectives, 36*(4), 255–256.

Beck-Coon, K. (2010). Mindfulness: Implications for safety, self-care, and empathy in nursing education. Quality and Safety Education for Nurses. Retrieved from http://www.qsen.org/modules/module3/index.php

Beddoe, A. E., & Murphy, S. O. (2004). Does mindfulness decrease stress and foster empathy among nursing students? *Journal of Nursing Education, 43*(7), 305–312.

Bein, A. (2008). *The zen of helping: Spiritual principles for mindful and open-hearted practice*. Hoboken, NJ: John Wiley & Sons.

Black, D. (2010). Incorporating mindfulness within established theories of health behavior. *Complementary Health Practice Review, 15*(2), 108–109.

Bodhi, B. (1994). *The noble eightfold path: The way to the end of suffering.* Kandy, Sri Lanka: Buddhist Publication Society.

Bolton, G. (2005). *Reflective practice: Writing and professional development.* London, UK: Sage.

Burton, A., Burgess, C., Dean, S., Koutsopoulou, G. Z., & Hugh-Jones, S. (2016). How effective are mindfulness-based interventions for reducing stress among healthcare professionals? A systematic review and meta-analysis. *Stress and Health, 33*(1), 3–13. doi:10.1002/smi.2673

Bybee, R. W., Buchwald, C. E., Crissman, S., Heil, D. R., Kuebis, P. J., Matsumoto, C., & McInerney, J. D. (1989). *Science and technology education for the elementary years: Frameworks for curriculum and instruction.* Washington, DC: National Center for Improving Science Education.

Cohen-Katz, J., Wiley, S. D., Capuano, T., Baker, D. M., & Shapiro, S. (2004). The effects of mindfulness-based stress reduction on nurse stress and burnout. *Holistic Nursing Practice, 18*(6), 302–308.

Cohen-Katz, J., Wiley, S. D., Capuano, T., Baker, D. M., & Shapiro, S. (2005). The effects of mindfulness-based stress reduction on nurse stress and burnout, part II. *Holistic Nursing Practice, 19*(1), 26–35.

Cozolino, L., & Sprokay, S. (2006). Neuroscience and adult learning. *New Directions for Adult & Continuing Education, 2006*(110), 11–19.

Cronenwett, L., Sherwood, G., Barnsteiner, J., Disch, J., Johnson, J., Mitchell, P., . . . Warren, J. (2007). Quality and safety education for nurses. *Nursing Outlook, 55*(3), 122–131.

Drew, B. L., Motter, T., Ross, R., Goliat, L., Sharpnack, P. A., Govoni, A.L., . . . Rababah, J. (2016). Care for the caregiver: Evaluation of mind-body self-care for accelerated nursing students. *Holistic Nursing Practice, 30*(3), 148–154.

Freshwater, D. (2008). Reflective practice: The state of the art. In D. Freshwater, B. Taylor, & G. Sherwood (Eds.), *International textbook of reflective practice in nursing* (pp. 1–18). Oxford, UK: Blackwell Publishing.

Gibbs, G., Farmer, B., & Eastcott, D. (1988). *Learning by doing: A guide to teaching and learning methods.* Birmingham, UK: FEU.

Greeson, J. M. (2008). Mindfulness research update: 2008. *Complementary Health Practice Review, 14*(1), 10–18.

Hayes, S. C., Luoma, J. B., Bond, F. W., Masuda, A., & Lillis, J. (2006). Acceptance and commitment therapy: Model, processes and outcomes. *Behaviour Research & Therapy, 44*(1), 1–25.

Hensel, D. (2011). Relationships among nurses' professional self-concept, health, and lifestyles. *Western Journal of Nursing Research, 33*(1), 45–62.

Hernandez, G. (2009). The HeART of self-C.A.R.I.N.G.: A journey to becoming an optimal healing presence to ourselves and our patients. *Creative Nursing, 15*(3), 129–133.

Hölzel, B. K., Lazar, S. W., Gard, T., Schuman-Olivier, Z., Vago, D. R., & Ott, U. (2011). How does mindfulness meditation work? Proposing mechanisms of action from a conceptual and neural perspective. *Perspectives on Psychological Science, 6*(6), 537–559.

Institute of Medicine. (2008). IOM report: Evidence-based medicine and the changing nature of healthcare: Workshop summary. Washington, DC: National Academies Press.

Jha, A. P., Krompinger, J., & Baime, M. J. (2007). Mindfulness training modifies subsystems of attention. *Cognitive Affective Behavioral Neuroscience, 7*(2), 109–119.

Kramer, G. (2007). *Insight dialogue: The interpersonal path to freedom.* Boston, MA: Shambhala Publications.

Leary, M. R., Tate, E. B., Adams, C. E., Allen, A. B., & Hancock, J. (2007). Self-compassion and reactions to unpleasant self-relevant events: The implications of treating oneself kindly. *Journal of Personality & Social Psychology, 92*(5), 887–904.

Lutz, A., Dunne, J. P., & Davidson, R. J. (2007). Meditation and the neuroscience of consciousness: An introduction. In P. Zelazo, M. Moscovitch, & E. Thompson (Eds.), *The Cambridge handbook of consciousness* (pp. 499–554). New York, NY: Cambridge University Press.

Motter, T., & Drew, B. L. (2011, October). Care for the caregiver: Implementing a self-care module for accelerated nursing students. Poster presented at New Careers in Nursing Annual Summit, Washington, DC.

Najjar, N., Davis, L. W., Beck-Coon, K., & Carney-Doebbeling, C. (2009). Compassion fatigue: A review to date and relevance to oncology healthcare providers. *Journal of Health Psychology, 14*(2), 267–277.

National Academies of Sciences, Engineering, and Medicine. (2015). Assessing progress on the Institute of Medicine report *The future of nursing*. Washington, DC: National Academies Press.

Neff, K. D. (2003). Development and validation of a scale to measure self-compassion. *Self and Identity*, 2(12), 223–250.

Neff, K. D., & Lamb, L. M. (2009). Self-compassion. In S. Lopez (Ed.), *The encyclopedia of positive psychology* (pp. 864–867). West Sussex, UK: Blackwell.

Noddings, N. (2013). *Caring: A relational approach to ethics and moral education.* Berkeley, CA: University of California Press.

Office of Disease Prevention and Health Promotion. (2016). 2020 topics and objectives. Healthy People 2020. Retrieved from https://www.healthypeople.gov/2020/topics-objectives

Parsons, E., Drew, B. L., Motter, T., Bozeman, M. C., & Rababah, J. (2015, April). Student experiences with mind-body self-care during their first nursing course: Content analysis of focus groups. Poster presented at the 39th annual Research Conference of the Midwest Nursing Research Society, Indianapolis, IN.

Praissman, S. (2008). Mindfulness-based stress reduction: A literature review and clinician's guide. *Journal of the American Academy of Nurse Practitioners*, 20(4), 212–216.

QSEN Institute. (2014). Competencies. Retrieved from www.qsen.org/competencies

Quality and Safety Education for Nurses (QSEN). (2008). Robert Wood Johnson Foundation. Retrieved from http://qsen.org/about-qsen

Riley, J. B., & Yearwood, E. L. (2012). The effect of a pedagogy of curriculum infusion on nursing student well-being and intent to improve the quality of nursing care. *Archives of Psychiatric Nursing*, 26(5), 364–373.

Rush, K., Kee, C., & Rice, M. (2005). Nurses as imperfect role models for health promotion. *Western Journal of Nursing Research*, 27(2), 166–183.

Schön, D. A. (1983). *The reflective practitioner: How professionals think in action.* New York, NY: Basic Books.

Shapiro, S. L., Astin, J. A., Bishop, S. R., & Cordova, M. (2005). Mindfulness-based stress reduction for health care professionals: Results from a randomized trial. *International Journal of Stress Management*, 12(2), 164–176.

Shermis, S. (1992). *Critical thinking: Helping students learn reflectively*. Bloomington, IN: EDINFO Press.

Siegel, D. J. (2007a). *The mindful brain: Reflection and attunement in the cultivation of well-being*. New York, NY: Norton, W.W. & Company, Inc.

Siegel, D. J. (2007b). Mindfulness training and neural integration: Differentiation of distinct streams of awareness and cultivation of well-being. *Social Cognitive and Affective Neuroscience, 2*(4), 259–263.

Smythe, E. A., Ironside, P. M., Sims, S. L., Swenson, M. M., & Spence, D. G. (2008). Doing Heideggerian hermeneutic research: A discussion paper. *International Journal of Nursing Studies, 45*(9), 1389–1397.

Tang, Y-Y., Hölzel, B. K., & Posner, M. I. (2015). The neuroscience of mindfulness. *Nature Reviews: Neuroscience, 16*(4), 213–225.

Tully, A. (2004). Stress, sources of stress and ways of coping among psychiatric nursing students. *Journal of Psychiatric & Mental Health Nursing, 11*(1), 43–47.

Urban Zen Foundation. (2011). Kent State University nursing program. Retrieved from http://www.urbanzen.org/news/kent-state-university-nursing-program/

Watson, J. (2008). *Nursing: The philosophy and science of caring*. Boulder, CO: University of Colorado Press.

Yearwood, E., & Riley, J. B. (2010). Curriculum infusion to promote nursing student well-being. *Journal of Advanced Nursing, 66*(6), 1356–1364.

Part III
Supporting Reflective Learning: In Didactic and Clinical Practice Contexts

Chapter 7

Learning Through Reflection and Reflection on Learning: Pedagogies in Action

–Sara Horton-Deutsch, PhD, RN, FAAN, ANEF
–Chantal Cara, PhD, RN
–With Learning Activities by Meg Moorman, PhD, RN, WHNP-BC;
Jamie Evancio, MEd, BN, RN; Jasmine Graw, MSN, RN, CPNP;
and Laura Sisk, DNP, RN

The moment-to-moment, purposeful, nonjudgmental awareness of mindful practice supports the development of reflexivity and encourages a genuine appreciation and mutual respect demonstrated through listening, attending, and being present with the patient. Reflective pedagogies are concerned with learning through everyday experiences with patients and aim to realize a desirable practice (Johns, 2006). Reflective approaches are deliberative and intuitive and can take place before, during, or after patient encounters. Mindful practice and reflective practices are consistent with a caring philosophy (Boykin, 1998; Cara et al., 2016; Cara & O'Reilly, 2008; Watson, 2002; Watson & Foster, 2003) and contribute to students' apprenticeship of their future practice of caring by inviting them to reflect on how to offer the best quality of nursing care.

According to Enzman Hines (2011), "Reflective practice assists the nurse in capturing the essence of caring in practice and relationship" (p. 206). Indeed, Watson (2012) states that a "higher sense of consciousness and valuing of inner self can cultivate a fuller access to the intuitive […] experiences, modes of thoughts, feelings, and actions" (p. 58). If caring is a moral ideal, as Watson (2005, 2012) upholds, then reflective practice seems a valuable approach to aim for this essence. Mindful practices encourage patient-centered care and human-to-human connections and support the collaboration and open dialogue that fosters a culture of professionalism, quality, and safety. Mindful practices also promote the development of self-awareness, interpersonal relationships, and leadership skills (Horton-Deutsch & Sherwood, 2008).

The attributes of reflective pedagogies correspond to the complexity of nurses' work and the continually changing dynamics of healthcare (Horton-Deutsch & Ironside, 2010). Reflective practices support educational strategies that are innovative, flexible, and aligned with clinical practice in response to the profound changes in science, technology, and healthcare (Benner, Sutphen, Leonard, & Day, 2010; Enzman Hines, 2011; Hills & Watson, 2011; Watson & Foster, 2003), and further support the call from the Institute of Medicine (2008) for patient-centered care, teamwork, and collaboration. For example, Hills and Watson argue that reflection "assists students to become reflective practitioners and to develop insight into their learning and practice" (p. 154). More specifically, Enzman Hines (2011) describes integration of various reflective strategies into the nursing classes within a university curriculum to promote student-teacher interactions, getting to know self as future advanced practice nurses, and reflecting on caring encounters with patients and families.

Over the past 30 years, a growing body of knowledge has supported the concept of reflection and its use as a pedagogical approach. Philosophers introduced the idea of reflective education to develop practice knowledge, autonomy, critical thinking, and open-mindedness. Other scholars contributed to the growing body of literature to facilitate student learning through reflection.

Learning through reflection and reflective practice is more effective when it's linked to specific goals or outcomes and when it follows a framework, particularly in the beginning, to guide learner thinking (Esterhuizen & Freshwater, 2008). Therefore, this chapter provides a brief historical overview of prominent definitions of reflection, reviews a number of reflective frameworks, incorporates relevant issues to nursing practice, and demonstrates how they can be integrated into contemporary education as well as Caring Science.

Learning Through Reflection: Theoretical Philosophy Perspectives

As a leader in the progressive movement in education and a distinguished philosopher, Dewey's work is useful in defining and describing the relationships among experience, learning, and reflection. As educators facilitate learning within their respective disciplines, reflection on didactic and clinical experiences is essential. Dewey defined what experiences are educative, how learning proceeds, and what role reflection plays.

Dewey (1933) states that experience is an interaction between the individual and the environment. Experience includes reading, taking notes, discussion, and participating in activities. An experience also contains *continuity,* a continuous flow of knowledge from previous experiences. Dewey mentions:

> What [a person] has learned in the way of knowledge and skill in one situation becomes an instrument of understanding and dealing effectively with the situations that follow. The process goes on as long as life and learning continue. (1938, p. 44)

Dewey describes learning as a continuous and cumulative process. Earlier learning becomes the basis for further understanding and insight. In his 1933 work, *How We Think,* he defines reflection as:

> ... an active, persistent and careful consideration of any belief or supposed form of knowledge in the light of the grounds that support it and the further conclusions to which it tends. (Dewey, 1933, p. 9)

Reflection is an activity that calls the learner to examine prior beliefs and assumptions and their implications. Reflection is also intentional. It demands a solution for a perplexity. The function of reflection is to transform a situation in which doubt, conflict, or disturbance is experienced into one that is clear, coherent, and harmonious (Dewey, 1933). Dewey suggests that reflection leads to increased control by directing the learner to deeper insight and freeing the learner from merely impulsive and routine activity. Reflective thinking takes time and requires engaging in several phases of thought (Dewey, 1933, pp. 106–115):

- **Perplexity:** Responding to suggestions and ideas that appear when confronted with a problem

- **Elaboration:** Referring to past experiences that are similar

- **Hypothesis:** Developing several potential hypotheses

- **Comparing hypotheses:** Finding some coherence within these hypotheses

- **Taking action:** Experiencing "mastery, satisfaction, enjoyment when selecting and then acting on these hypotheses"

Dewey claims these are not steps but aspects of reflective activity. You might need to stop at any given point, to go back, or to collect more experiences. The key is that informed thought follows a reflective thinking process. To Dewey, reflective thinking fosters the development of three attitudes that further reinforce the habit of reflection: open-mindedness, whole-heartedness, and responsibility to facing consequences.

Kolb's (1984) theory of experiential learning expands the process by which adults learn from their experience. Kolb's work sets experience in the context of learning. Kolb's model exemplifies four stages of learning from experience:

1. Concrete experience
2. Reflective observation
3. Abstract conceptualization
4. Active experimentation

The first phase of the Kolb cycle, *concrete experience*, means practical experience that results in knowledge. *Reflective observation*, the next phase, involves focusing on what the experience means and its associations in light of past learning. In the third phase, *abstract conceptualization*, learners relate their reflective observations to what they already know: theories, notions, and assumptions. During the final phase, *active experimentation*, the learner applies new concepts and theories to the real world. The cycle then begins again, because for Kolb (1984), learning perpetuates more learning. Reflection is viewed as the engine that moves the learning cycle along a path to further learning, action, and more reflection.

> *"Reflection is a learning tool that grew out of the limitations of knowledge derived from technical rationality and research-based knowledge alone."*

Schön (1983, 1987) was interested in how and when learners use reflection to build professional knowledge and expertise. Schön's work fits well for educators because he differentiates between static knowledge found in textbooks and the dynamic, adaptive knowledge used in clinical and professional settings. To bridge this gap, learners need guided practice. Given the dynamic and complex nature of healthcare settings in which nurses work, developing reflective capacity is essential. Schön described two processes that contribute to the development of expertise: *reflection-in-action* and *reflection-on-action*. The former refers to professionals reflecting while they are engaged in an experience, and the latter refers to reflecting after the experience is completed.

Though many have defined reflection, no one, universally accepted definition of reflection exists. Yet, the definitions that do exist share a number of similarities, including the exploration of experience and analysis of thoughts and feelings (of self) to inform learning. Also, an element of critical theory suggests that reflection will involve a change in perspective or transformation in thinking that leads to action. In short, you need to review the perspectives on reflection given throughout this chapter and apply them to your own thinking and practice to determine a meaningful definition of reflection.

As we emphasize throughout this book, the ability to reflect on experience is an essential aspect of learning. Reflection is a learning tool that grew out of the limitations of knowledge derived from technical rationality and research-based knowledge alone. Schön (1983) argues that practitioners face difficulties in using this knowledge because it is generated in situations that are context-free. As a rule, practitioners make decisions based on the context of the practice situation and their experience. Reflective practice allows learners to access and build upon their clinical experiences and emerging knowledge. Through this form of intentional practice, learners can become more fully aware of issues such as safety. They learn to think more about creating a safe environment for their patient, other patients, and other staff and the ways in which their practice contributes to this.

According to Watson (2012), reflective practice is crucial to a human caring approach with individuals experiencing health-illness-healing experiences; it honors the person's uniqueness and human dignity. Likewise, Boykin (1998) trusts that reflective practice enhances nurses' caring practice. In explaining the humanist model, Cara and her colleagues (2016) suggest that reflective practice helps nurses to better grasp the relational nature of the caring relationship with patients and families, which helps develop the humanist competency as well as to renew one's own caring practice.

Beyond theories, numerous frameworks have been developed for facilitating reflection. The Gibbs Reflective Cycle (1988) takes the nurse through six stages:

1. Describe what happened.

2. If it happened again, what would you do?

3. What were you thinking/feeling?

4. What else could you have done?

5. What was good/bad about the experience?

6. What sense can you make of the situation?

At each stage, nurses consider a question or cue to help them reflect on the experience. Because the cues are broad, this model can be applied to clinical situations with patients or in professional interactions with others. The Boyd and Fales (1983) model is similar to the Gibbs one in that they both conclude with deliberate consideration of whether or not to act on the reflective process. The Boyd and Fales model considers the following:

- A sense of inner discomfort

- Identification or clarification of concerns

- Openness to new information for external and internal sources

- Establishing continuity of self with past, present, and future

- Deciding whether to act on the outcome of the reflective process

Further, Mezirow's work examines the depth of reflection through a number of processes spanning from *consciousness* (the way we think about something) to *critical consciousness* (in which we pay attention and analyze our thinking processes). Stage and cyclical models can be particularly useful with novice nurses to help them grasp the essence of reflection. Mezirow's levels of reflectivity are outlined in Table 7.1. The Boyd and Fales (1983) and Mezirow (1981) models do not ask questions but present stages or levels of reflection that can be observed by others or through our own reflection-on-practice.

TABLE 7.1 Mezirow's Levels of Reflectivity (1981)

CONSCIOUSNESS LEVEL	CRITICAL CONSCIOUSNESS LEVEL
Affective reflectivity: Becoming aware of how we feel	Conceptual reflectivity: Questioning the adequacy or morality of concepts
Discriminant reflectivity: Perceiving the relationships between things	Psychic reflectivity: Recognizing our own prejudices and the impact on judgment and action
Judgmental reflectivity: Becoming aware of how we make value judgments	Theoretical reflectivity: Understanding self in the context of desirable action

Learning Through Reflection: Theoretical Nursing Perspectives

More recently, Johns (2006) describes reflection as a pedagogical approach in which students learn through inquiry rather than being prepared for inquiry. According to Johns, it:

- Is a way of being, an attitude, and an approach

- Is a systematic way of learning from experience by examining what we think about an experience and how we think others perceive it

- Involves opening an experience to the inquiry of others and studying the experience from a broader point of view

The Johns model for structured reflection offers nurses a way to access reflection in a non-prescriptive way—thus moving away from the idea that reflection is a technical or linear task—and emphasizes using the model creatively to guide and see self within the context of an experience. It offers cues to access the depth and breadth of reflection necessary for learning through experience. According to Johns (2006), the cues are internalized over time and are constantly being refined. The cues correspond to the four fundamental ways of knowing in nursing illuminated in Carper's (1978) work: aesthetic, ethical, empirical, and personal. Viewed through a reflective lens, the cues provide a systematic mode of reflective inquiry.

Johns (2006) also created a Model of Structured Reflection (MSR) map to guide learners to reflect on their clinical reasoning and action. The map can be viewed in Johns (2006) and guides learners to frame learning through reflection. At the core of the map is aesthetic response and includes four key processes:

1. The way the learner appreciated the pattern of the particular situation.

2. The way the learner made clinical judgments in terms of care needed.

3. The way the learner responded within the situation.

4. The judgment about the efficacy of response to meeting care needs.

Outlined in the periphery of the map, the learner must then ask the three following questions:

1. Did I act for the best? (ethical)

2. What did I know or should have informed my practice? (empirical)

3. What factors were influencing me? (personal)

Through questioning, the learner can illuminate the meaning of the interaction, including what went well and what might be done differently in the future. Through the use of Johns' MSR and MSR map (see Table 7.2), learners are guided to form and frame ideas as well as emerging insights by reflecting on the uniqueness and context of the story. Through this process, learners critique and assimilate theories and research to inform their future caring practice.

The list is not exhaustive, and other models may have value for nursing faculty and students. However, these works, along with those of Freshwater (2002, 2008), are the foundation of the scholarship of reflective practice in nursing as outlined in Chapters 1 and 2.

Reflection is an essential skill implicit in professional nursing practice. For example, the work of Benner (1984) and Benner et al. (2010) has provided a foundation for reflecting on nursing practice worldwide, in terms of the developing expertise of nurses in action. Other nursing scholars have linked caring as a foundation of reflective practice (Boykin, 1998; Cara et al., 2016; Cara & O'Reilly, 2008; Enzman Hines, 2011; Hills & Watson, 2011; Horton-Deutsch, 2016; Watson & Foster, 2003). Both reflection and caring reflective practice require the ability to make clinical judgments and intervene in nursing care contexts. Effective nursing practice, education, research, and leadership are grounded in the complexity of human relationships and, therefore, require systematic and careful thinking acquired through caring reflective practices to achieve meaningful and successful outcomes.

TABLE 7.2 Johns' Model of Structured Reflection (2006)

REFLECTIVE CUE	AESTHETICS	ETHICS	EMPIRICS	PERSONAL	REFLEXIVITY
Bring the mind home					
Focus on a description of an experience that seems significant	x				
What particular issues seem significant to pay attention to?	x				
How were others feeling, and what made them feel that way?	x				
How was I feeling, and what made me feel that way?				x	
What was I trying to achieve, and did I respond effectively?	x				
What were the consequences of my actions on the patient, others, and myself?	x				
What influenced the way I was feeling, thinking, or responding?				x	
What knowledge did or might have informed me?			x		
To what extent did I act for the best and in tune with my values?		x			
How does this situation connect with previous experiences?				x	x
How might I respond more effectively given this situation again?					x
What would be the consequences of alternative actions for the patient, others, myself?					x
What factors might constrain me from responding in new ways?				x	
How do I now feel about this experience?				x	
Am I better able to support myself and others as a consequence?					x
What insights have I gained?					x
Am I more able to realize desirable practice?					
What have I learned through reflecting?					

Reflective Learning Assessments: Exemplars of Reflective Pedagogies in Action

Success in higher education requires different, innovative approaches to teaching. Nursing education has the challenge of offering various clinical situations to help students reflect, learn, and understand the wholeness of human health-illness experiences to develop caring reflective practice. The remainder of this chapter describes and provides exemplars of three reflective learning assessments. The reflective learning assessments are as follows:

- Aesthetic knowing through Visual Thinking Strategies

- Reflective practice through Caring Science in service learning

- Student journaling in the clinical setting utilizing the Caritas Processes™

AESTHETIC KNOWING THROUGH VISUAL THINKING STRATEGIES (VTS), By Meg Moorman, PhD, RN, WHNP-BC

As educators seek out innovative learning experiences, the use of arts and humanities in nursing education provides rich learning opportunities for students and can broaden their horizons as well as develop critical thinking. Aesthetics as a way of knowing in nursing has been broadly studied in nursing education. Carper described aesthetic knowing as an appreciation for a situation and the ability to use creative resources to transform experiences and see beyond to connect with human experiences (Chinn & Kramer, 2015).

A good nurse must not only develop technical expertise; he or she must also have the ability to work with other members of the healthcare team and engage with patients to understand their needs. Educators need to help students develop aesthetic knowing and nurture understanding during their educational experiences. Johns (2004) articulates the importance of practitioners developing clinical judgments—that is, the ability to grasp and interpret clinical situations through their aesthetic response. "Reflexivity acknowledges both the influence of previous experience on clinical judgment and response, and the impact of applying new insights about practice through reflection on future experience" (Johns, 2004,

continues

continued

p. 4). Providing educational opportunities for nursing students to collaborate with other healthcare workers can help students enhance communications and lower anxiety related to hierarchy in healthcare.

Visual Thinking Strategies (VTS) was developed by Housen, a cognitive psychologist, and Yenawine (2002), an art educator, for visitors to art museums to study aesthetic meaning. Later it was studied as a teaching technique to develop aesthetic meaning in primary education. Mainly done in an art museum, a group of learners gathers around a work of art and, led by trained VTS facilitators, discusses the work of art in a prescribed way.

Works of art are preselected by the trained VTS facilitator. Visual Understanding in Education (VUE) is a not-for-profit organization that does workshops across the country for educators interested in becoming trained VTS facilitators. The works of art that are chosen are ones that can be interpreted without any prior knowledge of art or technique. Often, the selected art is slightly abstract so as to elicit multiple interpretations, yielding a deep, rich discussion.

UNDERSTANDING VISUAL THINKING STRATEGIES

Visual Thinking Strategies is a school curriculum and teaching method used to:

- *Develop critical thinking skills*
- *Engage learners in observations and meaning-making*
- *Facilitate learner-centered interactions*
- *Encourage students to socially construct knowledge through thoughtful discussions about art*

First, the facilitator asks, "Tell me what is going on in this painting." All learners are encouraged to participate, one at a time. The art provides a starting point for the experience and allows the learners to tell a story and personalize their experiences. The learners come to the work of art. As learners give their individual interpretations of the work of art, the facilitator paraphrases back what has been said and asks for clarification.

Next the facilitator asks, "What do you see that makes you say that?" This clarifies and asks the learners to give evidential reasoning for their opinions. The learners then respond by giving more detail and clarification about their interpretation of the work of art. No one learner's opinion is considered right or better than another's. The facilitator asks the learners to give visual evidence for what they are seeing. This continues until all the students have given their interpretation of the work of art. Often the interpretations are very different based on learners' varying experiences. Sometimes learners will scaffold off other student comments, considering another point of view and interpretation.

The final question asked by the facilitator is, "What more can you find?" This pushes learners to look again in a non-threatening way and consider what the work of art means to them. Some learners have shared interpretations of what the work of art means, and others have individual interpretations. A discussion about what occurred completes the discussion. At the end of this experience, learners often ask, "Who was right?" The facilitator reveals that no one right answer exists and encourages students to consider all possibilities.

REFLECTING ON . . . QUESTIONS FOR VISUAL THINKING STRATEGIES

- *What's going on in this picture?*
- *What do I see that makes me say that?*
- *What more can I find?*

EXAMPLE OF A VTS CONVERSATION

Facilitator: So what's going on in the painting?

Participant 1: It is a little boy who looks sad.

Facilitator: So you think this figure here is a boy and you think he is sad?

Participant 1: Yes. Or he is tired . . . I'm not sure which.

Facilitator: What are you seeing that makes you think he is sad?

continues

continued

Participant 1:	*Well, he is looking down with his head dropped like he is sad.*
Facilitator:	*So the position of his head lowered is what makes you think he looks sad.*
Participant 1:	*Yes, that's it.*
Facilitator:	*What more can you find?*
Participant 2:	*I also think he looks sad.*
Facilitator:	*What makes you say that?*
Participant 2:	*Well, he is painted in a blue color.*
Facilitator:	*So the blue color gives you the impression of sadness.*
Participant 2:	*Yes, that color represents sadness for me. If he was painted in red or orange, I would associate that with happiness.*
Facilitator:	*So blue represents sadness for you both and red or orange represent happiness or joy?*
Participants 1 and 2:	*Yeah.*
Participant 3:	*I think it might be a girl with short hair, and I think she is reading, not sad.*
Facilitator:	*What makes you say that?*
Participant 3:	*Well, I think it is a girl because she has longer hair and it looks like that is a bow around her neck. She is looking down because that is a book in her hands and she is reading it.*
Facilitator (pointing to the object in the painting the subject is holding):	*So you think this is a girl because of the length of the hair and this object looks like a book to you . . . did I understand that right?*

Participant 3:   Yes, that's right.

Participant 1:   I didn't even notice that book.

Facilitator: What more can you find?

Participant 1:   I still think it is a sad boy hanging his head, maybe sitting in the corner.

Facilitator: Can you tell me more?

Participant 1:   Well, I used to have to sit in the corner when I was young after I got in trouble. I also happened to have a really bad day in clinical today and didn't know the side effects of one of my meds, so my instructor wasn't very happy with me. I guess I am feeling like I got in trouble today.

Facilitator: So you had a bad day at the hospital today, and you projected your feelings about that onto this figure in the painting? Did I understand you correctly?

Participant 1:   Yeah, I guess I did. I didn't really think it was bothering me that much, but I guess it is.

We have been using VTS in an obstetrics BSN nursing program for 3 years, and now medical students have asked to join our discussions. We meet at the local art museum with a trained facilitator for the one-time experience. Responses have been extremely positive. Learners are given an opportunity to sign up for the experience in an obstetrics course and meet at a predetermined time with participants from the medical school and one of their educators. We limit the number of students to 10–12. A facilitator trained in VTS meets the group and takes them to a pre-chosen work of art.

The art museum is a neutral territory for nursing and medical students to meet, with no hierarchy, no uniforms or lab coats, and no expectations or roles. The facilitator does not know who is a nursing or medical student and is completely present and neutral in her response to them. Nursing students have reported feeling safe to respond without judgment or critique, and medical students have

continued

stated they have a deeper appreciation for the roles of nurses in patient care. Students often report active listening and improved communication skills after the VTS experience. Learners are able to link the importance of providing visual evidence and reasoning with their interpretations and find that the experience relates well with their clinical experiences in patient care. "I feel like I can give a more thorough report to other members of the healthcare team and find myself looking closer and looking again for more detail to support my observations of patients," reported one student after his VTS trip.

> *"Listening sounds easy but is often distorted as we contemplate what we will say next or how we relate to what someone is telling us."*

Other learners have noticed that they feel more present in discussions, both with patients and other healthcare members:

I notice that I listen more intensely now and try to really understand what someone is saying instead of thinking about what I am going to say next. I find my discussions are much deeper and more meaningful if I try to be present and really pay attention to what someone is telling me. I watched the facilitator do this in our VTS experience, and she really seemed to care about what we were saying. She kept clarifying and genuinely seemed to be interested. I know that took so much concentration on her part, but it made me feel really understood and respected. If I can do that with my patients and co-workers, it will make me a better nurse and communicator.

VTS honors past experiences and memories that viewers bring to a work of art. As learners reflect and share their personal thoughts about a work of art, deeper insights are brought about, and students manage to communicate more clearly. Listening sounds easy but is often distorted as we contemplate what we will say next or how we relate to what someone is telling us. " . . .Talk reflects patterns of power relationships and rivalry, where people jostle for control typified by people lining up to get their point across and win the argument. Very little genuine listening takes place. People partially listen to what they want to hear, seeking feedback to reinforce their position rather than be open to new possibility through dialogue" (Johns, 2004, p. 205).

As the VTS facilitator listens, he or she is modeling the art of being completely present with the student and must pay close attention so that he or she can repeat back and paraphrase what was said. Students then have the opportunity to agree or clarify what they said. After the experience, the facilitator asks the students to discuss what they noticed he or she was doing. Students comment on the facilitator's ability to clarify and discuss what it was like to have someone really listen to them and not judge them. They value the notion of having someone honor what they say and really pay attention to their words, an experience that they say does not often happen in nursing school. Student discussions often then turn to how this experience would benefit their clinical practice:

> Sometimes, like after a cancer diagnosis, a patient might just need the nurse to be there with them, to be completely present. It isn't about saying the right thing to fix the situation, but just knowing that their nurse is present and attentive is enough. This VTS experience helps me to realize the importance of that. That is a gift I can give my patients, the gift of being present. This changed the way I listen to people, not just patients.

Other learners find that their ability to notice detail is enhanced after a VTS experience:

> I find I am much more articulate after experiencing VTS. I not only notice more detail, but feel like I am more descriptive in recounting experiences or impressions to others. When I have to give a report to another nurse, I really back up what I am saying by giving examples and using visual evidence to back me up. I can see that this would be helpful when calling a report to a physician or other member of the healthcare team.

continues

continued

VTS offers a form of reflection in a group setting that allows participants to hold several possibilities at once. No one except the artist knows exactly what a work of art is trying to convey. It is up to the viewer to attach meaning to a work of art. Viewers often bring past experiences to the work of art, and these influence their interpretations. As interpretations are shared, all learners listen. No one interpretation is deemed correct. All interpretations are considered at the same time and held as possible.

REFLECTING ON . . . VISUAL THINKING STRATEGIES CONCEPTS

- *All students have the opportunity to participate.*

- *Students receive positive affirmations for their contributions.*

- *Students learn to value viewpoints of all comments as a means for viewing the art with multiple meanings.*

- *Teachers encourage active participation.*

- *Facilitators continually point at the painting, maintaining the group's focus on the work of art in front of them.*

VTS can be used in a myriad of ways to help teachers meet learning objectives. This teaching method encourages self-confidence and participation and offers students a chance to speak without being judged. Learners often bring their past experiences to the learning environment, and this is true in VTS as well. Learners often discover this as they reflect on the questions asked by the facilitator. As learners dig deeper for more meaning, they discuss and scaffold on each other's comments. As the facilitator paraphrases what each learner said, other learners reflect and discover deeper meaning in their own comments. Learners frequently state, "I didn't realize that I felt that way, but I guess I do." Learners feel safe—no one holds the right answer, and all interpretations are given equal attention and affirmation. Learners appreciate that the facilitator listens attentively and seeks understanding for what is said. Applied to the classroom, as learners respond to questions, the teacher listens attentively and paraphrases back what is said. Learners feel heard, and teachers gain valuable insight into how students are processing information, fostering mutual respect, and sharing a sacred learning space.

The arts and humanities have been used in medical education to improve visual acumen and diagnostic skills, as well as to improve communications. The arts provide unique opportunities for students to develop aesthetic knowing. This experience with art also helps learners and health professionals work in teams and develop communication skills (Moorman, Hensel, Decker, & Busby, 2016). Working in teams with other learners at the art museum provides an opportunity to learn in a safe, neutral territory and can help build self-confidence. Medical students have noted that they have a new appreciation for the work that nurses do after deep discussions about patient care and the importance of listening. They also report being able to note more detail and relate this to better diagnostic skills. Learners also report an appreciation for working together in a neutral environment and working collaboratively without the stress of being "right" or judged.

> *It was so refreshing to work together in an art museum and feel like we were really collaborating and not trying to impress anyone. I loved the chance to work together here. I think it will make future encounters less threatening, and it really highlighted the importance of giving visual evidence, which will permeate all of our work.*

REFLECTIVE PRACTICE THROUGH CARING SCIENCE IN SERVICE LEARNING, By Laura Sisk, DNP, RN, and Jasmine Graw, MSN, RN, CPNP

The practice of caring is central to all of nursing. Regardless of nursing specialty or patient population, caring is foundational to nursing. Caring supports patients and families in crisis and serves as the inspiration that bonds communities and society together. Nursing and caring are synonymous with one another and maintain the core ingredients of hope and commitment. As stated above, Jean Watson's Theory of Human Caring is based on the Science of Caring (Watson, 2008a). Watson's theory (and the Caritas Processes that help explain the theory) is illustrated in a unique student-led pregnancy and parenting program developed for childbearing teens. The word caritas comes from a Latin word meaning to cherish, appreciate, and to give special loving attention (Watson, 2008b).

continues

continued

The core principles are illustrated here to explain how it was integrated into a childbearing family course, specifically with a student-led program involving pregnant and parenting teen mothers.

- *Practice of loving-kindness and equanimity: Creating an environment where the teens felt comfortable speaking without judgment was essential. Exploring principles of social justice with nursing students and demonstrating genuine loving-kindness with this vulnerable population paved the way for future prenatal education and positive student interaction. An environment of trust and care was formed.*

- *Authentic presence: Enabling deep belief of other (patient, colleague, family, etc.): Being present in the moment included acceptance and active listening to address the many needs of the teen mother. This included introducing educational activities that encouraged the teen mothers to gain self-confidence while promoting a positive self-esteem. In addition, the nursing students participated in debriefing to encourage this authentic presence.*

- *Cultivation of one's spiritual practice toward wholeness of mind/body/ spirit: To embrace one's inner-self, strategies of self-care were used. Activities such as painting, aromatherapy, coping mechanisms, manicures, and yoga were introduced to the teens to enhance the totality of the mind, body, and spirit.*

- *"Being" the caring-healing environment: Nursing students were sources of information for the teen moms. The childbearing teens could see that the nursing students cared about them and felt their "being" presence. The student-to-student bond that was created promoted a caring-healing environment, prompting conversations that allowed the teen moms to speak freely.*

- *Allowing miracles (openness to the unexpected and inexplicable life events): Celebrating and recognizing the miracle of birth and the unexpected life changes experienced by the teen mothers was important. Additionally, providing flexible classes based on the needs of the teen mothers and being open to their unique life events was essential to the success of the project.*

Service learning combined with Watson's Theory of Human Caring as the underpinning for the student-led teen pregnancy and parenting program. Billings and Halstead (2012) described the ultimate goal of service learning as providing opportunities for civic engagement, development of cultural competence, and serving to develop a more caring society while fostering social justice. Service offers opportunities for learning that cannot be obtained in any other way. It provides for a truly meaningful act in the student's life. Service learning is not volunteering, nor is it a substitute for a nursing clinical experience, because the focus is on meeting the needs of the community, not of the nursing curriculum (Billings & Halstead, 2012).

Service learning is a teaching strategy that enhances learning experiences through reflective learning and reciprocal relationships. Reflection is a critical part of service learning; reflective practices promote learning and link service to the course objectives. The method used in a childbearing family course was the 6-word/55-word reflection, a reflective writing activity often used for healthcare professionals and students. It is based on two literary formats, the 6-word and the 55-word story. The writing activity is not just a story—the purpose is to reflect. The guiding principle is to choose your words carefully, as each reflection may only have 6 words or the expanded reflection of 55 words. The focus is on clarity and message.

Examples of Reflection

Helpful Steps for Implementing the 6-Word Reflection

1. *Learners make a list of three or four memorable experiences they had when they participated in a service-learning project.*

2. *Learners write their memories or experiences into a 6-word reflection (story).*

3. *Learners are reminded to choose their words wisely. There is power in words, and only six may be used.*

4. *Encourage learners to focus on being clear and complete to accurately encompass the impression of the event with a short phrase.*

Examples of 6-Word Reflections

Once they have selected the most memorable 6-word reflection, take that story and extend it into a 55-word story.

Rules for the 55-Word Reflection

Number one rule: The reflection must be exactly 55 words, tell a story, and be reflective of the service-learning experience.

> ***Tip for getting started:*** *Focus on clarity and the power of the words selected. Consider the things that make this story significant or special.*

continues

continued

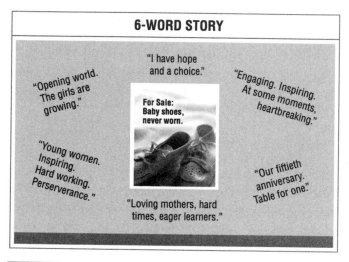

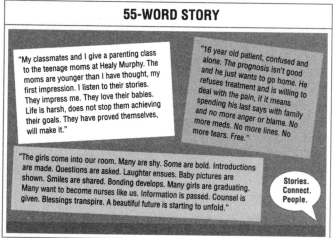

This form of reflection worked well for the childbearing family course and allowed nursing students to reflect and carefully consider their experience. Student nurses were able to see the importance of building a relationship and nurturing a caring environment for the pregnant and parenting teens. The integration of caring, reflection, and service learning created a significant impact on society by promoting positive health outcomes and assisting populations of need.

UTILIZING THE CARITAS PROCESSES™ TO GUIDE STUDENT JOURNALING IN THE CLINICAL SETTING, BY JAMIE EVANCIO, MED, BN, RN

Student Journaling While on Practicum

The purpose of this teaching modality is to help learners to grow in their ability to respond to the human condition, and to become reflective practitioners who are skilled in self-care and the therapeutic use of self. Learners come to practicum with limited life experience and need to quickly find the skills to cope with elderly persons experiencing multiple losses, including the loss of their ability to live on their own and the loss of the home they may have lived in for most of their adult life. When they come to the hospital and get the news they can't return to their previous living situation, their future immediately becomes uncertain. Where will they go? What will happen to their home and possessions? Whom can they trust to help them through this transition? Will they ever feel "at home" again in their new setting? This is a time of painful loss and life review accompanied by spiritual loneliness and social isolation for many older patients.

Learners traditionally arrive at clinical with a list of psychomotor skills they have learned/are learning and expect to practice in their assigned setting. They are often very focused on those skills, and this regularly spills over into their "reflective" journaling. When this happens, the value of reflection is lost along with the professional growth opportunity that should accompany the reflecting. Of even greater concern is that an important opportunity for professional growth and socialization is lost because learners may not have the guidance they need to provide the persons in their care with a truly therapeutic response. The potential for this to develop into a situation where learners see the clinical experience in a negative light cannot be overlooked.

Clinical educators who facilitate practicum must provide guidance to a diverse group of learners, some of whom have never been in a hospital or spoken to people who are experiencing loss. Learners invariably say they are nervous and uncertain as they anticipate their upcoming practicum days. Many report sleep challenges at this time and may have had to make special arrangements for others to take over their family responsibilities. In consideration of these realities, the instructor must support the students as they navigate the expectations of their new learning environment. It is the instructor's job to facilitate the learning that takes place in this precious time. The Caritas Processes provide an excellent foundation to help learners deepen their practice and strengthen their therapeutic impact.

continues

continued

Learners are guided to journal reflectively using the Caritas Processes:

On the first day of the practicum, which typically includes orientation, the clinical educator can review Caring Science basics and the Caritas Processes with the learner, focusing on learners' self-care plans for the practicum (and beyond). Clinical educators are important role models for self-care practices and can share their own ideas at this time. Learners are given questions to prompt their journal entries over the practicum experience. For added effectiveness, the instructor reads the questions to the learners and the learners write the questions into their journal, where they can remain as a permanent prompt.

The first journal entry that learners write focuses on the question, "What is my plan for self-care while on clinical practicum?" Learners are encouraged to think of how they would care for their own mind, body, and spirit during the practicum. Topics such as sleep needs, eating a healthy breakfast, and making time for renewal of energy are included in this discussion.

As the Caritas Processes are the essence of nursing, this way of guiding student journaling contributes to the nurturing of a deeper, more intentional experience for nursing learners. Any of the Caritas Processes can easily be turned into questions. The questions listed here are not exhaustive. Depending upon the client population being served (the patients/residents/clients to whom learners are assigned), learners are encouraged to consider prompts such as these to guide their journaling:

- *How did I care for my resident's mind/body/spirit today?*

- *How does my own wellness influence those whom I work with and those who are in my care?*

- *What does a healing environment look like?*

- *How can I contribute to my patient's healing by modifying his/her environmental experience?*

- *How is it that the nurse can be the patient's environment?*

- *What contributes to the development of a trusting, caring relationship?*

- *What can I do to alleviate my resident's suffering?*

- *What mysteries or miracles have I witnessed today?*

- *What does it mean to listen authentically?*

- *What is it like for me (and why is it important) to be able to listen to negative feelings from my resident? (Alternative wording could be: What therapeutic value is gained from listening to residents' negative feelings?)*

Note: Although learners may initially find it difficult to listen without attempting to redirect the conversation to positive topics, with the clinical educator's guidance they recognize the therapeutic value of the residents' expression of negative feelings. At some point the story ends, and learners can see that disclosure itself can lead to an unburdening.

Through my practice of using the Caritas Processes as prompts for journaling, it became clear that learners struggle to listen to negative feelings from patients, especially when the negative feelings are not within the power of the student to ameliorate in any way. As a result of their own discomfort, they reported that they would try to redirect the conversation by changing the topic in their belief that this is in fact a therapeutic intervention. Clinical educators can positively guide learners through this experience by helping them to see they are being therapeutic by listening authentically and not intervening in the client's story. With experience, learners do see that the act of attentively listening to the client as he tells his story provides relief for the client. Once learners understood the importance of allowing that expression, it was evident that they were much more satisfied with their role in the encounter, and this new awareness contributed to their confidence to communicate on a professional level.

Final Reflections

Educators often engage learners with teaching approaches on critical and analytical thinking where the primary focus is on others. More recently, this approach has expanded to include self-thinking and the importance of learner development through reflective practices. Beyond this, reflection is also an important part of professional lifelong learning, particularly when working through challenging and difficult situations. Reflective practice leads to the ability to step back and look at issues from a broader perspective, to see a situation from each person's unique perspective and meaning, an indispensable aspect within a caring philosophy (Cara et al., 2016; Mayeroff, 1990; Watson, 2012).

Ultimately, integrating reflective practices into nursing education and professional development has a significant impact on the quality of work processes and their outcomes. Reflective practices influence learners in their search to become caring professionals. Reflection as a learning strategy helps increase awareness of perceptions. When viewed as learning from experience, reflection is an important aspect of knowledge development and skill acquisition, which is essential to professional development. Reflection involves thinking about experience, which leads learners to a fuller understanding about what they know and increases their capacity for human-to-human connection, compassion, caring, and mindful leadership (Horton-Deutsch & Sherwood, 2008; Horton-Deutsch, 2016; Johns, 2016; Watson, 2008a).

References

Benner, P. (1984). *From novice to expert: Excellence and power in clinical nursing practice.* Menlo Park, CA: Addison-Wesley.

Benner, P., Sutphen, M., Leonard, V., & Day, L. (2010). *Educating nurses: A call for radical transformation.* San Francisco, CA: Jossey-Bass.

Billings, D. M., & Halstead, J. A. (2012). *Teaching in nursing: A guide for faculty* (4th ed.). St. Louis, MO: Elsevier.

Boyd, E. M., & Fales, A. W. (1983). Reflective learning key to learning from experience. *Journal of Humanistic Psychology, 23*(2), 99–117.

Boykin, A. (1998). Nursing as caring through the reflective lens. In C. Johns & D. Freshwater (Eds.), *Transforming nursing through reflective practice* (pp. 45–50). Malden, MA : Blackwell Science, Inc.

Cara, C., Gauvin-Lepage, J., Lefebvre, H., Létourneau, D., Alderson, M., Larue, C., . . . Mathieu, C. (2016). Modèle humaniste des soins infirmiers—UdeM: Perspective novatrice et pragmatique [The humanistic model of nursing care—UdeM: An innovative and pragmatic perspective]. *Recherche en Soins Infirmiers [Research in Nursing Care], 125*(2), 20–31.

Cara, C., & O'Reilly, L. (2008). S'approprier la Théorie du Human Caring de Jean Watson par la pratique réflexive lors d'une situation clinique [Embracing Jean

Watson's Theory of Human Caring through a reflective practice within a clinical situation]. *Recherche en Soins Infirmiers* [*Research in Nursing Care*], *95*, 37–45.

Carper, B. (1978). Fundamental patterns of knowing in nursing. *Advances in Nursing Science, 1*(1), 13–23.

Chinn, P. L., & Kramer, M. (2015). *Integrated theory and knowledge development in nursing* (9th ed.). St. Louis, MO: Mosby Elsevier.

Dewey, J. (1933). *How we think: A restatement of the relation of reflective thinking to the educative process.* Boston, MA: D. C. Heath and Co.

Dewey, J. (1938). *Experience and education.* New York, NY: Collier Books, Macmillan.

Enzman Hines, M. (2011). Caring in advance practice education: A new view of the future. In M. Hills & J. Watson (Eds.), *Creating a Caring Science curriculum: An emancipatory pedagogy for nursing* (pp. 203–216). New York, NY: Springer.

Esterhuizen, P., & Freshwater, D. (2008). Using critical reflection to improve practice. In D. Freshwater, B. J. Taylor, & G. Sherwood (Eds.), *International textbook of reflective practice in nursing* (Chapter 5). Oxford, UK: Blackwell Publishing.

Freshwater, D. (Ed.). (2002). *Therapeutic nursing: Improving patient care through reflection.* London, UK: Sage Publications.

Freshwater, D. (2008). Reflective practice: The state of the art. In D. Freshwater, B. J. Taylor, & G. Sherwood (Eds.), *International textbook of reflective practice in nursing* (pp. 1–18). Oxford, UK: Blackwell Publishing.

Gibbs, G. (1988). *Learning by doing: A guide to teaching and learning methods.* Oxford, UK: Further Education Unit, Oxford Polytechnic, now Oxford Brookes University. Retrieved from https://thoughtsmostlyaboutlearning.files.wordpress.com/2015/12/learning-by-doing-graham-gibbs.pdf

Hills, M., & Watson, J. (2011). *Creating a Caring Science curriculum: An emancipatory pedagogy for nursing.* New York, NY: Springer.

Horton-Deutsch, S. (2016). Open and visionary: Remaining open to the possibilities of nursing praxis. In W. Rosa (Ed.), *Nurse leaders: Evolutionary visions of leadership* (pp. 311–322). New York, NY: Springer.

Horton-Deutsch, S., & Ironside, P. (2010). Teaching patient-centered care using narrative and reflective pedagogies. Quality and Safety Education for Nurses. Retrieved from http://qsen.org/courses/learning-modules/module-six/

Horton-Deutsch, S., & Sherwood, G. (2008). Reflection: An educational strategy to develop emotionally competent nurse leaders. *Journal of Nursing Management, 16*(8), 946–954.

Housen, A., & Yenawine, P. (2002). Aesthetic thought, critical thinking and transfer. *Arts and Learning Research Journal, 18*(1), 99–131.

Institute of Medicine (IOM). (2008). IOM report: Evidence-based medicine and the changing nature of healthcare: Workshop summary. Washington, DC: National Academies Press.

Johns, C. (2004). *Becoming a reflective practitioner* (2nd ed.). Carlton, Victoria, Australia: Blackwell Publishing, Ltd.

Johns, C. (2006). *Engaging reflection in practice: A narrative approach.* Oxford, UK: Blackwell.

Johns, C. (2016). *Mindful leadership. A guide for health care professionals.* London, UK: Palgrave Macmillan.

Kolb, D. A. (1984). *Experiential learning: Experience as a source of learning and development.* Englewood Cliffs, NJ: Prentice Hall.

Mayeroff, M. (1990). *On caring.* New York, NY: HarperPerennial (Original work published 1971).

Mezirow, J. (1981). Critical theory of adult learning and education. *Adult Education, 3*(1), 3–24.

Moorman, M., Hensel, D., Decker, K., & Busby, K. (2016). Learning outcomes with visual thinking strategies in nursing education. *Nursing Education Today.* Advance online publication. doi:10.1016/j.nedt.2016.08.020

Schön, D. A. (1983). *The reflective practitioner: How practitioner professionals think in action.* New York, NY: Basic Books.

Schön, D. A. (1987). *Educating the reflective practitioner.* San Francisco, CA: Jossey-Bass.

Watson, J. (2002). Intentionality and caring-healing consciousness: A practice of transpersonal nursing. *Holistic Nursing Practice, 16*(4), 12–19.

Watson, J. (2005). *Caring Science as sacred science.* Philadelphia, PA: F. A. Davis Company.

Watson, J. (2008a*). Nursing: The philosophy and science of caring* (Rev. ed.). Boulder, CO: University Press of Colorado.

Watson, J. (2008b). Core concepts of Jean Watson's Theory of Human Caring/Caring Science. Retrieved from https://watsoncaringscience.org/

Watson, J. (2012). *Human Caring Science: A theory of nursing.* Sudbury, MA: Jones & Bartlett Learning.

Watson, J., & Foster, R. (2003). The Attending Nurse Caring Model: Integrating theory, evidence and advanced caring-healing therapeutics for transforming professional practice. *Journal of Clinical Nursing, 12*(3), 360–365.

Yan, C., & Berggren, R. (2016). Project 6-55: Workshop trainer [Presentation]. University of Texas Health Science Center, San Antonio, TX.

Chapter 8

Narrative Pedagogy: Co-Creating Engaging Learning Experiences With Students

–*Pamela Ironside, PhD, RN, FAAN, ANEF*

–*Marie Hayden-Miles, PhD, RN, CNE*

Despite calls for transformation in nursing education (Benner, Sutphen, Leonard, & Day, 2010; Institute of Medicine [IOM], 2011), nursing faculty continue to teach as they were taught, relying heavily (if not exclusively) on conventional pedagogy. This pedagogy emphasizes cognitive gain and skill acquisition as the basis for all learning encounters occurring in classrooms, labs, and clinical settings (Ironside, 2001). As the knowledge and skills required for practice continue to grow exponentially, however, the limits of this approach are becoming increasingly pronounced. New, research-based pedagogies, such as *Narrative Pedagogy*, are now available for faculty to use to address these limitations.

In this chapter, we explore ways faculty can use Narrative Pedagogy to co-create different kinds of courses with students—courses in which reflecting on experiences, thinking from multiple perspectives, questioning assumptions, and exploring new possibilities for nursing education and practice are co-equal to learning and applying content.

Narrative Pedagogy

Narrative Pedagogy, a research-based, phenomenological pedagogy, was discovered during a longitudinal study of the experiences of nursing students, teachers, and clinicians (Diekelmann, 1995, 2001; Diekelmann & Diekelmann, 2009). Narrative Pedagogy is a way of thinking about nursing education and practice *with* students and teachers, and at times with clinicians and patients (Ironside et al., 2003), and of communally and collaboratively exploring new possibilities for improving schools of nursing and the care being learned and provided (Ironside, 2015). Co-creating experiences in which teachers and students think together and seek new ways to understand their experiences extends and enhances conventional pedagogy. When using Narrative Pedagogy, teachers focus on developing students' interpretive skills (skills related to reflecting on experiences, thinking in new ways and from multiple perspectives) and the ways students engage in questioning inherited practices and processes in nursing (Ironside, 2006, 2015).

For example, when teachers ask students questions in settings where conventional pedagogy is used, these often are questions that have one right or "best" answer, and rarely is the complexity of the practice encounter preserved in the question (Ironside, 2014; Ironside, Brown, & Wonder, 2015; Ironside, Diekelmann, & Hirschmann, 2005a, 2005b). To respond to such questions, students search their memory for the required piece of information (e.g., the side effects of a medication being administered or the injection sites for appropriate administration) (Ironside, 2005).

In Narrative Pedagogy, teachers focus on engaging students in understanding a situation, the assumptions they are making about it, and what might be wrong with the typical or habitual way of responding (e.g., How do patients experience this medication regimen? How might this patient's experience facilitate or inhibit his or her willingness to take this medication as prescribed? How is this patient's response similar to or different from others with whom you have worked?).

Students and teachers consider the context in which the question came up and the options for care that are and are not relevant, safe, appropriate, or desirable in a specific situation or across several situations (Scheckel & Ironside, 2006).

Because the use of Narrative Pedagogy is contextual through and through, the complexity of the practice (and patient situations) students encounter is central to the dialogue. Indeed, without understanding the context of the experience, the experience cannot be understood at all (Gadamer, 1989).

When teachers and students share and interpret their experiences in nursing education using Narrative Pedagogy, what is working and what is not working well in their school of nursing or a given clinical setting becomes apparent, and new possibilities can be collectively explored. Thought of in this way, using Narrative Pedagogy enables teachers and students to co-create learning encounters in which to collectively explore, critique, and question their nursing knowledge and their understanding of the situations they encounter. They also challenge assumptions, critique prevailing perspectives and the limits of current knowledge, and explore the meaning and significance of their interpretations for the emerging practice (Ironside, 2015; Ironside et al., 2015). Such thinking is not separated from content knowledge as it is in conventional pedagogy, with content on a particular condition being presented by the teacher prior to the interpretive encounter. Rather, when students and teachers co-create learning encounters using Narrative Pedagogy, they bring their current knowledge and questions to the conversation and, through dialogue with others, the gaps, oversights, and misunderstandings are explored co-equally with the new knowledge, insights, and "ah-ha" moments (Ironside, 2006, 2014).

Enacting Narrative Pedagogy begins when teachers, students, and clinicians share their experiences, which might be derived from practice, life experience, or experiences in the school of nursing. This is the first sense in which learning encounters are co-created by students and teachers. The importance of sharing stories of their experiences isn't about merely sharing (or hearing) the story, but on communally striving to bear witness to the experience, to understand the experience as experience, to question the prevailing interpretation of it (how it is understood as being an experience of this or that), and to elicit thinking from multiple perspectives.

During each class, clinical, or lab session, teachers and students focus their conversation on exploring students' (or patients') experiences, and the conversation follows the questions that arise as they collectively explore the meaningfulness of the experience. Though the teacher might ask students to bring and share particular types of experiences or encounters, the conversations that ensue are always situated in experience, with all the ambiguity, uncertainty, limits, and disruptions inherent in day-to-day nursing practice intact (Ironside et al., 2015). This is in stark contrast to teacher-centered pedagogies in which the issues to be discussed are preplanned by the teacher, and students take up only the questions or concerns the teacher raises.

When using Narrative Pedagogy, teachers also engage in the conversation with students. Teachers themselves work with students to learn more about the experiences being described. This is important because teachers and students work together to understand the experience in new, different, or more complex and nuanced ways. This means the teacher learns right along with the students rather than waiting for students to discover what the teacher has already determined is important. For example, the experience being shared is not considered "an example" of diabetes or heart failure. The experiences are not directed merely at pointing out particular content knowledge in the situation (e.g., "This is a good example of why delegation is important."). Rather, the experience itself is a call to thinking about everything present and absent in the experience from multiple perspectives, with the only end in view being that teachers and students actively engage in reflecting on, thinking through, and questioning these experiences.

The Concernful Practices of Schooling Learning Teaching

During the course of her research to understand Narrative Pedagogy and the common experiences that emerge when students and teachers gather to communally explore their experiences, Diekelmann (2001) described the *Concernful Practices of Schooling Learning Teaching*. The Concernful Practices shift teachers' and students' attention away from merely the acquisition of content knowledge or skill proficiency to a co-equal focus on how they understand and experience the situations they encounter as they learn and practice nursing.

Importantly, the Concernful Practices co-occur and can be experienced positively or negatively (Diekelmann & Diekelmann, 2009). For example, schools of nursing can be experienced (by teachers and students) as caring places, where a sense of community infuses school activities and brings out the best in everyone. But they can also be experienced as uncaring places where competition and isolation prevail, bringing out the worst in everyone.

When teachers and students consider the Concernful Practice of Caring: Engendering of Community (Diekelmann & Diekelmann, 2009, p. 343), they are made mindful of their community—of what is working well and what isn't—and they begin to discover new ways to learn and work together (Young, Hayden-Miles, & Brown, 2010). Although a detailed explication of the Concernful Practices is beyond the scope of this chapter, these practices will be emphasized throughout the remainder of the chapter to draw readers' attention to the possibilities that arise by shifting our focus from a language of strategies, methods, goals, and objectives/outcomes to these common practices.

REFLECTING ON . . . THE CONCERNFUL PRACTICES OF SCHOOLING LEARNING TEACHING

Presencing: *Attending and Being Open*

Assembling: *Constructing and Cultivating*

Gathering: *Welcoming and Calling Forth*

Caring: *Engendering of Community*

Listening: *Knowing and Connecting*

Interpreting: *Unlearning and Becoming*

Inviting: *Waiting and Letting Be*

Questioning: *Sense and Making Meanings Visible*

Retrieving Places: *Keeping Open a Future of Possibilities*

Preserving: *Reading, Writing, Thinking-Saying, and Dialogue*

Source: Diekelmann & Diekelmann, 2009

Getting Started With Narrative Pedagogy

Using Narrative Pedagogy is very familiar to nurses. As we practice, we continually encounter patients with different stories to tell, and we *listen* differently when we are taking a health history, exploring a new symptom, or responding to a patient's grief or great joy. We know the stories of the patients for whom we *care,* and this knowledge guides our ongoing development and study as we advance our practice. Getting started in using Narrative Pedagogy is about infusing our encounters with students with stories in which to communally explore and understand nursing practice and learning to be a nurse.

However, though experienced nurses are very at home in stories, many students are not. Co-creating learning experiences with students using Narrative Pedagogy requires that teachers talk with students about the kind of experience they (collectively) are creating in the course and why this is important in *becoming* a nurse. They also need to spend time talking about the importance of creating fair, safe, and respectful *gathering*s where everyone's voice is heard and respected. Of course, confidentiality and trust between teachers and students and among students, so crucial to *engendering community,* must also be discussed.

Using Narrative Pedagogy, faculty often *welcome* and *gather* students into the course by helping them reflect on the experiences they bring into the course; *connect* with other students (many of whom they have yet to meet); and focus on common experiences shared by teachers, other students, and practicing nurses. *Inviting* students to share these reflections publicly provides a rich context for *dialogue* and sets the stage for *attending* to reflective thinking, *listening* to each other, and *thinking* and learning in new ways. For example, faculty might introduce their courses to students by conveying how passionate they are about nursing, by sharing with students how exciting they hope the course will be, and by enlisting students' assistance in making the course a meaningful one for everyone (Ironside, 2014).

Teachers can also *construct* short classroom activities to *cultivate* students' ability to reflect on the teaching practices that have helped them learn in the past and then share them with the class. For example, students might respond to a prompt such as, "The thing I have liked most about this school of nursing is . . ."

or "Since I've been a nursing student, I've learned that the most important thing a teacher can do to help me learn is . . ." The teacher does the assignment too, responding to similar prompts: "The thing I have liked most about this school of nursing is . . ." or "Since I've been a teacher, I've learned that the most important thing students can do to help me be the best teacher I can be is . . ."

Communally discussing (dialogue) responses to these prompts engenders community as students begin to recognize how common their experiences are to other nursing students. This activity can be a very important learning experience when students believe their feelings of being overwhelmed by the work to be done in the course or their questions about their ability to be successful in the nursing program are indicative of a personal failing or deficit rather than a common experience of becoming a nurse. Similarly, students also begin to understand and explore some of the dilemmas of teaching (e.g., what one student finds most meaningful is what another student wants to avoid) and how similar students' and teachers' concerns often are (e.g., teachers too are often overwhelmed by all the work to be done in a course and so forth).

Another faculty member uses two prompts as a way of engendering community in her courses: "The thing I worry most about in coming to nursing school is . . ." and "The worst thing that could happen to me as a nursing student is . . ." She finds that spending time reflecting on and discussing these issues creates a meaningful way for her to know and connect with students and for students to begin knowing and connecting with each other. After providing the prompts, she gives the students a few minutes to reflect and then to write a short paragraph they will read aloud to the class. Again, as the instructor, she also does the assignment and shares her reflections with the students.

As each member of the class reads his or her concerns, students begin to identify (or the teacher might point out) the common themes that emerge. For example, students often share worries of not being successful, of having no personal life because of the demands of the program, or of harming a patient.

Dialogue among class members highlights how these are common concerns. Indeed, students and faculty share many of these concerns: They are more alike than they are different. As part of this dialogue, the teacher can also highlight how many of these struggles are common to nurses in practice. For example, students might share how overwhelming the amount of reading is as they learn nursing. Pointing out how nurses often struggle with these issues (i.e., what to read, how much to read) as they try to keep up with changes in practice offers students new ways to think about different reading strategies. When teachers draw attention to practices like reading in ways that exceed merely giving reading assignments or quizzing for comprehension, students begin to understand how they are learning skills that will help them be successful in nursing throughout their careers, not just in school. Together, teacher and students can discuss strategies for managing large amounts of reading.

The teacher can also engage students in identifying the resources that are available to help them be successful and how to access these resources. Similarly, dialogue might include specific information about how to handle a clinical error, how to communicate with teachers or clinicians when they have concerns about the quality of care or their ability to handle a particularly clinical situation, how teachers and clinicians provide backup for students as they learn in clinical settings, and so forth. Such dialogue helps students realize their common concerns and collectively devise ways to engender communities in which to work together to deal with the risks, anxiety, stress, or workload they share as students, teachers, and clinicians.

Using Narrative Pedagogy

Teachers use Narrative Pedagogy to create learning encounters that invite reflecting on experiences, thinking from multiple perspectives, questioning assumptions, and exploring new possibilities for learning and providing care (Ironside, 2014). Rather than assembling handouts or study guides, or PowerPoint slides for presentation, teachers focus on calling forth experiences that can create compelling dialogue with students within which the practice of nursing can be explored. Many teachers have found it helpful to construct an example of the assignment (in this case, an account of an experience) so students understand clearly what they are being asked to do. Other teachers find that providing students with prompts or "things to think about" as they write this assignment is helpful. Tatiana, an experienced teacher of pre-clinical students, created the following exercise to engage students in exploring communication.

JOURNALING ABOUT COMMUNICATION

For our next class, please write about an experience that has meaning for you, describing a time when you and another person communicated well (or didn't communicate well). Try to tell the story in as much detail as possible so that as you read it to us, we can see and hear the situation. It might be helpful to think about the following as you get started:

- *What was going on at the time? (Time of day, setting, individuals involved, etc.)*

- *How did you know the communication was going well, or not going well? What did you see or hear that told you this?*

- *What were you concerned about at the time?*

- *What was going through your head as the situation unfolded?*

- *What were you feeling during and after the experience?*

- *Did anything surprise you in the experience?*

I would anticipate your story will be 1–2 pages long. When you have finished writing your story, please write a second story from the perspective of another person who shared this same experience. Again, try to include as much detail as possible—describe as clearly as you can what the situation looked like to that other person. What were that person's concerns? What do you suppose was running through his or her head as the situation unfolded? Please try to keep this story to 1 page. Remember, we will be reading our stories aloud in class.

Here is how one pre-clinical student responded to these prompts:

While I was working as an assistant at a gym, a man who was severely hearing-impaired tried to speak with me using hand signals. When I did not understand him, he began to gesture more quickly and tensely, making things even worse. I could see the frustration and tension on his face. I felt completely helpless and tried to imagine how a patient would feel if he couldn't communicate his needs to his nurse. I knew I had to find a way to help him, and I remembered some signs from my high school American Sign Language class. I signed "hello" and the man completely relaxed, a big smile coming across his face. He signed that he spoke Spanish and knew little English—another challenge! I had also taken high school Spanish, and slowly, we found a way to communicate, which gave me a great sense of satisfaction. Each time he returned to the gym, he looked for me. I learned from that experience that sometimes just trying to help people communicates caring and makes a big difference in a person's life.

Attending to Students' Learning

When teachers use Narrative Pedagogy, they often report noticing changes in students' abilities to reflect on their experiences, think from multiple perspectives, question assumptions, and explore new possibilities for nursing education and practice. Yet these changes aren't readily captured in conventional assessment strategies like forced-choice exams. Indeed, research in nursing education has drawn attention to the importance of pedagogically consistent evaluation mechanisms (Ironside, 2003). Therefore, an important aspect of using Narrative Pedagogy is to assemble an array of ways to notice and attend to students' thinking and learning.

Roger, a new teacher in a prelicensure program, asks students to respond to the following prompts each class period before leaving:

- One thing I learned today that I did not know before is . . .

- One thing I knew before, but now understand in a different way . . .

- I still have questions or concerns about . . .

These prompts invite students to reflect on what they have learned and the questions that remain for them before the session ends, providing an important opportunity for students to think through and articulate what they have learned—for themselves and the teacher—and to evaluate their own learning and needs for further study. These are important skills that can be cultivated through these seemingly simple strategies and can spark dialogue among teachers and students, creating further opportunities for learning. It also makes evaluation a shared responsibility in which teachers and students work together to evaluate the learning accomplished and plan the next steps to accomplish further learning. In addition, by reading all students' responses, the teacher is better able to intentionally expand on particular issues, respond to misunderstandings, or direct students to further areas for discussion or study as the course progresses.

The following are examples of student responses to Roger's prompts.

One Thing I Learned Today That I Did Not Know Before Is . . .

Today I learned how critical it is to consider multiple perspectives. The patient's plan of care can't be decided on just one factor. There are many variables that have to be taken into account in order to formulate the best possible interventions. I also learned how vital it is to monitor the plan of care as it is being applied. For example, is it effective? What can we do to make it more effective?

One Thing I Knew Before But Now Understand in a Different Way . . .

Today I learned different aspects of critical thinking. Through everyone's stories, I was able to identify certain traits and skills required for critical thinking. First, critical thinking [grows] with experience. Also, nurses not only need to think clearly and plan the best care, but be able to put thoughts . . . into action and accomplish a goal. Not only do nurses need to think and communicate effectively, but understand effectively as well. If nurses don't know how to interpret information properly, they won't be able to provide the best care.

Final Reflections

Narrative Pedagogy provides a research-based approach for teachers to use to co-create engaging learning experiences with students. By focusing on developing and practicing their interpretive skills (reflecting on experiences, thinking in new ways and from multiple perspectives, and questioning their typical or inherited way of listening and responding to the situations they encounter), teachers and students can envision and enact new possibilities for understanding and working with each other and those for whom they care. Indeed, in the context of these conversations, students often say, "I never thought of it that way before," and become adept at asking, "Is there another way to think about this situation?" Given the complexity of the current healthcare environment and the challenges of preparing the future workforce, Narrative Pedagogy challenges the ubiquitous teacher-centered approaches to nursing education and opens new possibilities for dialogue among teachers and students toward improving nursing practice and education.

References

Benner, P., Sutphen, M., Leonard, V., & Day, L. (2010). *Educating nurses: A call for radical transformation.* Stanford, CA: Jossey-Bass.

Diekelmann, N. L. (1995). Reawakening thinking: Is traditional pedagogy nearing completion? *Journal of Nursing Education, 34*(5), 195–196.

Diekelmann, N. L. (2001). Narrative pedagogy: Heideggerian hermeneutical analyses of lived experiences of students, teachers, and clinicians. *Advances in Nursing Science, 23*(3), 53–71.

Diekelmann, N., & Diekelmann, J. (2009). *Schooling learning teaching: Toward narrative pedagogy.* Bloomington, IN: iUniverse Press.

Gadamer, H. G. (1989). *Truth and method* (Rev. ed.) (J. Weinsheimer & D. G. Marshall, Trans.). New York, NY: Continuum.

Institute of Medicine (IOM). (2011). *The future of nursing: Leading change, advancing health.* Washington, DC: National Academies Press.

Ironside, P. M. (2001). Creating a research base for nursing education: An interpretive review of conventional, critical, feminist, postmodern, and phenomenologic pedagogies. *Advances in Nursing Science, 23*(3), 72–87.

Ironside, P. M. (2003). Trying something new: Implementing and evaluating narrative pedagogy using a multi-method approach. *Nursing Education Perspectives, 24*(3), 122–128.

Ironside, P. M. (2005). Teaching thinking and reaching the limits of memorization: Enacting new pedagogies. *Journal of Nursing Education, 44*(10), 441–449.

Ironside, P. M. (2006). Using narrative pedagogy: Learning and practising interpretive thinking. *Journal of Advanced Nursing, 55*(4), 478–486.

Ironside, P. M. (2014). Enabling narrative pedagogy: Inviting, waiting, and letting be. *Nursing Education Perspectives, 35*(4), 212–218.

Ironside, P. M. (2015). Narrative pedagogy: Transforming nursing education through 15 years of research in nursing education. *Nursing Education Perspectives, 36*(2), 83–88.

Ironside, P. M., Brown, E. C., & Wonder, A. H. (2015). Narrative teaching strategies to foster quality and safety. In G. Sherwood & J. Barnsteiner (Eds.), *Quality and safety in nursing: A competency approach to improving outcomes*, 2nd ed. (pp. 221–232). Hoboken, NJ: Wiley-Blackwell.

Ironside, P. M., Diekelmann, N. L., & Hirschmann, M. (2005a). Learning the practices of knowing and connecting: The voices of students. *Journal of Nursing Education, 44*(4), 153–155.

Ironside, P. M., Diekelmann, N. L., & Hirschmann, M. (2005b). Student voices: On listening to experiences in practice education. *Journal of Nursing Education, 44*(2), 49–52.

Ironside, P. M., Scheckel, M., Wessels, C., Bailey, M., Powers, S., & Seeley, D. (2003). Experiencing chronic illness: Co-creating new understandings. *Qualitative Health Research, 13*(2), 167–179.

Scheckel, M. M., & Ironside, P. M. (2006). Enacting narrative pedagogy: Cultivating interpretive thinking. *Nursing Outlook, 54*(3), 159–165.

Young, P., Hayden-Miles, M., & Brown, P. (2010). Narrative pedagogy. In L. Caputi (Ed.), *Teaching nursing: The art and science* (Vol. 2) (pp. 804–836). Dupage, IL: College of DuPage Press.

Chapter 9
Reflective Practice in Simulation-Based Learning

–Kathryn R. Alden, EdD, MSN, RN, IBCLC
–Carol F. Durham, EdD, MSN, RN, ANEF, FAAN

Reflective practice and simulation-based learning (SBL) and are two well-known and widely used instructional strategies in nursing education. Reflection and SBL are a perfect partnership, working synergistically to promote effective learning. Reflection is integral and essential to maximizing the effectiveness of simulation learning experiences.

In the nursing literature, reflection and reflective practice are recognized as transformational tools for individuals and for the practice of nursing (Johns & Freshwater, 2005). Similarly, in contemporary nursing education, simulation-based learning (SBL) or simulated clinical experiences (SCE) might also be deemed transformational. The popularity, versatility, and effectiveness of this experiential, learner-centered instructional strategy has transformed clinical teaching in both academic and practice settings, including opportunities for the various types of health professions to learn together in interprofessional simulation. Furthermore, the educators and nursing programs that use this interactive, learner-centered teaching strategy find it transformational as well (Parker & Myrick, 2010).

Reflection as it relates to simulation-based learning is most often focused on the debriefing that occurs immediately following a simulated clinical experience. Upon further examination, it is clear that reflection and reflective practice are inherent to all phases of simulation learning activities for the individuals and for the small groups of learners who typically participate together in SBL, as well as for the educators who facilitate the activities. To maximize the effectiveness of simulation as a learning strategy, educators should carefully consider how to deliberately promote reflective practice among learners during all phases of simulated clinical experiences.

Situated cognition theory, also known as *situated learning*, is foundational to simulation-based learning (Onda, 2012). According to the theory, learning is influenced by the situation in which it occurs and is most effective if the environment is authentic. Learning requires engagement by the learner in authentic activities resembling the real world. The result is transformation of knowledge from theoretical and abstract to practical application (Brown, Collins, & Duguid, 1989). Reflection is critical to situated cognition theory, which proposes that as learners participate in authentic activities, there must be time for them to step back and reflect on the experience (Gieselman, Stark, & Farruggia, 2000). Reflection occurs throughout every phase of simulation: before, during, and after the simulated clinical experience (Onda, 2012).

According to Tanner's Model of Clinical Judgment (2006), reflection is the key component for nurses to develop clinical judgment. One of the goals of simulation activities is to help learners develop *clinical judgment,* which can be defined as "an interpretation or conclusion about a patient's needs, concerns, or health problems, and/or the decision to take action (or not), use or modify standard approaches, or improvise new ones as deemed appropriate by the patient's response" (Tanner, 2006, p. 204). Tanner proposes that the development of clinical judgment begins with noticing, proceeds to interpreting and responding, and concludes with reflecting. She refers to "reflection-in-action" that occurs during the patient interaction and "reflection-on-action" that occurs after the interaction. This reflective process helps learners develop tacit knowledge as they meld their experiences into what they have learned didactically (Armstrong & Sherwood, 2012).

Simulation as an Instructional Strategy in Nursing Education and Practice

Simulated clinical experiences are an essential component of nursing education. The Institute of Medicine (IOM, 2011) report, *The Future of Nursing,* recommends the use of simulation and emphasizes its value for interprofessional learning opportunities.

In *Educating Nurses: A Call for Radical Transformation*, Benner and associates cite the need to move nursing education from an emphasis on critical thinking to teaching multiple ways of thinking. They propose teaching "clinical reasoning clinical imagination, critical, creative, scientific and formal criterial reasoning" (Benner, Sutphen, Leonard, & Day, 2010, p. 85). *Clinical reasoning* is the ability to reason as a clinical situation changes, taking in context patient trends and expected trajectories, as well as patient and family wishes and concerns (Benner et al., 2010). They recommend experiential learning strategies such as simulation to create situated learning experiences where learners can develop and refine their thinking like a nurse in preparation for patient care. Connors and Tally (2015) emphasize that simulation requires integration across the curriculum to enhance patient safety.

Simulation is defined as a technique that creates a situation or environment to allow persons to experience a representation of a real event for the purpose of practice, learning, evaluation, testing, or to gain understanding of systems or human actions (Lopreiato et al., 2016). In nursing education programs, simulated clinical experiences (SCE) are designed to augment or complement the clinical practicum. Systematic reviews of the literature have identified the value of SCE in improving cognitive, affective, and psychomotor skills. Simulation learning experiences can increase knowledge; improve critical thinking and clinical reasoning abilities; enhance communication skills with patients, families, and interprofessional team members; and increase self-efficacy or self-confidence. Students report high levels of satisfaction with SCEs (Cant & Cooper, 2010; Foronda, Liu, & Bauman, 2013; Franklin & Lee, 2014; Yuan, Williams, & Fang, 2012).

Prelicensure nursing education programs use simulation throughout their curricula, beginning with early courses such as physical assessment and fundamentals, in specialty courses such as pediatrics or obstetrics, and in capstone courses where students engage in complex scenarios requiring synthesis of knowledge, skills, and attitudes they have gained during the nursing program. Simulation is a strategy for remediation when students are having difficulties in the clinical setting and as makeup time for students who were absent from clinical.

Simulated clinical experiences can effectively substitute for a portion of prelicensure clinical practicum hours in hospitals and other healthcare settings (Larue, Pepin, & Allard, 2015). The National Council of State Boards of Nursing (NCSBN) supports the use of simulation learning experiences for up to 50% of clinical practicum hours (Hayden, Smiley, Alexander, Kardong-Edgren, & Jeffries, 2014).

In 2015, the NCSBN provided guidelines for the use of simulation in pre-licensure nursing programs (Alexander et al., 2015). These guidelines include commitment to simulation from the institution, appropriate facilities and equipment, and faculty development. The International Nursing Association for Clinical Simulation and Learning (INACSL) has developed *Standards of Best Practice: Simulation*[SM] to guide the development of quality simulation. These standards were cited in the NCSBN report as resources and are available without cost from http://www.inacsl.org/i4a/pages/index.cfm?pageid=3407. The *INACSL Standards of Best Practice: Simulation*[SM] *Simulation Design* provides an overview of developing simulations that will provide the framework necessary for program development (Lioce et al., 2015).

Simulation is used in graduate nursing education programs to teach advanced practice skills and concepts to clinical nurse specialist, nurse practitioner, nurse anesthetist, and doctorate of nursing practice students (Garnett, Weiss, & Winland-Brown, 2015; Haut, Fey, Akintade, & Klepper, 2014; Mompoint-Williams, Brooks, Lee, Watts, & Moss, 2014; Pittman, 2012). Graduate students in nursing education programs engage in simulated clinical experiences as they are learning about the roles and responsibilities of clinical supervision (Shellenbarger & Edwards, 2012).

In nursing education programs, simulated clinical experiences can be used to facilitate transition into the role of clinical instructor. Through the use of simulation, new clinical instructors can practice facilitating student learning in the clinical area and receive immediate feedback from experienced faculty members and student volunteers who participate in the simulations (Hunt, Curtis, & Gore, 2015; Hunt, Curtis, & Sanderson, 2013; Shellenbarger & Edwards, 2012). Experienced clinicians who transition from practice to academic roles as clinical faculty can also benefit from participating in simulated experiences (Grassley & Lambe, 2015; Reid, Hinderer, Jarosinski, Mister, & Seldomridge, 2013).

Healthcare agencies utilize simulation learning activities with nursing staff and other healthcare professionals to assess competency; to educate about new policies, procedures, or equipment; to practice management of patients experiencing critical events; and to promote collaboration and teamwork. Simulation exercises in hospital settings have been shown to improve the technical performance of healthcare teams during critical events and procedures (Schmidt, Goldhaber-Fiebert, Ho, & McDonald, 2013). *In situ* simulation refers to SCEs that take place in actual patient care environments such as a patient room, emergency department, hospital lobby, or prehospital site. These simulations provide enhanced realism, are convenient for staff, and can be done in existing space without the expense of a simulation center. In situ simulation can be done routinely or as "just in time" training to promote individual, team, unit, and organizational learning within and across clinical and nonclinical areas to improve patient outcomes (Fent, Blythe, Farooq, & Purva, 2016; Rosen, Hunt,

Pronovost, Federowicz, & Weaver, 2012). Healthcare system improvements can be supported at a higher level of relevance and detail through the use of in situ simulation compared with simulations occurring in simulation centers (Lockman, Ambardekar, & Deutsch, 2015).

Simulation-based learning is incorporated effectively into the experiential learning component of advanced life support courses such as Pediatric Advanced Life Support (PALS) and Advanced Cardiac Life Support (ACLS) (Cheng et al., 2015). Simulations are used to allow learners to demonstrate competence after having completed online modules or face-to-face classes.

Simulation can ease the transition to practice for new graduates of nursing education programs. SCEs during nurse residency programs help new nurses and their instructors to identify gaps in knowledge and skills (Everett-Thomas et al., 2015).

Intraprofessional collaboration between nursing educators in academic settings and educators or staff in healthcare institutions can provide unique and beneficial learning opportunities. This type of collaboration may involve sharing of simulators, equipment, and personnel, as well as sharing of expertise to enhance SCEs for learners. Liaw, Palham, Chan, Wong, and Lim (2014) found strong collaboration between faculty and practicing nurses was important to successful SCEs. For example, nurses from a labor and delivery unit at a university hospital collaborated with faculty in prelicensure maternity courses to create and implement simulated clinical experiences around intrapartum care. Experienced staff nurses from the hospital acted as facilitators and assumed roles as charge nurses or healthcare providers in simulation scenarios with pre-licensure students. Reciprocally, nursing faculty collaborated with educators from the labor and delivery unit to offer simulated clinical experiences for new nurse orientees on the labor and delivery unit (Alden, Coulombe, & Alderman, 2013).

Interprofessional education is increasingly being recognized as an essential component of professional healthcare education programs. *Interprofessional education* is defined by the World Health Organization (WHO) as occurring when "students from two or more professions learn about, from, and with each other to enable effective collaboration and improve health outcomes" (WHO, 2010, p. 7). Interprofessional education involves teams of learners representing a variety of professions whose interactions influence patient care outcomes. George Thibault remarked at the Interprofessional Education for Collaboration conference (IOM, 2013) that "working in groups is not the same as learning in teams." Many healthcare educators continue to confuse those two activities. For interprofessional education to be effective, educators must be well prepared to deliver IPE course content, manage the interprofessional groups of learners, develop appropriate learning objectives, and adapt instructional strategies to address the diversity among the learners (Palaganas & Rock, 2015).

Interprofessional simulation in healthcare may include a variety of learners representing practice disciplines such as nursing, medicine, and pharmacy. Participants may be enrolled in educational programs or they may be licensed professionals, or a combination of both. For example, at a public university and medical center, prelicensure nursing students enrolled in a maternal/newborn nursing course participate in interprofessional simulations with medical students from obstetric and pediatric courses and pharmacy students enrolled in a Pharm D program. The primary focus of the simulations is teamwork, communication, and collaboration; the secondary focus is on the content of the simulation scenarios and patient care interventions (see Table 9.1).

Meaningful learning must be strategically designed to create opportunities for interprofessional teams to collaborate in the care of patients. Simulation provides such a platform for interprofessional education—providing opportunities for learners from various healthcare professions to engage with one another in meaningful interactions that promote effective collaboration and improved patient care outcomes (Murdoch, Bottorff, & McCullough, 2014). Decker and colleagues (2015) reported that interprofessional simulation is associated with "perceived improvement in: 1) knowledge, skills, attitudes, and behaviors related to teamwork; 2) appreciation of other professionals, their patient care roles, and skills; 3) awareness regarding the effective use of resources; 4) communication and collaboration; 5) self-confidence as it relates to teamwork; 6) clinical reasoning; (7) shared mental model; and 8) understanding the importance of patient safety initiatives" (p. 294).

It is highly desirable that learners in health professions have the opportunity to interact with and learn from individuals in other professions. Interprofessional simulations should integrate the *Interprofessional Collaborative Practice Competencies*: Interprofessional Teamwork and Team-based Practice; Interprofessional Communication Practices; Roles and Responsibilities for Collaborative Practice; and Values/Ethics for Interprofessional Practice, as outlined in the "Core Competencies for Interprofessional Collaborative Practice" report (Interprofessional Education Collaborative [IPEC], 2016).

Interprofessional education is ideally accomplished through multiple opportunities for learners to engage in simulated clinical experiences. Repeated interactions allow participants from varied professions to learn from and about each other and to learn how to interact, communicate, and collaborate. There are myriads of methods to accomplish this work, but it is important to have an interprofessional team of educators to plan, implement, evaluate, and refine the IPE activities. For example, a semester-long interprofessional course focusing on teamwork, communication, and patient safety is offered to nursing, medicine, and pharmacy students. The course integrates simulation-based learning activities in the majority of the weekly classes. This provides multiple opportunities for students to integrate more fully as an interprofessional team and to turn their focus on quality of care required by the simulated patient. Students participating in this course report improvement in: interprofessional communication, collaboration, and team function; understanding of roles and responsibilities; collaboration with a patient- and family-centered approach; and how to manage conflict resolution (Baker & Durham, 2013).

Simulation and Reflection: Making Sense of the Experience

The authors of this chapter developed a model that integrates concepts of reflective practice and simulation-based learning (Durham & Alden, 2013) (see Figure 9.1). The two processes are sequential and parallel. Stages or phases of each process occur simultaneously and in tandem with one another. Foundational and inherent to the processes are knowledge, skills, attitudes, experiences, and emotions.

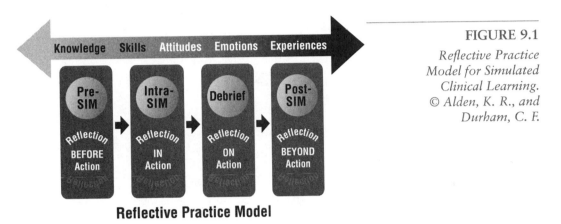

Reflective Practice Model

FIGURE 9.1

Reflective Practice Model for Simulated Clinical Learning. © Alden, K. R., and Durham, C. F.

This model acknowledges that learners are not a blank slate when they enter a simulated clinical experience. Instead, they come with a repertoire of knowledge, skills, attitudes, experiences, and emotions that influence the learning outcomes of the simulation experience. More importantly, throughout the phases of simulation, learners are reflecting on their knowledge, skills, attitudes, experiences, and emotions; they are using reflective practice to help them make sense of the experience (see Table 9.1).

TABLE 9.1 Strategies for Reflective Practice in Simulated Clinical Experiences

REFLECTIVE PRACTICE	SIMULATION PHASE	SUGGESTED STRATEGIES
Before Action	Pre-simulation: Preparation	Reflect on knowledge, skills, attitudes, experiences, and emotions
	Pre-briefing	Orientation to environment and simulator
		Review of learning objectives
		Explanation of process (pre-briefing/scenario/debriefing)

continues

TABLE 9.1 (continued)

REFLECTIVE PRACTICE	SIMULATION PHASE	SUGGESTED STRATEGIES
		Expectations of learners
		Evaluation or not
		Assurance of confidentiality
		"Fiction contract"
		Assigning roles
		Presentation of case
		Team huddle
In Action	Intra-simulation	Thinking on your feet: individual/group contemplation before acting
		Team "time-out"; huddle
		"Freeze frame"
On Action	Debriefing	Debriefing: reflection on individual and group performance, teamwork, communication, confidence, decision-making, emotions
		Group discussion led by facilitator(s)
		Review of select segments of video-recorded simulation
Beyond Action	Post-simulation	Guided reflection written assignments 1 week later/end of course/end of program; review of video and critique of individual performance in SCE

Phases of Simulated Clinical Experiences

In the model, simulated clinical experiences are conceptualized as occurring in four phases: (1) pre-simulation: preparation for the experience and pre-briefing or briefing that immediately precedes the simulation; (2) intra-simulation: active engagement in the simulation scenario; (3) post-simulation: debriefing that occurs immediately following the SCE; and (4) post-simulation: beginning as soon as debriefing ends and extending indefinitely into professional practice.

Stages of Reflective Practice

Reflection is inherent to well-known theories of experiential learning. Kolb's theory of experiential learning emphasizes the importance of reflection. He proposes that adults learn from their experiences through four stages (Kolb, 1984):

- *Concrete observation:* Observing during the actual learning experience

- *Reflective observation:* Exploring the meaning of the experience in light of previous learning

- *Abstract conceptualization:* Relating one's reflective observations to existing knowledge, theories, and assumptions

- *Active experimentation:* Applying new concepts and theories to future experiences

David Schön recognized the importance of reflection for professional knowledge. He referred to teachers as reflective practitioners. Schön proposed that there are two types of reflection that occur in a learning situation: one during and one after an activity or event. He presented the concepts of reflection-in-action and reflection-on-action. *Reflection-in-action* takes place during a learning activity and requires "thinking on your feet" and deciding what to do next. He noted that when faced with a new situation, the learner allows himself to feel surprised, puzzled, or confused; he then reflects on the current situation and on previous understanding. The next step is to proceed with an experiment to change the situation and to generate a new understanding. During *reflection-on-action*, the learner spends time examining what occurred, trying to make sense of it, and then generating perspectives, theories, and understandings (Schön, 1983).

The connection between reflective practice and simulated clinical experiences is widely recognized. The debriefing that occurs immediately following the SCE is a reflective exercise. As learners reflect on the simulation learning activity, facilitators (faculty or clinical educators) guide the discussion to help participants examine their actions and thinking. This is consistent with "reflection-on-action" as theorized by Schön (1983). While debriefing constitutes the most obvious reflective process in simulation, we need to consider the other aspects or stages of simulation and how reflection is integral to learning before, during, and after learner participation in simulation scenarios.

Recognizing the parallel between simulation-based learning and reflective practice, the authors propose that "reflection-before-action" occurs in the pre-simulation period when learners engage in structured activities and individual contemplation in anticipation of the simulation session. "Reflection-in-action" occurs during the simulation scenario as learners engage actively as participants, or vicariously as observers. "Reflection-on-action" is the time immediately following the simulation when debriefing occurs with the group of learners who participated in the learning activity. "Reflection-beyond-action" refers to reflective practice beyond the simulation activity and debriefing session, extending indefinitely as learners attempt to assimilate the knowledge, skills, and attitudes and apply them in other clinical situations.

Factors Influencing Reflective Practice and Simulated Clinical Experiences

Knowledge, skills, attitudes, emotions, and experiences influence how learners respond, react, and learn from simulation activities. These same factors affect reflective processes. Knowledge, skills, and attitudes are key to nursing education. According to the Quality and Safety Education for Nurses (QSEN) project, the goal of nursing educators is to prepare future nurses with the knowledge, skills, and attitudes (KSAs) necessary to continuously improve the quality and safety of the healthcare systems within which they work (Cronenwett et al., 2007; 2009).

With each simulated clinical experience, learners bring previous knowledge, skills, and attitudes. However, they also bring experiences and emotions, which are less objective, but nonetheless important to reflective practice and learning outcomes of simulation. For example, a student who will be caring for a simulated patient with congestive heart failure reflects on the pathophysiology of the disorder, skills for auscultating cardiac and lung sounds, and attitudes that convey caring and professionalism. It is reasonable to expect that the learner will also reflect on previous clinical experiences with cardiac patients and think about related emotions such as feelings of loss and grief over having lost a grandparent because of CHF.

The same knowledge, skills, attitudes, emotions, and experiences affect how the student thinks and performs during the simulation and how she processes and reflects on the experience during the immediate post-simulation debriefing and the time beyond the simulation.

Pre-Simulation: Reflection-Before-Action

Pre-simulation refers to the time prior to the beginning of the actual simulation scenario. Other terms used to describe this phase of simulation are *briefing, pre-simulation, prescenario, introduction,* or *preparation.* In actuality, the pre-simulation phase of an SCE occurs in two stages: first, there is preparation for the SCE that may occur hours, days, or even weeks prior; and secondly, there is pre-briefing that occurs when learners arrive at the simulation lab. Experts acknowledge that pre-briefing is critical to the success of the learning activity and greatly influences participation and engagement of learners in the scenario, debriefing, and reflection (McDermott, 2016; Rudolph, Raemer, & Simon, 2014). Pre-simulation, and more specifically, pre-briefing, has received little attention in the literature, and there is minimal empirical evidence related to this phase of simulation (Chamberlain, 2015; McDermott, 2016; Page-Cutrara, 2015).

Preparation for the SCE lays the foundation for learning. It provides the learner with an opportunity to gain new knowledge and review existing knowledge; learn new skills and review and practice familiar ones; examine attitudes and beliefs; consider previous experiences with similarities to the upcoming SCE; and think about emotions related to any aspect of the SCE.

Pre-briefing sets the stage for the actual SCE. Pre-briefing is critical to the success of the learning activity and greatly influences participation and engagement of learners in the scenario, debriefing, and reflection (McDermott,

2016; Rudolph et al., 2014). It is a time for orienting learners to the environment, demonstrating the properties of the simulator, providing learners with hands-on opportunities to become familiar with the simulator, and pointing out the location of various supplies and equipment that may be used in the scenario. During pre-briefing, facilitators clarify learning objectives and expectations, explain the process and timing of the scenario and debriefing, and describe the role of the facilitators. It is a time for creating psychological safety, stating whether or not learner performance is being evaluated, explaining how mistakes will be handled, emphasizing confidentiality, and appealing to the learners to suspend disbelief and to engage fully in the scenario (Janzen et al., 2016; Rudolph et al., 2014).

Reflection-before-action is consistent with the pre-simulation phase of simulated clinical learning experiences. Interestingly, the literature contains little mention about reflection prior to action. Boud and colleagues acknowledge the timing of reflective activities with the three stages of experiential learning activities: preparation, engagement, and processing (Boud, Keogh, & Walker, 1985). These stages are consistent with the three recognized phases of simulation: pre-simulation, scenario, and debriefing. Reflection-before-action involves examination of knowledge, skills, attitudes, experiences, and emotions prior to engaging in the simulation activity. Reflection occurs during the preparation and pre-briefing that precede the actual SCE. Reflection-before-action may be deliberate, serendipitous, or a combination of both.

In *preparation* for the SCE, participants may be presented with specific learning objectives for the upcoming scenario and asked (or required) to complete an assignment designed to prepare them to enter the learning activity with foundational knowledge and information to enhance the effectiveness of the simulation scenario. The assignment may be designated as the learner's "admission ticket" to the SCE. For example, prior to participating in a simulated clinical experience about a patient experiencing adult respiratory distress syndrome (ARDS), students enrolled in a capstone medical/surgical nursing course might be assigned readings on ARDS, followed by an online quiz. A web-based or virtual simulation on ARDS may be assigned. Students may be asked to review specific psychomotor skills they will use in the simulation activities, such as intravenous catheter insertion or medication administration.

Open-ended questions in the pre-simulation assignment guide reflection as students consider any similar patients they have encountered in the clinical setting, any friend or family member with the condition/disease/disorder in the upcoming SCE, or any personal experience with such conditions. To encourage reflection on previous experiences, attitudes, and emotions, learners may be asked to respond to open-ended questions that guide their reflection. Guided reflection in the pre-simulation assignment or activity can promote a sense of confidence, reduce anxiety, and prepare the learner to maximize the educational value of the simulation scenario. An example is: "If you or anyone in your family has ever been hospitalized in an intensive care unit, what was that like?"

The psychological aspects of SCEs and the emotions that are evoked before, during, and afterward influence participation and outcomes of the SCE. The element of the unknown and the associated anxiety that may precede the actual simulation experience can involve reflective practice. Consciously or subconsciously, learners consider their previous experiences with SCEs and how they felt in those sessions. If it is the first experience in the simulation lab, learners may fear the unknown; they do not know what to expect, and "insights" from peers who have previously done SCEs can help to diminish or accelerate their concerns. Learners may also reflect on clinical practicum experiences where they provided care for patients with similar conditions. They might recall their interventions, how they performed clinical skills, administered medications, interacted with the patient and family, recorded in the patient record, and how they felt during the experience. If they have had personal experience related to the learning activity, reflection may involve positive or negative emotions, including joy and satisfaction, or grief and disappointment. For example, a learner who is studying about high-risk pregnancy prior to simulation might have personally experienced a high-risk pregnancy that ended in the birth of a healthy infant, or one that resulted in a devastating perinatal loss. This may evoke an emotional reaction that can enhance or deter learning and participation in the simulation. Educators need to be sensitive to the potential for these reactions to occur and should respond appropriately in a very caring manner.

The pre-briefing component of pre-simulation begins when learners arrive for the simulation activities. They enter a "pre-entry" phase where they are briefed about how the activities will proceed. If it is the learners' first encounter with the manikin, they attend an orientation time in which the facilitator describes the features and functions of the simulator and allows learners to touch the manikin, listen to breath and heart sounds, to palpate pulses, and to hear the voice of the manikin. They are also oriented to the environment, equipment, medications, and other items, such as a telephone or computer that they can use in the scenarios. The learners are informed if the simulation is being recorded, and they are told whether or not they are being evaluated.

In group simulations, roles are assigned to participants in an effort to delineate responsibilities in the scenarios. Roles vary but can include primary nurse, secondary nurse, communicator, and recorder. Learners are provided a brief description of the expectations for each role, and they are encouraged to ask questions of the facilitator if they need clarification. To be time-efficient, lanyards can be created with the role in big letters on the front and a brief description of the role on the back. This allows the facilitator to quickly know who is functioning in what role during the simulation and provides learners a moment to quickly review the key responsibility of that role as they center themselves to assume those responsibilities.

Prior to entering the patient room in an SCE, learners are presented with a report on their patient. The report is likely to resemble a shift report or "hand-off" and includes the patient's history, presenting problem, current status, and healthcare provider orders. Presenting the information in SBAR format is helpful in reinforcing the concepts of teamwork and communication as set forth by the TeamSTEPPS program (King, Toomey, Salisbury, Webster, & Almeida, 2006). The primary nurse leads the team in a "huddle" to reflect on the data from the report and to plan the approach to patient care. As learners anticipate and plan their actions in the scenario, they necessarily reflect on their knowledge of the particular problem the patient presents, any experience they have had with other patients, and on their knowledge of the nursing process. Tasks are delegated by the primary nurse, and the team prepares to enter the patient room.

Intra-Simulation: Reflection-in-Action

During the actual simulation learning activity, participants are engaged in reflection-in-action, whether or not they realize or acknowledge doing so. As learners encounter a new situation in the SCE, their responses and actions are based on their repertoire of experiences, knowledge about the specific situation, attitudes, emotions, and expectations. The frame of reference is also important. Learners frame the problem of the situation, determine the desired goal, and plan appropriate actions to reach that goal. In SCEs, learners must utilize the nursing process as they assess, plan, intervene, and evaluate the patient care. They apply knowledge, employ various psychomotor skills, and interact with the simulated patient and family as they attempt to provide care that optimizes outcomes.

Facilitators can promote reflective practice (reflection-in-action) during simulated clinical experiences by allowing learners to pause if needed to evaluate interventions and/or to contemplate next steps. This reflection-in-action might be called "freeze frame" or "time-out." Learners may be allowed to call for these periodic pauses in the action, or facilitators may notice that learners are struggling or frustrated and call for a needed pause in the action. This can allow individuals or groups of learners in SCEs to reflect on previous and current knowledge, skills, attitudes, experiences, and emotions as they decide how to proceed in caring for the patient in the scenario. If the learners are participating in the SCE as a group, a team huddle to discuss the plan of care can clarify next steps in the scenario for all the participants. Facilitators or observers can note where in the SCE the pauses occurred and include discussion about this in the debriefing.

Debriefing: Reflection-on-Action

Debriefing is the process following a clinical simulation during which facilitators and learners review and analyze selected actions and thoughts from the learning activity. Ideally, debriefing occurs immediately following the simulation and is led by one or more facilitators of the SCE (Cantrell, 2008; Wotton, Davis, Button, & Kelton, 2010). With interprofessional simulations, it is important that facilitators from each of the professions participate in the debriefing.

Facilitators should devote adequate time to this activity. Some experts have proposed that the length of debriefing should be at least equal to the time of the actual scenario while others suggest debriefing should be double the simulation time (Fanning & Gaba, 2007). It is ideally held in close proximity to the simulation room (Arafeh, Hansen, & Nichols, 2010; Fanning & Gaba, 2007); learners are seated in a circle or around a table so that all are at the same level without a sense of someone being in charge. When debriefing begins, learners are informed about role delineation, time frame, and format (Arafeh et al., 2010; Mayville, 2011). If the simulation session was videotaped, facilitators can include review and critique of select video clips in the debriefing.

Debriefing is critical to the learning experience of clinical simulation. Because simulation involves cognitive, psychomotor, and affective aspects, debriefing necessarily addresses all these components of the learning experience. It is a time to evaluate the thinking processes, interventions, and behaviors that occurred and to consider the emotions that were evoked by the scenario and by involvement in the learning activity. Designing the debriefing around a familiar framework such as the nursing process enhances assimilation of the knowledge, skills, and attitudes into practice and helps the learner transfer the learning to future clinical situations (Dreifuerst, 2009).

Debriefing is an opportunity for intentional critical reflection on the simulated patient care experience. Schön (1987) refers to "reflection-on-action," which aligns with Kolb's (1984) experiential learning cycle; debriefing is the time for reflective observation, which follows engagement in a concrete experience (simulation session).

There are many different models for debriefing. It is evident from the NCSBN Simulation Study (Hayden et al., 2014) that facilitators need to select and follow a model to provide the best possible reflective experience for the learners. The knowledge about debriefing continues to evolve as we integrate Schön's work on reflection. There is no recommendation for one best model or process for debriefing; however, it is evident that the plus-delta technique alone is not sufficient to create the depth of reflection necessary to improve practice. Plus-delta is an easily adaptive technique, and most facilitators use this method as a component of debriefing. Three columns are drawn with the left-hand column listing selected actions from the SCE; the second column, labeled "plus," lists the effective actions; and the third column, labeled "delta" (change), lists the improvement opportunities (Littlewood & Szyld, 2015).

Debriefing commonly has three phases: reactions, analysis, and summary. The reactions phase allows for release of emotions, reviews facts, and reinforces the supportive learning environment. Debriefing provides an avenue for learners to experience emotional release. Simulation learning activities can trigger a variety of emotions for the learner. According to Schön (1983), emotion can enhance learning as it frames the experience, yet it can impede learning if it causes the learner not to fully engage in the experience. The nature of simulation asks learners to suspend disbelief and to treat the scenario and manikin as if they were real. Some learners find it more difficult than others. Some learners encounter anxiety when participating in clinical simulation, which can interfere with learning. Learners need the opportunity to express their feelings about participating in the scenario. This emotional release can help clear the pathway back to reflective learning (Dreifuerst, 2009).

The analysis phase examines the experience, makes connections, and considers ways that these reflections can influence practice. This reflection-on-action is a retrospective process that promotes development of clinical reasoning and clinical judgment skills through reflective learning processes (Dreifuerst, 2009). Although reflection is considered an innate activity, great variability exists among learners in terms of the consistency and thoughtfulness in reflection that influence the value of the learning experience. Debriefing is a time to facilitate reflective processes for learners so that they gain maximum benefit from the learning experience (Decker, 2007). The dialogue among the participants is important because it helps the individual increase awareness of his or her own thinking and rationale and exposes each person to the ideas of others, which helps develop professional boundaries and identity (Esterhuizen & Freshwater, 2008).

The summary phase of debriefing allows learners to consider the interconnectedness of issues in relation to practice, review key points, and discuss newly generated ideas (Littlewood & Szyld, 2015). As a part of debriefing, facilitators can review key points related to care of the patient with the particular problems encountered in the scenario. They can focus the discussion on a specific disease or condition, pertinent nursing assessments and interventions, lab tests, medications, or other key issues. Additionally, they should guide learners to reflect on patient safety concerns and how well they accomplished the related QSEN competencies, such as patient-centered care, teamwork and collaboration, and/or safety. Facilitators should prompt learners to consider if they dismissed important patient data because they had already made a decision about what was going on, which is defined as *premature closure*. Debriefing is a rich environment for reflective practice and can be as simple or complex as demanded by the educational design. The facilitator can use this phase to set the stage or as a springboard for reflection-beyond-action.

The atmosphere of the debriefing should be nonthreatening and nonjudgmental to encourage learners to share openly and honestly without fear of recrimination. In order to improve open communication and sharing emotions and points of view among interprofessional learners, the importance of a psychologically safe environment (Littlewood & Szyld, 2015) cannot be over-emphasized, because we are laying down foundations for future practice.

Post-Simulation: Reflection-Beyond-Action

Though reflection is commonly considered to occur during ("reflection-in-action") or immediately following ("reflection-on-action") the simulation, Dreifuerst (2009) proposes that a critical aspect of reflection occurs much after the experience. "Reflection-beyond-action" represents the process of assimilating and integrating the knowledge, skills, and attitudes into one's conceptual framework for nursing practice. Kolb's active experimentation phase of experiential learning is consistent with reflection-beyond-action.

Reflection-beyond-action begins as soon as the learners leave the simulation setting. It can occur hours, days, weeks, months, or even years after the SCE. Reflection may focus on the content of the scenario and how it increased understanding or awareness of disease process, assessments, interventions, communication, etc. Reflection may include evaluation of individual and/ or group performance in the simulations, with thoughts of what one might do next time to improve performance. For students who feel they "failed" or their performance was inadequate, the reflection may evoke painful emotions. Students who perceived their participation in the SCE as positive are likely to experience increased self-esteem and improved self-confidence. There is no time limit on this stage of reflection; as learners move on to professional roles, they may reflect back to the learning experiences in simulation.

Educators can assign reflective activities following simulation as an adjunct exercise. Reflective journaling about the clinical simulation provides written evidence of learner responses to simulation. Learners might be asked to answer specific questions, such as those used in debriefing, to guide their written reflection (Mayville, 2011). An assignment to "finish the story" encourages further reflection on the patient's point of view about his/her health and caregiver responsibilities. Learners might be asked to complete a self-assessment following clinical simulation, such as the one developed by Lasater (2007). The Lasater Clinical Judgment Rubric is based on the Tanner Model of Clinical Judgment (Tanner, 2006) and provides a frame of reference for learners to organize their thoughts in response to the clinical simulation. Clinical faculty can incorporate reflection about the SCE into discussions of actual patient care situations that occurred on the hospital unit.

As learners' repertoires of experiences continue to grow, they have greater opportunity for reflection and intellectual growth. Beyond prelicensure education, as students transition to roles as professional nurses and during their years of practice, they will engage in reflection. Through reflection, nurses make sense of their work, and it becomes a transformative process that leads to improvements in practice, increased meaning and satisfaction as a nurse, and ultimately fosters retention.

Reflective Practice and Simulated Clinical Learning: Exemplar

The phases of simulation and stages of reflective practice can be strategically and intentionally integrated into an interprofessional simulated clinical learning activity. The primary focus of the SCE is teamwork, communication, and collaboration. Teamwork, collaboration, and communication are essential to improving patient care (IPEC, 2011, 2016). Interprofessional simulation provides immersive activities for learners to work together around the care of patients. The secondary focus of the SCE is the content and skills in the scenario.

Faculty from the schools of nursing, medicine, and pharmacy at a large public university collaborated to create and implement an interprofessional SCE around obstetrics and neonatal care (see Table 9.2). Participants include prelicensure nursing students in a maternal/newborn nursing course, medical students in obstetrics and pediatric courses, and pharmacy students. Nursing students and obstetric medical students provide intrapartum care for a woman who gives birth to a compromised neonate. The infant requires full resuscitation by the pediatric medical students and nursing students. The pharmacy students act as consultants for the healthcare providers as they decide on pharmacological interventions. Additionally, the pharmacy students assist with preparation of medications during the neonatal resuscitation.

Pre-Simulation (Reflection-Before-Action)

Preparation: Simulation experiences are augmented by integrating different activities into the pre-simulation phase. Film provides an excellent platform to situate the scenario. In the simulation example provided in Table 9.2, film is used for training on TeamSTEPPS concepts and also serves as a stimulus for reflection. Through collaboration of faculty across two major universities and their respective schools of nursing and medicine, a concise film was developed about key concepts from TeamSTEPPS (http://www.med.unc.edu/csc/resources/for-faculty/teamstepps). In the pre-simulation preparation, learners are directed to watch the TeamSTEPPS video. In addition, the TeamSTEPPS program offers brief "opportunity" and "success" videos on intrapartum care; students are asked to view these short videos and to reflect on what they observed. Through open-ended questions, learners reflect on their experiences working with other healthcare professionals and with patients and families in labor and delivery units. They are also asked to reflect on their emotions related to those experiences. Prior to arriving at the simulation lab, students complete a brief online survey about teamwork, communication, and collaboration. Because the

SCE involved neonatal resuscitation, students are asked to review the current guidelines from the American Heart Association.

TABLE 9.2 Reflective Practice and Simulated Clinical Learning: Exemplar

REFLECTIVE PRACTICE	SIMULATION PHASE	SUGGESTED STRATEGIES
Before Action	Pre-simulation	Preparation: 1) View TeamSTEPPS video (50 minutes) to review teamwork, communication, and collaboration skills. http://www.med.unc.edu/csc/resources/for-faculty/teamstepps 2) View Labor and Delivery Opportunity video (3 minutes, 12 seconds): Mrs. Keys admitted for induction of labor. http://www.ahrq.gov/teamstepps/instructor/videos/ts_vig004a/vig004a.html Notice verbal and nonverbal behavior and reflect on where there are opportunities for improvement on teamwork, communication, and collaboration. 3) Watch Labor and Delivery Success video (5 minutes, 3 seconds). http://www.ahrq.gov/teamstepps/instructor/videos/ts_vig004b/vig004b.html Reflect on your solutions and how they align with the successes noted in this version of Mrs. Keys's story. 4) Reflect on your experiences and attitudes toward labor and delivery. 5) Reflect on how you feel about working and communicating as a member of healthcare teams.

continues

TABLE 9.2 (continued)

REFLECTIVE PRACTICE	SIMULATION PHASE	SUGGESTED STRATEGIES
		Pre-briefing: Orientation to environment; explanation of process, objectives, expectations; assigning roles; presenting case; team huddle.
		Case: Ms. Smith is a 36-yr-old gravida 2 para 1 at 41 weeks gestation. She is A+ and rubella immune; prenatal history is negative and all admission labs are normal. She was admitted 4 hours ago in active labor. At last check 1 hour ago she was 6 cm dilated, 100% effaced, and 0 station. Contractions are coming every 3 minutes and last 50–60 seconds. She wants to have a "natural birth" and has had no medications. She has an IV of Lactated Ringer's at 125ml/hr. Her mother is her support person; she has gone home to take the 2-year-old to a neighbor and will return soon.
In Action	Intra-simulation	Immerse interprofessional students in simulation. Part 1: Care of woman during labor and birth Part 2: Neonatal resuscitation; immediate postpartum care and support for mother
On Action	Debriefing	Debriefing: Reflection on individual and group performance, teamwork, communication, confidence, decision-making, emotions. Group discussion led by interprofessional team of facilitators.

REFLECTIVE PRACTICE	SIMULATION PHASE	SUGGESTED STRATEGIES
Beyond Action	Post-simulation	1-week post simulation

- Complete two-page paper on what were the most challenging components of this simulation and how you imagine applying lessons learned into your practice.

End of course

- Rewatch Labor and Delivery Success video (5 minutes, 3 seconds). http://www.ahrq.gov/teamstepps/instructor/videos/ts_vig004b/vig004b.html

- Complete one-page reflection, compare/contrast clinical experiences, noting the healthcare practitioners collaboration for the benefit or determent to woman/baby/family.

- Compare/contrast simulation and clinical experiences with communication, teamwork, and collaboration noted in the care of Mrs. Keys in the success video.

- Reflect about content learned in class, application in simulation, and outcomes in scenario compared to high-risk patients cared for in clinical experiences. What was similar? Different? Briefly describe the patient care situation.

continues

TABLE 9.2 (continued)

REFLECTIVE PRACTICE	SIMULATION PHASE	SUGGESTED STRATEGIES
		End of program
		• Complete two-page reflection paper.
		• Reflect throughout your experiences, whether in clinical or simulation; apply lessons learned about teamwork and communication.
		• Describe how your experiences align with high-functioning team demonstrated in the Labor and Delivery Success video.
		• Indicate lessons learned and insights gained, specifically skills, teamwork, communication, and collaboration around the care of obstetric patients and their families.

Pre-briefing: When all students are gathered in the conference room adjacent to the simulation lab, introductions are made by the students and the facilitators who represent the three schools. One facilitator explains the objectives of the SCE and the process that will be followed. Roles are assigned, followed by distribution of lanyards with color-coded cards specifying the school and the role for each participant. The students enter the simulation lab where they are oriented to the maternal and infant high-fidelity simulators, the equipment, and supplies. The school of nursing facilitator then presents the case to the nursing students (usually three to four) who will provide care for the laboring woman. This is done as a shift report or "hand-off" using SBAR (situation, background, assessment, recommendation) format. The nursing team "huddle" is led by the primary nurse, and when the team is ready, they enter the patient's room to begin the SCE.

Intra-Simulation (Reflection-in-Action)

After performing hand hygiene and making introductions, the nurses assess the patient and fetal heart tracing. The fetal heart pattern suddenly changes to a nonreassuring (category 3) pattern of late decelerations, which prompts the nurses to intervene by repositioning the woman, applying oxygen, increasing the IV rate, and calling the obstetric care provider (i.e., medical student) who answers the cell phone from a nearby room. The late deceleration resolves as a result of the interventions. Soon thereafter, the laboring woman starts to complain of feeling "pressure" like she needs to have a bowel movement. The nurses assess her perineum and see that the baby's head is crowning. They call for the OB provider, and the OB medical students (usually two) enter the room. Birth is imminent, and the OB provider delivers the baby as the nurses coach the mother. The neonate is flaccid and is not breathing. The nurses dry and stimulate the baby and notify the pediatric team, who appear quickly and begin to assess the newborn. The pediatric medical students and two of the nursing students work together in neonatal resuscitation. The newborn is intubated and chest compressions are performed. The pharmacy student assists with determining appropriate dosages and preparing medications needed during the resuscitation. Meanwhile, the OB medical students and the primary nurse for the mother are providing immediate postpartum care for the mother, who is extremely distressed and worried about her baby. The resuscitation is successful; the neonate begins to breathe spontaneously and the apical pulse is strong and regular. The team decides to transport the infant to the neonatal intensive care unit. One of the pediatric students gives report to the mother. At that point, the SCE ends and the students are dismissed to the conference room for debriefing.

Debriefing (Reflection-on-Action)

The facilitators from the three schools engage the learners in reflection-on-action during debriefing as they proceed through the phases of reactions, analysis, and summary. The debriefing discussion first centers around teamwork, collaboration, and communication. Care of the mother and neonate is discussed and key points are emphasized. At the conclusion of the debriefing, the students complete the post-simulation survey about teamwork, collaboration, and communication.

Post-Simulation (Reflection-Beyond-Action)

Reflection-beyond-action begins the moment that the students leave the debriefing. Much of the reflection occurs unintentionally as students recall the experience. Educators can design intentional reflective activities to be completed at specific times; for example, at 1-week post-simulation, end of course, and end of program. A brief assignment at 1 week may be to reflect on the most challenging and rewarding aspects of the simulation experience and how to apply lessons learned to clinical practice. At the end of the course, students may be asked to view the labor and delivery "success" video once again, considering the teamwork, collaboration, and communication strategies that were used and to compare those strategies with what they observed in their clinical practicum. A synthesis reflection assignment at the end of the program might ask students to reflect on all their clinical experiences in terms of their observations and perceptions of teamwork, collaboration, and communication among various healthcare professionals. They can identify lessons learned and how they will incorporate the concepts from TeamSTEPPS into their professional practice.

Final Reflections

Learning is complex; it is not adequate to just complete a simulation scenario. Simulation is a fertile field for changing practice when reflection is designed as an inherent part of the learning experience. To maximize the impact of educational experiences to build knowledge, educators must give learners the opportunity to reflect *before action* (pre-simulation), *in action* (intra-simulation), *on action* (immediately post-simulation debriefing), and *beyond action* (integration of knowledge following simulation which can occur in days, weeks, or longer). Training professional learners to utilize reflection can transform their clinical practice and improve the effectiveness of their patient care.

References

Alden, K. R., Coulombe, L., & Alderman, J. T. (2013). You scratch my back, I'll scratch yours: Reciprocal intraprofessional collaboration for OB simulation. *Journal of Obstetrics, Gynecologic and Neonatal Nursing, 42*(Suppl. 1), S9.

Alexander, M., Durham, C. F., Hooper, J. I., Jeffries, P. R., Goldman, N., Kardong-Edgren, S., . . . Tillman, C. (2015). NCSBN simulation guidelines for prelicensure nursing programs. *Journal of Nursing Regulation, 6*(3), 39–42. doi:http://dx.doi.org/10.1016/S2155-8256(15)30783-3

Arafeh, J. M., Hansen, S. S., & Nichols, A. (2010). Debriefing in simulated-based learning: Facilitating a reflective discussion. *Journal of Perinatal and Neonatal Nursing, 24*(4), 302–309.

Baker, M. J., & Durham, C. F. (2013). Interprofessional education: A survey of students' collaborative competency outcomes. *Journal of Nursing Education, 52*(12), 713–718. doi:10.3928/01484834-20131118-04

Benner, P., Sutphen, M., Leonard, V., & Day, L. (2010). *Educating nurses: A call for radical transformation.* San Francisco, CA: Jossey-Bass.

Boud, D., Keogh, R., & Walker, D. (Eds.). (1985). *Reflection: Turning experience into learning.* London, UK: Kogan Page.

Brown, J. S., Collins, A., & Duguid, P. (1989). Situated cognition and the culture of learning. *Educational Researcher, 18*(1), 32–42.

Cant, R. P., & Cooper, S. J. (2010). Simulation-based learning in nurse education: Systematic review. *Journal of Advanced Nursing, 66*(1), 3–15.

Cantrell, M. A. (2008). The importance of debriefing in clinical simulation. *Clinical Simulation in Nursing, 4*(2), e19–e23.

Chamberlain, J. (2015). Prebriefing in nursing simulation: A concept analysis using Rodger's methodology. *Clinical Simulation in Nursing, 11*(7), 318–322.

Cheng, A., Lockey, A., Bhanji, F., Lin, Y., Hunt, E. A., & Lang, E. (2015). The use of high-fidelity manikins for advanced life support training: A systematic review and meta-analysis. *Resuscitation, 93*(Aug. 2015), 142–149.

Connors, H. B., & Tally, K. (2015). Integrating technology in education. In M. Oermann (Ed.), *Teaching in nursing and role of the educator: The complete guide to best practice in teaching, evaluation, and curriculum development* (pp. 61–81). New York, NY: Springer Publishing Company.

Cronenwett, L., Sherwood, G., Barnsteiner, J., Disch, J., Johnson, J., Mitchell, P., . . . Warren, J. (2007). Quality and safety education for nurses. *Nursing Outlook*, *55*(3), 122–131.

Cronenwett, L., Sherwood, G., Pohl, J., Barnsteiner, J., Moore, S., Taylor Sullivan, D., . . . Warren, J. (2009). Quality and safety education for advanced practice nursing practice. *Nursing Outlook*, *57*(6), 338–348.

Decker, S. (2007). Integrating guided reflection into simulated learning experiences. In P. R. Jeffries (Ed.), *Simulation in nursing: From conceptualization to evaluation* (pp. 73–85). New York, NY: National League for Nursing.

Decker, S. I., Anderson, M., Boese, T., Epps, C., McCarthy, J., Motola, I., . . . Lioce, L. (2015). Standards of best practice: Simulation standard VIII: Simulation-enhanced interprofessional education (Sim-IPE). *Clinical Simulation in Nursing*, *11*(6), 293–297. Retrieved from http://dx.doi.org/10.1016/j.ecns.2015.03.010

Dreifuerst, K. T. (2009). The essentials of debriefing in simulation learning: A concept analysis. *Nursing Education Perspectives*, *30*(2), 109–114.

Durham, C. F., & Alden, K. R. (2013). *Innovative reflective practice model for simulation.* Podium presentation, International Nursing Simulation/Learning Resource Centers Conference, Orlando, FL.

Esterhuizen, P., & Freshwater, D. (2008). Using critical reflection to improve practice. In D. Freshwater, B. J. Taylor, & G. Sherwood (Eds.), *International textbook of reflective practice in nursing* (pp. 99–118). Oxford, UK: Blackwell Publishing.

Everett-Thomas, R., Valdes, B., Valdes, G. R., Shekhter, I., Fitzpatrick, M., Rosen, L. F., . . . Birnbach, D. J. (2015). Using simulation technology to identify gaps between education and practice among new graduate nurses. *Journal of Continuing Education in Nursing*, *46*(1), 34–40.

Fanning, R. M., & Gaba, D. M. (2007). The role of debriefing in simulation-based learning. *Simulation in Healthcare*, *2*(2), 115–125.

Fent, G., Blythe, J., Farooq, O., & Purva, M. (2016). In situ simulation as a tool for patient safety: A systematic review identifying how it is used and its effectiveness. *BMJ Simulation and Technology Enhanced Learning*, *1*(5), 103–110.

Foronda, C., Liu, S., & Bauman, E. B. (2013). Evaluation of simulation in undergraduate nurse education: An integrative review. *Clinical Simulation in Nursing*, *9*(10), e409–e416.

Franklin, A. E., & Lee, C. S. (2014). Effectiveness of simulation for improvement in self-efficacy among novice nurses: A meta-analysis. *Journal of Nursing Education, 53*(11), 607–614.

Garnett, S., Weiss, J. A., & Winland-Brown, J. E. (2015). Simulation design: Engaging large groups of nurse practitioner students. *Journal of Nursing Education, 54*(9), 525–531.

Gieselman, J. A., Stark, N., & Farruggia, M. J. (2000). Implications of the situated learning model for teaching and learning in nursing research. *Journal of Continuing Education in Nursing, 31*(6), 263–268.

Grassley, J. S., & Lambe, A. (2015). Easing the transition from clinical to nurse educator: An integrative literature review. *Journal of Nursing Education, 54*(7), 361–366.

Haut, C., Fey, M. K., Akintade, B., & Klepper, M. (2014). Using high-fidelity simulation to teach patient safety behaviors in undergraduate nursing education. *Journal of Nursing Education, 49*(1), 48–51.

Hayden, J. K., Smiley, R. A., Alexander, M., Kardon-Edgren, S., & Jeffries, P. R. (2014). Supplement: The NCSBN National Simulation Study: A longitudinal, randomized, controlled study replacing clinical hours with simulation in prelicensure nursing education. *Journal of Nursing Regulation, 5*(2), S1–S64.

Hunt, C. W., Curtis, A. M., & Gore, T. (2015). Using simulation to promote professional development of clinical instructors. *Journal of Nursing Education, 54*(8), 468–471.

Hunt, C. W., Curtis, A. M., & Sanderson, B. K. (2013). A program to provide resources and support for clinical associates. *Journal of Continuing Education in Nursing, 44*(6), 269–273.

Institute of Medicine (IOM). (2011). *The future of nursing: Leading change, advancing health.* Washington, DC: The National Academies Press.

Institute of Medicine (IOM). (2013). Interprofessional education for collaboration: Learning how to improve health from interprofessional models across the continuum of education to practice: Workshop summary. Washington, DC: The National Academies Press.

Interprofessional Education Collaborative (IPEC). (2011). Core competencies for interprofessional collaborative practice: Report of an expert panel. Washington, DC: Interprofessional Education Collaborative. Retrieved from http://www.aacn.nche.edu/education-resources/IPECReport.pdf

Interprofessional Education Collaborative (IPEC). (2016). Core competencies for interprofessional collaborative practice: 2016 update. Washington, DC: Interprofessional Education Collaborative. Retrieved from http://www.aacn.nche.edu/education-resources/IPEC-2016-Updated-Core-Competencies-Report.pdf

Janzen, K. J., Jeske, S., MacLean, H., Harvey, G., Nickle, P., Norenna, L., . . . McLellan, H. (2016). Handling strong emotions before, during, and after simulated clinical experiences. *Clinical Simulation in Nursing, 12*(2), 37–43.

Johns, C., & Freshwater, D. (2005). *Transforming nursing through reflective practice* (2nd ed.). Oxford, UK: Blackwell Science.

King, H. B., Toomey, L., Salisbury, M., Webster, J., & Almeida, S. (2006). TeamSTEPPS [Team Strategies and Tools to Enhance Performance and Patient Safety]. Retrieved from http://teamstepps.ahrq.gov/

Kolb, D. A. (1984). *Experiential learning*. Englewood Cliffs, NJ: Prentice Hall.

Larue, C., Pepin, J., & Allard, E. (2015). Simulation in preparation or substitution for clinical placement: A systematic review of the literature. *Journal of Nursing Education and Practice, 5*(9), 132.

Lasater, K. (2007). Clinical judgment development: Using simulation to create an assessment rubric. *Journal of Nursing Education, 46*(11), 496–503.

Liaw, S. Y., Palham, S., Chan, S. W., Wong, L. R., & Lim, F. P. (2014). Using simulation learning through academic-practice partnership to promote transition to clinical practice: A qualitative evaluation. *Journal of Advanced Nursing, 71*(5), 1044–1054. doi:10.1111/jan.12585

Lioce, L., Meakim, C. H., Fey, M. K., Chmil, J. V., Mariani, B., & Alinier, G. (2015). Standards of best practice: Simulation standard IX: Simulation design. *Clinical Simulation in Nursing, 11*(6), 309–315. Retreived from http://dx.doi.org/10.1016/j.ecns.2015.03.005

Littlewood, K. E., & Szyld, D. (2015). Debriefing. In J. C. Palaganas, J. C. Maxworthy, C. A. Epps, & M. E. Mancini (Eds.), *Defining excellence in simulation programs* (pp. 558–572). Philadelphia, PA: Wolters Kluwer.

Lockman, J. L., Ambardekar, A., & Deutsch, E. S. (2015). Optimizing education with in situ simulation. In J. C. Palaganas, J. C. Maxworthy, C. A. Epps, & M. E. Mancini (Eds.), *Defining excellence in simulation programs* (pp. 90–98). Philadelphia, PA: Wolters Kluwer.

Lopreiato, J. O. (Ed.), Downing, D., Gammon, W., Lioce, L., Sittner, B., Slot, V. (Associate Eds.), . . . Terminology & Concepts Working Group. (2016). *Healthcare simulation dictionary*. Retrieved from http://www.ssih.org/dictionary

Mayville, M. L. (2011). Debriefing: The essential step in simulation. *Newborn and Infant Nursing Reviews, 11*(1), 35–39.

McDermott, D. S. (2016). The prebriefing concept: A Delphi study of CHSE experts. *Clinical Simulation in Nursing, 12*(6), 219–227.

Mompoint, D., Brooks, A., Lee, L., Watts, P., & Moss, J. (2014). Using high-fidelity simulation to prepare advanced practice nursing students. *Clinical Simulation in Nursing, 10*(1), e5–e10.

Murdoch, N. L., Bottorff, J. L., & McCullough, D. (2014). Simulation education approaches to enhance collaborative healthcare: A best practices review. *International Journal of Nursing Education Scholarship, 10*(1), 307–321.

Onda, E. L. (2012). Situated cognition: Its relationship to simulation in nursing education. *Clinical Simulation in Nursing, 8*(7), e273–e280.

Page-Cutrara, K. (2015). Prebriefing in nursing simulation: A concept analysis. *Clinical Simulation in Nursing, 11*(7), 335–340.

Palaganas, J. C., & Rock, L. K. (2015). Simulation-enhanced interprofessional education: A framework for development. In J. C. Palaganas, J. C. Maxworthy, C. A. Epps, & M. E. Mancini (Eds.), *Defining excellence in simulation programs* (pp. 108–119). Philadelphia, PA: Wolters Kluwer.

Parker, B., & Myrick, F. (2010). Transformative learning as a context for human patient simulation. *Journal of Nursing Education, 49*(6), 326–332.

Pittman, O. A. (2012). The use of simulation with advanced practice nursing students. *American Academy of Nurse Practitioners, 24*(9), 516–520.

Reid, T. P., Hinderer, K. A., Jarosinski, J. M., Mister, B. J., & Seldomridge, L. A. (2013). Expert clinician to clinical teacher: Developing a faculty academy and mentoring initiative. *Nurse Education in Practice, 13*(4), 283–293.

Rosen, M. A., Hunt, E. A., Pronovost, P. J., Federowicz, M. A., & Weaver, S. J. (2012). In situ simulation in continuing education for the health care professions: A systematic review. *Journal of Continuing Education in the Health Professions, 32*(4), 243–254.

Rudolph, J. W., Raemer, D. B., & Simon, R. (2014). Establishing a safe container for learning in simulation. *Simulation in Healthcare, 9*(6), 339–349.

Schmidt, E., Goldhaber-Fiebert, S. N., Ho, L. A., & McDonald, K. M. (2013). Simulation exercises as a patient safety strategy: A systematic review. *Annals of Internal Medicine, 158*(5Pt2), 426–432.

Schön, D. A. (1983). *The reflective practitioner: How professionals think in action.* New York, NY: Basic Books.

Schön, D. A. (1987). *Educating the reflective practitioner.* Hoboken, NJ: Jossey-Bass.

Shellenbarger, T., & Edwards, T. (2012). Nurse educator simulation: Preparing faculty for clinical nurse educator roles. *Clinical Simulation in Nursing, 8*(6), e249–e255.

Tanner, C. A. (2006). Thinking like a nurse: A research-based model of clinical judgment in nursing. *Journal of Nursing Education, 45*(6), 204–211.

World Health Organization (WHO). (2010). *Framework for action on interprofessional education & collaborative practice.* Geneva, Switzerland: World Health Organization.

Wotton, K., Davis, J., Button, D., & Kelton, M. (2010). Third-year undergraduate nursing students' perceptions of high-fidelity simulation. *Journal of Nursing Education, 49*(11), 632–639.

Yuan, H. B., Williams, B. A., & Fang, J. B. (2012). The contribution of high-fidelity simulation to nursing students' confidence and competence: A systematic review. *International Nursing Review, 59*(1), 26–33.

Chapter 10

Reflection in Clinical Contexts: Learning, Collaboration, and Evaluation

–Gail Armstrong, PhD, DNP, RN, ACNS-BC, CNE
–Sara Horton-Deutsch, PhD, RN, FAAN, ANEF
–Gwen D. Sherwood, PhD, RN, FAAN, ANEF
–With Learning Activity by Kristina Thomas Dreifuerst, PhD, RN, CNE, ANEF

Reflective practice is based on the fundamental principle of continuous learning through a process of self-assessment and integration of knowledge with experience. As such, it highlights the responsibility of professional nurses to adopt an open attitude and lifelong commitment to assessing and continuously improving their work. Helping professional nurses develop these qualities requires educational approaches that include open, interactive dialogue between learners and teachers. Learners need opportunities to tell their stories, especially about clinical events, in order to meld experiential learning with theoretical learning. Reflective exercises in clinical learning environments can build mental habits that carry over into professional nurse roles, whether as a clinical nurse, nurse educator, or nurse leader. Fostering a reflective philosophy of self-assessment and learning from all experiences is a habit of the mind essential to sense-making in practice and establishes lifelong learning.

There is little evidence to guide nursing clinical curricula to best implement reflective learning. Reflective learning shifts from a teaching paradigm to a learning paradigm. Traditional clinical evaluative methods that rely on objective measures might not reveal the changes in attitude and behavior that derive from reflective learning. In reflective paradigms, the learner engages in self-monitoring, so there is an assessment value even within the learning experience. Educators and learners maintain openness and flexibility in the dialogue that emerges from reflective journaling and other means of feedback.

This chapter will explore ways to facilitate reflection, primarily in the clinical learning context, and provide feedback to learners that is consistent with reflective learning. We will discuss how the increasing application of reflection in higher education challenges us to rethink clinical assessment and evaluation. The philosophy of learner-centered education promotes co-creating the learning environment in a partnership between learners and educators. We will explore ways to develop a reflective clinical learning environment open to inquiry and continuous learning as the foundation of self-monitoring and evaluation.

Reflection, Learning, and Assessment: Building Partnerships Between Educators and Learners

Self-management and learner engagement are basic tenets of reflective practice; thus, involvement in co-creating the learning environment helps establish habits of self-management and engagement in monitoring outcomes. This creates a partnership between clinical educators and learners rather than the educator determining the experience without learner input.

"Commitment is the fluid dialogue that moves between learners and educators in a manner that nurtures the development of professional identity."

Drawing heavily on work from Dewey, Shulman (2002) engaged in a longitudinal study of knowledge growth. Through this work he created a table of learning that includes engagement, understanding, action, reflection, judgment, and commitment. The relationship of these concepts to one another is outlined as follows:

Learning begins with student engagement, which in turn leads to knowledge and understanding. Once someone understands, he or she becomes capable of performance or action. Critical reflection on one's practice and understanding leads to higher-order thinking in the form of capacity to exercise judgment in the face of uncertainty and to create designs in the presence of constraints and unpredictability. Having skills to think in the middle of unpredictability is particularly valuable in nursing students' clinical development. Ultimately, the exercise of judgment makes possible the development of commitment. In commitment, we become capable of professing our understandings and our values, our faith and our love, our skepticism and our doubts, internalizing those attributes and making them integral to our identities. These commitments, in turn, make new engagements possible—even necessary (Shulman, 2002, p. 38).

Educators, including clinical preceptors, can apply Shulman's table of learning to assessment (competency achievement) and evaluation (judgment); this philosophy recognizes that both assessment and evaluation are part of the commitment educators make to learners in a mutually unfolding learning process. By providing feedback through a lens of commitment, educators shift from what learners missed to what learners understand and facilitate further critical reflection. This way of providing feedback models our engagement in the learning experience and a way of being professionally in the practice world with others (including other members of the healthcare team). Educators might view commitment as the sole responsibility of the learner; however, commitment is the fluid dialogue that moves between learners and educators in a manner that nurtures the development of professional identity.

A growing sense of professional identity is a critical element of effective clinical development. Learner outcomes are demonstrated through a change in the quality and focus of interactions and discussions with team members, patients, and educators/teachers. Learners begin to demonstrate greater awareness of self and others.

Collaboratively Structuring Reflection in Clinical Learning

Clinical learning experiences take place within complex healthcare environments and require alternative types of assessment of performance (Day & Sherwood, 2017a). Reflecting-before-action can be observed in clinical situations, for example, through teamwork briefings to reflect on what should be done; reflecting-in-action by huddling to problem-solve in the middle of a situation; and reflecting-on-action during debriefing to learn from actions taken (Schön, 1983).

Educators can use clinical learning agreements to document and assess reflective assignments. Learning contracts have sometimes been associated with weak learner performance to detail the terms of the agreement between learners and educators. However, a shift to using learning contracts in a positive way with all learners sets clear guidelines for reflecting on practice and experiences and clearly identifies what must be achieved in program or course competencies. The following is an example of a learning agreement adapted from Bulman and Schutz (2005):

1. Identify learning needs in the context of the educational objectives.

2. Identify resources and strategies to achieve expectations.

3. Gather evidence, integrating evidence-based practice, practice-based evidence, and a reflective narrative.

4. Seek comments and feedback from peer and preceptor.

These questions can also guide post-clinical conference discussions, either individually or as a group. Although reflecting-on-action is frequently the process used by educators following clinical experiences, both for students and for nurses working with preceptors in practice settings, guided questions can facilitate the process so that learners tease out deeper levels of what happened, how they responded, what they could do differently in the future, and how they are reacting emotionally. This debriefing time is often overlooked as a critical time for coping with the emotional aspects of caregiving. Reflecting-on-action can foster recognition of emotions and facilitate making sense of events. Failure to recognize and coach learners at such a significant time in their nursing journey places them at risk for emotional burnout, disengagement, and rote actions.

Partnerships to Create a Reflective Learning Environment

The dominant mode of instruction in nursing education (especially clinical education) has traditionally been an expert-novice relationship between educator and learner. Learning strategies that help develop an open learning partnership aligned with the goals and aims of reflection (Macfarlane, 2004) can prove challenging to educators seeking to change the clinical learning paradigm. Engaging learners in reflective practice requires mutual openness to examine new ideas and the ability to listen and act appropriately; both learners and educators must adopt an open attitude. We do not learn from experience alone; we learn from critically reflecting on experience. Educators can apply reflective evaluation to role-model the openness to learning from clinical experiences that undergirds the lifelong skill for continuously improving one's work.

Appreciative Inquiry (AI) can provide a foundation for creating an open and affirming educational process by including students in determining successful strategies for the learning environment (Cooperrider & Whitney, 2005). An appreciative approach focuses on what learners desire versus what learners do incorrectly; for example, focusing on desired practice versus a gap analysis. Rather than clinical educators setting rules for behavior in the clinical situation, together educators and learners follow the steps from AI to establish agreed-upon elements of engagement.

REFLECTING ON . . . APPRECIATIVE INQUIRY

Appreciative Inquiry (AI) is a narrative-based process to create positive change using open-ended questions, therefore easily adapted to assessment based on reflection. AI engages learners and educators in a deep dialogue about strengths, resources, capabilities, and assessment. Together, they develop a series of activities envisioned for future experiences by discussing and creating propositions that will guide future work together. Finally, it involves forming teams to carry out the work needed to realize the dreams and designs for the future. AI focuses on metaphor, narrative, and relational ways of knowing, thus encouraging the exploration of ideas through open-ended questioning that encompasses a reflective process. AI focuses on inquiry, imagination, and innovation rather than a gap analysis or problem-solving. Instead of negativism, criticism, and spiraling diagnoses, the emphasis is on discovery, dream, and design (Cooperrider & Whitney, 2005), an openness to the possibilities for the future.

Learners might be asked to reflect on what creates an environment conducive to learning, perhaps by completing a brief online survey or by answering open-ended questions about previous classroom or clinical experiences. The process of reflection involves letting go of control; both educators and learners must be willing to share in creating the learning experience. As an example, in a new clinical rotation, learners identify processes that they have found to be key to successful learning in the past, essentially assessing their past learning experiences. Through continuous discussion, they can reach consensus on their clinical aspirations for the rotation to achieve the course outcomes, in response to the clinical environment.

With this proactive process and advanced information, both learner and preceptor can focus clinical opportunities on experiences congruent with the learner's aims. In this way, preceptor and learner also understand the terminal objectives on which they will be evaluated. Educators and learners agree on the *elements of engagement* (sometimes called *rules of engagement*) that guide how the clinical learning is structured. These will likely vary from course to course, consistent with and depending on the clinical environment, course goals, and learning objectives. Outlining elements of engagement is a self-management strategy that allows learners to nurture and monitor their own professional and personal growth and enables them to help set clear expectations for performance, which can become part of assessment and evaluation. These are important lessons in learning so that they can continuously monitor their experiential learning throughout their practice and careers.

Horton-Deutsch and Ironside (2010) provide an example of working with learners to create elements of engagement at the beginning of each course so learners are clear on expectations and develop their capacity for self-regulation. Although this example came from an academic setting, educators in clinical settings can easily adapt it to working with clinicians and developing guidelines for post-clinical conferences.

REFLECTING ON . . . THE ELEMENTS OF ENGAGEMENT

- *Be present and on time.*
- *One person speaks at a time and encourages asking questions.*
- *Listen with compassion and curiosity; ask for what you need and offer what you can.*
- *Each learner takes responsibility for his or her own learning.*
- *Share ideas and experiences.*
- *Articulate positive expectations.*
- *Encourage three practices: listen with attention, speak with intention, and contribute to the well-being of the group (Horton-Deutsch & Ironside, 2010).*

Asking learners to set their own expectations for clinical learning sets the tone for professional behavior, encourages learners to hold each other accountable for their learning, develops self-monitoring, and builds a partnership between educators (or preceptors) and learners. Talking specifically about elements of engagement reminds learners and educators of the shared responsibility for the learning environment. Educators often feel so conscientious about creating a productive learning environment that all the details of the course are developed in advance, so learners have the "received view" that does not take into account the unique needs of each learning group. By letting go of the tight control of the learning process and asking learners to participate in identifying and designing their learning experiences, educators further sustain and facilitate the learners' learning. This process encourages students to draw on their existing knowledge, ask questions, and identify their learning needs in relation to their practice, thereby actively engaging them in the process. Educators become coaches, guides, and facilitators rather than the person delivering content, setting standards, and holding all the answers.

Quality and Safety as a Clinical Domain for Reflection

Reflective learning is also consistent with the focus on competency development that is replacing content-based curricula (Benner, Sutphen, Leonard, & Day, 2010; Day & Sherwood, 2017b). Competencies are assessed through the specific knowledge, skills, and attitude objectives that define each. Learners can demonstrate their achievement of a competency as they reflect on how they plan to integrate the knowledge into their work and can reveal changes in attitudes as they discuss how they would change their actions in future situations.

The domain of competency development is exemplified through the national initiative Quality and Safety Education for Nurses (QSEN), which has guided extensive curricula updates to incorporate quality and safety competencies for both prelicensure and graduate learners (Cronenwett et al., 2007, 2009). These competencies, first identified by the Institute of Medicine (2003), encompass patient-centered care, safety, teamwork, quality improvement, evidence-based practice, and informatics (see Appendix B) and are easily accessed at www.qsen. org. It was through the work of QSEN that awareness surfaced of the need for faculty, learner, and clinician development to integrate reflective practices in academic and clinical settings (Cronenwett, Sherwood, & Gelmon, 2009).

Inviting students to reflective practice during a clinical rotation is well facilitated when the QSEN KSAs (knowledge, skills, and attitude objectives) are used as the basis for clinical evaluation. There are several examples in the literature of using QSEN KSAs as the basis for clinical evaluation tools (Altmiller,

2013, 2017). Table 10.1 provides examples for clinical reflection for learners based on exemplar QSEN skills and attitude elements.

Table 10.1 Quality and Safety Education for Nurses Attitude Element Prompts for Clinical Reflection

QSEN COMPETENCY	COMPETENCY ELEMENT	PROMPT FOR CLINICAL REFLECTION
Patient-Centered Care	Value the patient's expertise with own health and symptoms (Attitude)	• What observable behaviors in your practice demonstrate this attitude? • How do you balance the need for efficiency in your practice and the time/space for this attitude and corresponding behaviors? • Are there clinical situations where this attitude is in conflict with another practice value?
	Value continuous improvement of own communication and conflict resolution skills (Attitude)	• Consider nurses you have observed who role-model this attitude in their practice and describe what it looks like. • What are the difficult or uncomfortable aspects of this attitude? How does your own self-awareness help with the improvement process included in this attitude?
Safety	Demonstrate awareness of own strengths and limitations as a team member (Skills)	• How do clinicians demonstrate this skill? How would this look to his/her colleagues? • How does this skill facilitate healthy teamwork?
	Respect the unique	• How might you gain awareness of

continues

Table 10.1 (continued)

QSEN COMPETENCY	COMPETENCY ELEMENT	PROMPT FOR CLINICAL REFLECTION
	attributes that members bring to a team, including variations in professional orientations and accountabilities (Attitude)	the "variations in professional orientations and accountabilities" of colleagues on your healthcare team? Why is this important? • What examples have you observed of "respect" acted out on the healthcare team? How has this attitude enhanced team functioning (from a colleague perspective)? From a patient perspective?
Evidence-Based Practice	Question rationale for routine approaches to care that result in less than desired outcomes or adverse events (Skills)	• This skill requires individuals or teams to speak up. What are your observations of an individual's or a team's comfort with speaking up to question rationale for routine approaches that are ineffective? • As a nursing leader, how can you impact the culture of a microsystem so that individuals and teams feel free to speak up about ineffective care?
Quality Improvement	Appreciate that continuous quality improvement is an essential part of the daily work of all health professions (Attitude)	• How is this attitude promoted among nurse leaders? • What is your experience of the adoption of this attitude among all team members? • What are supporting and disabling factors for this attitude in the work processes or habits you have observed? How do you integrate this attitude as a core part of your nursing practice?

Other Tools to Enhance Clinical Reflection

Emotional intelligence (EI) is defined by self-awareness and self-monitoring, which are core elements of clinical growth. Reflective practice is an essential skill in developing EI. By self-monitoring feelings and emotions, learners gain the ability to discriminate among them and use the information to guide their thinking, action, and thus practice. Self-assessments encourage learners to reflect on their actions, whether in practice or in relation to others (Horton-Deutsch & Sherwood, 2008), all of which are part of EI. EI takes into account consciousness of self, others, and the situational context or environment. These are requisite skills for effective practice.

Self-assessments, especially about clinical experiences, encourage self-thinking and provide an opportunity for learners to explore and attend to feelings and attitudes, promoting their accountability. They raise awareness about what a learner might do in his/her practice to make better choices in the future. Educator-facilitated self-assessments use open-ended questioning to help develop this self-awareness. Self-assessments can be crafted to give an opportunity to safely make sense of both positive and negative emotions. Helping nurses establish the practice of self-assessment during their clinical education encourages them to continue this practice and incorporate it as part of lifelong professional development, particularly when working through challenging or complex clinical situations. Nurses then develop the capacity to step back and look at their practice from a broader perspective, to see a situation from each participant's point of view. They gain the ability to ask questions about themselves, a first step in change. Reflection leads to self-awareness of how they fit into the situational context and how well they are doing and being, which in turn leads to improved practice. Reflection is a transformational tool for individuals and their professional practice (Horton-Deutsch & Sherwood, 2008; Johns & Freshwater, 2005).

REFLECTING ON . . . REFLECTIVE SELF-ASSESSMENT

- *Describe: Relate the clinical event in an objective way.*

- *Appreciate: What went well?*

- *Personal growth: What about the clinical event made me feel clinically effective?*

- *Professional knowledge: What did I learn from this event to inform my knowledge, skills, attitudes, or practice?*

- *Ethical comportment: What values and attitudes influence my actions?*

- *Self-assess: How is this different from how I have acted in previous events?*

- *Transform: What can I apply in the future?*

Educators can use examples of self-assessment at the onset of a class or learning activity and at the end. To help learners mindfully engage at the outset, help them consider the purpose and goals for learning. Asking them to identify why they are participating can lead them to a more focused presence.

- Why am I here?

- What is my goal for learning?

- What commitment do I make to engage in learning to achieve my goals?

At the end of class, learning activity, or clinical rotation, self-assessment exercises deepen learners' capacity to continually assess their professional development, which fosters lifelong learning. Learners are thus encouraged to own accountability for their development. Learners may submit an online or written response to three questions:

1. In what ways did the class/activity or clinical experience address my expectations?

2. What did I learn?

3. How will I use what I learned in my practice?

These questions facilitate reflecting-before-action, -in-action, and afterward, -on-action.

The focus on task-orientation in clinical learning and practice (Henderson, Cooke, Creedy, & Walker, 2012) creates time and space for reflection, which is critical for debriefing. Group discussions among learners are one way to evaluate critical reflection. Post-clinical conferences as well as small group discussions can be designed for learners to explore case analysis from the varied ways of knowing, including empirical, ethical, personal, and aesthetic, as discussed in Chapter 1.

Creating Space for Reflection in Clinical Settings: Debriefing for Meaningful Learning

Within clinical settings, learners are provided the context to bridge the theory-practice gap. Clinical instructors can facilitate learners to bridge this gap by employing consistent methods of reflective practices. For example, Debriefing for Meaningful Learning (DML) is one way clinical instructors can promote meaningful learning, to help learners reflect on clinical experiences and, in fact, help learners begin to think like nurses as demonstrated through a change in clinical reasoning (Dreifuerst, 2012).

DML is a method of reflective debriefing that instructors apply with learners to revisit clinical experiences in the context of a structured and mindful dialogue. DML promotes clinical reasoning, a desired attribute in nurses, by guiding learners to actively reflect-in-action and reflect-on-action as described by Schön (1983) and reflect-beyond-action (Dreifuerst, 2009) through a process in which learners discover, reveal, and discuss the thinking and actions that occur during patient care. This mindful method of debriefing clinical experiences helps learners to develop a thinking presence that engages them in active inquiry and shapes their future actions and decisions through a deeper understanding of the clinical situation they just experienced. Particular attention is paid to the relationship between thinking and actions. Although right thinking-right action is the goal, through Socratic dialogue, instances of wrong thinking and right action or wrong action and right thinking are also evident and discussed. These discoveries provide an opportunity for learners to reveal the frames that underpin their thinking, especially about clinical contexts, and offer intentional occasions to fuse experiential learning with theoretical learning. Clinical teachers can use

Socratic questioning prompts and guided reflection to teach students to challenge taken-for-granted assumptions and discuss relationships between thinking and actions that impact patient care and outcomes (Dreifuerst, 2015).

In this way, DML teaches learners complex reasoning processes that encompass thinking like a nurse by making visible the nursing assessments, actions, and decisions in relation to the patient responses (Dreifuerst, 2015). Using this debriefing dialogue and structure, the instructor and learners mindfully reflect on the clinical experience together, make sense of it, and prepare for future clinical encounters by reflecting-beyond-action. DML helps learners to build upon what was learned from the current clinical situation using an iterative yet consistent six-step method based on the educational model (Bybee et al., 1989) to anticipate actions and clinical decisions within future clinical encounters.

THE E6 PROCESS

Engage *in the debriefing dialogue about the clinical situation.*

Evaluate *what went well and the challenges the student encountered, including correction of inappropriate interpretation, decisions, and actions.*

Explore *and review the experience from the perspective of the student and the faculty and experience thinking like a nurse through faculty-guided thinking-in-action and thinking-on-action.*

Explain *the patient care elements (assessment, planning, intervention, and evaluation) through concept mapping.*

Elaborate *on the knowledge, skills, and attitudes that were evident, as well as those that were missing.*

Extend *what was learned from this clinical experience to the next through guided anticipation and active assimilation or accommodation depending on how the clinical situation is framed by the faculty to prepare the student for thinking-beyond-action and decision-making while encountering a different yet conceptually similar clinical situation. (Dreifuerst, 2009)*

DML also uses theoretical underpinnings from constructivism and the Reflective Cycle (Gibbs, 1988). Gibbs' Reflective Cycle is a circular representation of the elements of reflection, including a description of what happened, with specific attention to participant feelings, evaluation of the experience, and identification of what was good and bad. This is followed by a period of analysis and sense-making of the experience, determination of conclusions from the experience with particular consideration of alternative actions, and, finally, contemplation of an action plan should the experience occur again.

The following are two examples of student comments after using DML:

- "The students verbalized that the DML concept of thinking-in-action enabled critical reflection in the moment and allowed students the chance to advance their thinking during clinical experience instead of waiting until post-conference to discover what could be done differently next time. 'We look at it together and learn from it and move forward in post-conference, and now I can do that myself or with my instructor during the clinical day. It doesn't hinder my performance or confidence level for the rest of the day.' As the semester progressed, the students recognized how the DML model influenced their own critical reflection and mindfulness. They collectively agreed with one student's statement: 'I started assessing my own performance in real time throughout the day, recognizing what I was doing right or what I needed to improve upon.'"

- "After using DML to guide post-conference for a semester, students reflected on how its use enhanced their learning and helped them to be more mindful, thinking-on-action. Debriefing allowed students to share the highs and lows of the clinical day, and DML facilitated students to think conceptually about what they were walking away with at the end of each clinical experience. They verbalized, 'It (DML) helped us think about thinking in context' and 'recognize what's happening in the clinical setting based on what we had experienced before and could anticipate would come next, even if the circumstances were different, because we practiced that kind of thinking.'"

Allowing Reflection to Inform Evaluation

Educational approaches based on reflection have been explored throughout this book; this chapter explores how to integrate these approaches into students' formative and summative clinical assessments and evaluative feedback. Other examples in the literature illustrate the challenges and opportunities in using various reflective assignments to engage learners in developing reflective practice (Burns & Bulman, 2000; Esterhuizen, Freshwater, & Sherwood, 2008; Horton-Deutsch & Ironside, 2010; Horton-Deutsch, McNelis, & O'Haver Day, 2012; Horton-Deutsch & Sherwood, 2008). Educators can inspire learners to use their reflective lens to constantly combine analysis of their experiences with the goals and standards of care to improve their work, and ultimately their practice.

There are varied perspectives on assessing reflective assignments. Grading associated with reflective assignments is usually limited, although learners want regular formative feedback. Rubrics are a helpful way to offer feedback to learners so that they are able to write deeper, more direct reflections and apply evidence to how they are thinking about their practice. As such, reflective writing becomes a dialogue between educator and learner: The learner writes according to the assignment; the educator responds with additional questions for helping think through the next event, and so on. In this back-and-forth written dialogue, educator and learner mutually learn and grow. Effective prompts for clinical reflection are offered in Chapter 2.

Rubrics are particularly helpful in assessing online assignments and fostering development of the relationship between educator and learner. Pesut adapted a rubric by Bauer (2002) to evaluate learner participation in an online leadership course. Learners were given the following knowledge work questions for reflecting on their readings each week. The following framework guided weekly feedback.

- What concepts, theories, models, tools, techniques, and resources in the week's assigned readings did you find most valuable?

- How might you use this information in your practice?

- Why is the information important to your practice?

- How will the knowledge improve your effectiveness as a clinician?

- How does the knowledge and information help you understand the interdependence of system dynamics in terms of context, relationships, and trends?

- Why care about the knowledge? How does it help you clarify values and manage professional purpose?

- How does the knowledge gained advance your achievement of the nursing program outcomes and support your mastery of the essentials for preparation as a registered nurse?

- What other thoughts, reflections, or significant learning have influenced your personal and/or professional development these past few weeks?

- Create and pose a question of your own design to the members of your learning circle. Answer at least one question posed by a colleague in your learning circle.

New paradigms for learner-centered approaches in contemporary higher education create new challenges for assessment and evaluation. A review of the literature reveals increasing use of reflective assignments in nursing, yet there is little guidance on how to shift from traditional objective evaluation (judgment) and assessment (level of competence) to more appropriate methods that match the reflective philosophy. An appreciative philosophy applied to assessment and evaluation of learners is consistent with current views in higher education that balance the learner and educator relationship for mutual learning. Using power in a wise and just manner creates credibility and demonstrates fair assessment practices, which are at the heart of the pedagogic role in evaluation.

Reflective learning is predicated on openness between learner and educator; as such, educators need to pay greater attention to fairness and the exercise of academic power by being open to discussions on fair assessments, knowing when to be flexible on timelines, and adjudicating in disputes between students working in groups (Macfarlane, 2004). Reflective learning reduces the hierarchy between learners and educators by opening the dialogue for continuously analyzing and reframing learning goals. The focus shifts from achieving objectives to assessing how well learners are able to internalize what is learned and translate changes into practice behavior.

Assessing Reflective Work

Clear criteria for a reflective assignment enable learners to understand expectations and thus have a more meaningful reflective experience. These criteria should recognize the complex nature of practice, and they should not be rigid, but open and fluid for modification in meeting the needs of the learner and recognizing the complex nature of practice. The act of co-creating helps learners continue to think about the topic in new ways. Teachers can ask, "In this assignment, how would I know if you understood all that you needed to know?" If learners are struggling, teachers can ask probing questions to stimulate thinking, such as the importance of alternative possibilities. Learners feel empowered when they are asked to co-create and engage in dialogue about learning expectations.

Burns and Bulman (2000) identified four potential outcomes of reflection which can be reframed to assess if the learner: 1) developed a new perspective on experience; 2) changed behavior; 3) achieved readiness for application; and 4) committed to action. These four outcomes, which can be cognitive and affective in nature, can also be the foundation for developing a rubric.

Clark (2011) proposes a set of reflective questions for educators to ask in setting expectations for evaluation of learner activities that can be used in didactic or clinical learning experiences:

- Does the learner seek alternatives?

- Does the learner view the experience from various perspectives?

- Does the learner seek a framework, theoretical basis, or underlying rationale (of behaviors, methods, techniques, programs)?

- Does the learner compare and contrast?

- Does the learner put the experience into different or varied contexts?

- Does the student ask, "What if . . .?"

- Does the learner consider consequences?

These prompts are particularly effective for clinical reflection, because cognitive agility is often the hallmark of an effective clinician. Innovative assessment strategies include narratives, unfolding cases, simulation, focus groups, rubrics, reflection-on-action, and Appreciative Inquiry. Following a specific reflective model or guide can offer structure to reflective learning activities. Kirkpatrick (1995) developed a model using four levels of assessment that moves away from the focus on learner satisfaction and places greater emphasis on performance and impact and can include open-ended reflective questions:

- Level 1, Reaction: How did participants react to the learning experience?

- Level 2, Learning: To what extent did learners improve knowledge and skills and improve attitudes as a result of the learning experience?

- Level 3, Behavior: To what extent have learners changed how they do their work?

- Level 4, Results: What is the benefit of the learning?

Each level provides an assessment checkpoint and illustrates the usefulness of evaluating student progress at each level. All levels are important for effective and safe practice and are best accomplished with a variety of assessment methods. Where objective measures might not illustrate the nuances of a student's development, reflective journals or rubrics for reflection might reveal progress of the learner's development through Kirkpatrick's four levels. For example, if the learner did not gain the knowledge needed (Level 2), the reactions at Level 1 will reveal the barriers to learning. If learners do not use the skills gained in their work situations (Level 3), then they might not have actually achieved the skills in the first place (Level 2).

REFLECTING ON . . . USING THE FOUR LEVELS OF ASSESSMENT

How can educators determine learner achievement based on the four levels of assessment using unfolding case studies?

A Reflective Approach to Student Evaluations of Courses

In conventional pedagogy, student evaluation questionnaires are the principal means by which the quality of teaching/learning is gathered from students, typically at the end of the semester. Ideally, a variety of methods should be deployed for evaluating and reflecting on the quality of clinical teaching/learning. In an appreciative learning environment, learners are given the opportunity to provide ongoing evaluative feedback of their learning in all settings. This information is taken into consideration by educators, who then have the opportunity to immediately adjust learning activities to better meet the needs of learners. Appreciative questions that aid in ongoing evaluation of learners learning include:

- What went well for you in class (clinical) today?

- What do you want more of?

- What, if anything, is frustrating you?

- What are you still worried about?

This form of formative evaluation from students not only provides valuable feedback to teachers and preceptors, but it also further engages students in reflective practice. It encourages both students and clinical educators to adopt an open attitude and invest effort in the improvement of practice. It encourages an open learning partnership in which both students and teachers remain open to criticism and new ideas. It provides teachers and preceptors an opportunity to genuinely listen and act where appropriate, not submit unreflectively. Most importantly, when implemented with an appreciative stance, it promotes open and rigorous dialogue between students and teachers.

> **REFLECTING ON . . . APPLYING APPRECIATIVE INQUIRY TO COURSE ASSESSMENT OR LEARNING ACTIVITY**
>
> - *What gave energy to this learning activity, course, or clinical rotation?*
> - *What made it come alive for you?*
> - *What were the most successful experiences you had in this course, rotation, or activity?*
> - *What was happening?*
> - *Who was involved?*
> - *What did they do?*
> - *What was your role?*

Final Reflections

This chapter examined the way that reflective learning can enhance clinical education models. Incorporating reflective learning into clinical collaboration, clinical learning, and clinical assessment can change both educator and learner. Reflection itself is asking questions about what happened. By consciously adding an evaluative framework, learners develop the habit of continuously monitoring their work to establish lifelong learning. Applying principles of Appreciative Inquiry, Kirkpatrick's evaluation model, and reflective self-assessment to clinical education can stimulate changes in how learners grow into self-aware, reflective clinicians who can continue to grow and respond to a complex healthcare system.

References

Altmiller, G. (2013). Application of the quality and safety education for nurses competencies in orthopaedic nursing: Implications for preceptors. *Orthopaedic Nursing, 32*(2), 98–103.

Altmiller, G. (2017). Content validation of a quality and safety education for nurses-based clinical evaluation instrument. *Nurse Educator, 42*(1), 23–27. Advance online publication. Retrieved from https://www.ncbi.nlm.nih.gov/pubmed/27490313

Bauer, J. F. (2002). Assessing student work from chat rooms and bulletin boards. In R. S. Anderson, J. F. Bauer, & B. W. Speck (Eds.), *Assessment strategies for the on-line class: From theory to practice* (pp. 31–36). San Francisco, CA: Jossey Bass.

Benner, P., Sutphen, M., Leonard, V., & Day, L. (2010). *Educating nurses: A call for radical transformation.* Stanford, CA: Jossey-Bass.

Bulman, C., & Schutz, S. (2005). *Reflective practice in nursing* (3rd ed.). London, UK: Blackwell.

Burns, S., & Bulman, C. (2000). *Reflective practice in nursing: The growth of the professional practitioner* (2nd ed.). Oxford, UK: Blackwell Science.

Bybee, R., Buchwald, C., Crissman, S., Heil, D., Kucrbis, P., Matsumoto, C., & McInerney, J. (1989). *Science and technology education for the elementary years: Frameworks for curriculum and instruction.* Andover, MA: The National Center for Improving Science Education.

Clark, D. R. (2011). Learning through reflection. Retrieved from http://www.nwlink. com/~donclark/hrd/development/reflection.html

Cooperrider, D., & Whitney, D. (2005). *Appreciative Inquiry: A positive revolution in change.* San Francisco, CA: Berrett-Koehler.

Cronenwett, L., Sherwood, G., Barnsteiner, J., Disch, J., Johnson, J., Mitchell, P., . . . Warren, J. (2007). Quality and safety education for nurses. *Nursing Outlook, 55*(3), 122–131.

Cronenwett, L., Sherwood, G., & Gelmon, S. (2009). Improving quality and safety education: The QSEN Learning Collaborative. *Nursing Outlook, 57*(6), 304–312.

Cronenwett, L., Sherwood, G., Pohl, J., Barnsteiner, J., Moore, S., Sullivan, D. T., . . . Warren, J. (2009). Quality and safety education for advanced nursing practice. *Nursing Outlook, 57*(6), 338–334.

Day, L., & Sherwood, G. (2017a). Transforming education to transform practice: Using unfolding case studies to integrate quality and safety in subject centered classrooms. In G. Sherwood & J. Barnsteiner (Eds.), *Quality and safety in nursing: A competency approach to improving outcomes* (2nd ed.) (pp. 199–220). Hoboken, NJ: Wiley-Blackwell.

Day, L., & Sherwood, G. (2017b). Quality and safety in clinical learning environments. In G. Sherwood & J. Barnsteiner (Eds.), *Quality and safety in nursing: A competency approach to improving outcomes* (2nd ed.) (pp. 253–263). Hoboken, NJ: Wiley-Blackwell.

Dreifuerst, K. T. (2009). The essentials of debriefing in simulation learning: A concept analysis. *Nursing Education Perspectives, 30*(2), 109–114.

Dreifuerst, K. T. (2012). Using debriefing for meaningful learning to foster development of clinical reasoning in simulation. *Journal of Nursing Education, 51*(6), 326–333. doi:10.3928/01484834-20120409-0

Dreifuerst, K. T. (2015). Getting started with debriefing for meaningful learning. *Clinical Simulation in Nursing, 11*(5), 268–275. doi:10.1016/j.ecns.2015.01.00

Esterhuizen, P., Freshwater, D., & Sherwood, G. (2008). Developing a reflective curriculum. In D. Freshwater, B. Taylor, & G. Sherwood (Eds.), *International textbook of reflective practice in nursing* (pp. 177–196). Oxford, UK: Blackwell Publishing.

Gibbs, G. (1988). *Learning by doing: A guide to teaching and learning methods.* Oxford, UK: Oxford Polytechnic.

Henderson, A., Cooke, M., Creedy, D. K., & Walker, R. (2012). Nursing students' perception of learning in practice environments: A review. *Nurse Education Today, 32,* 299–302.

Horton-Deutsch, S., & Ironside, P. (2010). Learning module 6: Teaching patient-centered care using narrative and reflective pedagogies. Retrieved from http://qsen.org/courses/learning-modules/module-six/

Horton-Deutsch, S., McNelis, A., & O'Haver Day, P. (2012). Developing a reflection-centered curriculum for graduate psychiatric nursing education. *Archives of Psychiatric Nursing, 26*(5), 341–349. doi:10.1016/j.apnu.2011.09.006

Horton-Deutsch, S., & Sherwood, G. (2008). Reflection: An educational strategy to develop emotionally competent nurse leaders. *Journal of Nursing Management, 16*(8), 946–954.

Institute of Medicine (IOM). (2003). *Health professions education: A bridge to quality.* Washington, DC: The National Academies Press.

Johns, C., & Freshwater, D. (2005). *Transforming nursing through reflective practice* (2nd ed.). Oxford, UK: Blackwell.

Kirkpatrick, D. (1995). *Another look at evaluating training programs.* Alexandria, VA: ASTD.

Macfarlane, B. (2004). *Teaching with integrity: The ethics of higher education.* New York, NY: RoutledgeFalmer.

Pesut, D. J., & Herman, J. (1999). *Clinical reasoning: The art and science of critical and creative thinking*. Albany, NY: Delmar Publishers.

Schön, D. A. (1983). *The reflective practitioner: How professionals think in action*. New York, NY: Basic Books.

Shulman, L. (2002). Making a difference: A table of learning. *Change, 34*(6), 36–44.

Part IV

Deepening the Foundations of Professional Practice Through Reflection

Chapter 11
Attention to Self as Nurse: Caring for Patients, Caring for Self, Making Sense of Practice

–Gwen D. Sherwood, PhD, RN, FAAN, ANEF
–Sara Horton-Deutsch, PhD, RN, FAAN, ANEF
–Cheryl Woods Giscombe, PhD, RN, PNMNP-BC
–With Learning Activity by Cheryl Giscombe

As professionals, nurses are in a constant state of metamorphosis. By the very definition of nursing as the response to the diagnosis and treatment of human beings, the practice of nursing is influenced by society, economics, and political attitudes and events that are continually evolving. Because we care for human beings in all their dimensions, nursing then is more than a rational practice based on exploding scientific evidence; it carries an emotional labor as well, melding affective and empirical rationalities. Immersed daily in the drama of human lives and intervening in lives during times of vulnerability, how do nurses internally process events in their work so they sustain their own capacity for care, compassion, love, listening, acting, and responding even while continually building their own personal and professional development?

Reconnecting to our disciplinary roots through Caring Science serves as a moral-philosophical-theoretical foundation and a meaningful way to sustain the profession. When nursing, or any health profession, is grounded in the consciousness and clarity of Caring Science, it is clear that a relational ontology that honors the connectedness and belonging of all living things moves humanity closer to a moral community where we care for self and others; evidence has linked a focus on biomedical-technical science alone to over-emphasis on a separatist worldview that contributes to task orientation and behaviors often labeled noncaring (Watson, 2016). The integration of Caring Science in the discipline of nursing promotes interpersonal practice that complements Caring Science and thus transforms healthcare to a relational way of being that sustains our shared humanity.

> *"Registered nurse turnover in most countries is a serious economic issue in the healthcare industry, because nurses are necessary for the operation of almost every healthcare setting and constitute the largest group of employees. The loss of human capacity through emotional drain, however, is not measured in economic terms only."*

The increasingly complex practice environment requires evidence-based decisions to manage care. Nurses have a compelling need for an empirical knowledge base for practice, yet content overload in many curricula suppresses the opportunity to develop reflective and critical thinking skills to balance evidence with person-centered care needs. Reflection can be the first step in the evidence-based nursing process for weighing the evidence itself, making the crucial decision to honor patients' values and beliefs even in the light of evidence, or allowing answerable questions to surface to improve care (Ireland, 2008). To develop learners who become users of all forms of evidence, nurse educators must nurture habits of the mind that cultivate reflection in and on a practice within a person-centered framework. This framework puts people, their families, and communities at the center of care and decisions, seeing them as the experts working alongside healthcare professionals toward the desired outcome.

This is imperative because empirical knowledge alone cannot answer certain questions about humanity (people, families, communities) and what it means to care, to be human. Overall, conventional science is not concerned with specific individual responses and "does not offer insights into the depth of human experiences such as pain, joy, suffering, fear, forgiveness, love and so on. Such an in-depth exploration of humanity is expressed and pondered through the study of philosophy, drama and the arts, film, literature, humanistic studies in the liberal arts, humanities proper, and so on. This perspective is learned through self-knowledge, self-discovery, and shared human experiences, combined with the study of human emotions and relations that mirror our shared humanity" (Watson, 2008, p. 20).

Finding a balance of rational thinking with caring ideals in the real world of practice is critical to avoid burnout, a common cause of nurses changing jobs or leaving nursing altogether. Dissatisfaction often results from working in controlling environments that stifle questioning and limit the ability to find the balance within the rational and affective dimensions, to learn coping skills to make sense of the intensity of working with human beings, and to resolve frustrations from the gap between theory and actual practice. The cost of formal nursing education plus lengthy orientation to achieve proficiency in the transition to practice is a staggering waste when nurses leave the profession after a short tenure. Registered nurse turnover in most countries is a serious economic issue in the healthcare industry (Aiken, Clarke, & Sloane, 2012), because nurses are necessary for the operation of almost every healthcare setting and constitute the largest group of employees. The loss of human capacity through emotional drain, however, is not measured in economic terms only.

This chapter explores the importance of "attention to self as nurse"—the importance of continually finding restoration from the heavy work demands situated in a complex environment and systematically working to make sense of practice events in sustainable ways that help develop professional expertise to lead to improved care. The first section, "Making Sense of Practice," focuses on learning to think like a nurse as described in Tanner's Model of Clinical Judgment, explores how reflective practice helps develop clinical reasoning, and integrates multiple ways of knowing to contribute to an evidence base for practice.

The second part of the chapter, "Attending to Self as Nurse," focuses on attention to self as nurse through reflective practices in developing emotional intelligence (EI), mindful practice, Appreciative Inquiry (AI), and other forms of development that cultivate gratitude and loving-kindness toward self and others. The last section, "Bringing It Together: Professional Development Strategies," describes innovative ways to attend to self, for—to coin a phrase—"who we are is who we bring to practice." Later in this chapter, Cheryl Woods Giscombe describes an example of developing an institutional wellness program to channel nurses' application of reflective practices for self-care. In the integration of multiple perspectives, nurses develop clinical reasoning that builds a professional practice model, and they find sustenance and renewal to provide care for self and others in making sense of the complexities of their work.

Making Sense of Practice

Nurses are continually evolving. Nurses learn and grow throughout their careers as a mark of professionalism. The radical transformation of nursing education demands that dynamics of clinical practice be more fully integrated into didactic learning. Nurses often experience a shock when they move from the structured academic environment to the complex clinical environment. Day and Sherwood (2017a) describe ways to develop formal and informal learning gained from professional experience; the spirit of inquiry begins in the classroom through clinically focused learning that builds on reflective practices. Habits of questioning help nurses continually examine and develop insights into the real-world nurse role and ease the transition to practice. Content-based formal learning helps develop knowledge and skills, but nurses still must assimilate the norms, values, and attitudes that guide "thinking like a nurse" and help make sense of practice, and simultaneously develop their own self-care practices.

Developing Competence and Confidence to Think Like a Nurse

Nursing is a complex set of interactions, not only with patients and families but also with other members of the caregiving team. Nursing is characterized as a caring practice that is based on science but guided by the moral art and ethics of care and responsibility. Professional practice is based on melding multiple types of knowledge and multiple applications in practice. The complexity manifests in the need to adapt to evolving situations, participate in interprofessional teams, and work with patients and families from multiple cultures with differing health beliefs and values. During their academic education, nurses are taught ideal practice, but are they also taught how to cope with realities of practice that often do not match the textbook portrayal? How do nurses deal with contradictions in practice? Decision-making in nursing is not simply an objective, detached exercise; instead, nurses call on multiple ways of knowing to consider both objective science undergirding evidence of care standards, and knowing how and when to make exceptions to individualize care for a particular patient and family—a critical thinking process.

This relationship-centered moral and ethical view of nursing recognizes the "privileged place of nursing." Expert nurses describe this as the trust inherent in the caregiving relationship. In examining how expert nurses think, give care, and make a difference in patients' lives, Benner and Wrubel (1989) describe nurses' engagement and mindfulness in making care decisions based on knowing the individual patient. Their description of this "privileged place of practice" is quite different from the biomedical view that often dominates education and practice. Expert nurses have learned how to integrate knowledge of the anatomy of an illness combined with taking the time to understand what it means in the patient's experience; this process illustrates reflecting in- and on-action to provide patient-centered expert care (Walton & Barnsteiner, 2017).

How do nurses develop along the continuum from novice to an expert with a higher level of understanding practice? Novice nurses often feel disconnected or out of place because they do not yet fully understand the scope of their work with real patients. Learners and novice nurses are often more concerned about performance of technical skills and may have difficulty adapting what they learned in class and the skills-learning lab into care of a real patient. Novice nurses feel pressed to demonstrate their skill know-how; they often believe this can help them begin to feel comfortable in the work environment and gain acceptance as team members.

Indeed it is important for nurses to experience confidence in their technical skills to gain confidence and expand their awareness of the environment, appreciate the relevance of their actions in the overall care of the patient, and contribute as full members of the care team (Dearmin, 2000). Educators can explore other learning strategies that realign classroom and skills-lab learning so the subject focus is the patient; interactive, case-based learning may help speed the process of integrating content with practice-based situations (Day & Sherwood, 2017a). Reflective practice skills to make sense of practice take time to develop, and still nurses have to develop confidence in the technical aspects of care to begin to feel competent to meld objective and subjective knowing to understand the context of the patient's illness experience and develop trust in their decision-making. Reflection can be a valuable asset in the sense-making process and in approaching patient care with a sense of what is right and honoring the "privileged place of nursing."

Developing Clinical Judgment to Move Toward Expert Practice

The practice of nursing is based on reasoning through a process of analysis, recognizing, and then making decisions determined by existing knowledge applied to a particular situation (Benner, Kyriakidis, & Stannard, 2011). Understanding how nurses perform their work is a critical aspect of nurse development from novice to expert; integrating our multiple types of knowledge with our evolving experiences informs how we develop as practitioners. As nurses gain experience, they begin to develop practical or tacit knowledge— learning from everyday experience—that allows continuous adjustment and refinement of textbook knowledge.

Tanner (2006) examined the reasoning process nurses use to make clinical decisions, which she called *clinical judgment*. More than just applying a standardized set of actions for a given condition, clinical judgment is a more complex set of professional thinking skills. It is the "interpretation or conclusion about a patient's needs, concerns, or health problems" (Tanner, 2006, p. 205). It involves the decision on how or what action to take, using or modifying standard approaches, or improvising according to the patient's situation. Clinical judgment is more than objective knowledge; nurses bring knowledge from other experiences, what they know about the patient, their understanding of the context in which practice occurs, and the cultural dynamics of the nursing unit (Benner, 1984; Benner, Tanner, & Chesla, 1996; Tanner, 2006).

The Model of Clinical Judgment considers the human factors of the situation, taking into account the nurse's background, the situational context, and the nurse-patient relationship as central to how and what nurses notice, how they interpret findings to determine their response, and how they reflect on their responses. The nurse self is thus an important part of practice, and our development as a nurse is critical for how we make clinical judgments and make sense of practice.

REFLECTING ON . . . THE MODEL OF CLINICAL JUDGMENT

Developed by Tanner (2006), the Model of Clinical Judgment is a model of clinical judgment for nurses based on a form of engaged moral reasoning that guides nurses to think like a nurse based on four processes:

- **Noticing:** *Begins with a perceptual grasp of the situation*
- **Interpreting:** *Developing sufficient understanding to respond*
- **Responding:** *Deciding on what to do appropriate to the situation*
- **Reflecting:** *Attending to the patient's responses while caring for them and assessing the outcomes afterward*

Tanner includes both reflection-in-action and reflection-on-action as major components of how nurses develop clinical judgment. Reflection-in-action refers to how well the nurse assesses the patient response in the moment of practice; care is grounded in patient-centeredness in which nurses adjust their response to how the patient is responding. The ability to move back and forth in these responses develops tacit knowledge, the practical knowledge to know what to do in given situations beyond simply rational, objective knowledge. Reflection-on-action teases out what nurses learn from experience that contributes to ongoing knowledge development and influences future practice.

Nurses will always face judgment calls in situations of uncertainty; how nurses learn to deal with uncertainty is part of the evolution to expert practitioner by viewing every situation as an opportunity to learn. This openness and inquisitiveness develops within a supportive environment, one that encourages examination of context to reinforce the habit and skill for reflective learning and personal engagement. Reflective engagement in the Clinical Judgment Model derives from a sense of responsibility to connect actions with outcomes; building evidence-based practice requires knowing what occurred as a result of nursing actions (Nielson, Stragnell, & Jester, 2007).

The Model of Clinical Judgment helps build a spirit of inquiry for continued learning, a habit of the mind critical to professional practice. Developing clinical judgment replaces sole reliance on nursing processes based on standardized nursing diagnosis categories and embraces inclusive language across professions. Tanner (2006) argues that clinical judgment develops reasoning patterns that are more complex than the linear thinking displayed in the traditional nursing process; clinical judgment is influenced by the nurse's background, context for decision-making, and the nurse-patient relationship. To guide educators in helping learners develop clinical thinking, Lasater and Nielsen (2009) developed a *guide for reflection* based on the Clinical Judgment Model as well as a rubric for assessment. Day and Sherwood (2017b) pose strategies for transforming traditional pedagogy with subject-centered classrooms—in which patients are the center—to reframe how learners organize and analyze what they know to apply to real-world situations in ways that consider the full dimensions of care.

Knowing and Navigating the Context of Practice

The difficulty of making sense of practice is compounded by the context in which practice takes place, yet sense-making is critical to how nurses process care experiences and find satisfaction in work (Benner et al., 1996; Benner, Sutphen, Leonard, & Day, 2010; Ebright, Patterson, Chalko, & Render, 2003). The nursing practice environment has a social embeddedness expressed in the unit culture and work routines, the formal and informal way that work gets completed (Sherwood, 2003). New nurses on the unit might find it difficult to absorb both the social and political contexts that exist. To adapt to working in such complex situations, nurses must use a variety of reasoning patterns, including:

- The analytic, to separate the whole into its parts and to study the parts and its relations

- The intuitive, to embrace instinctive and unconscious knowing

- Narrative thinking, to incorporate the patterns and idiosyncrasies of the patient's story

Analytic and intuitive thinking might employ reflection-in-action, whereas narrative thinking relies on reflection-on-action. Helping learners improve clinical reasoning involves the multiple conditions of developing the skills and habits of reflection but, importantly, within a supportive environment (Johns, 2016; Kuiper, Pesut, & Arms, 2016). Novice nurses might find the multiple aspects of practice confusing and difficult to integrate into a practice framework that makes sense to them (Forneris & Peden-McAlpine, 2006). To instill the habit of inquiry, having nurses continually questioning through reflection-on-action can help them determine outcomes of work events by asking questions such as the following:

- What did I do?

- What should I have done that I did not do?

- How would I act differently? What could I do next time?

Dearmin (2000) includes an exemplar on the value of reflection to make sense of practice through a way to handle the stress of a particularly difficult day at work. Nurses can use reflection to sort out "the good and the bad bits of the day and the whole situation" (p. 163) and to integrate the evidence derived from research on which to base interventions. "Rather than just do things," it is "integrating research, theory and practice. If I am not happy about a certain way of doing something, I'll go read about it, get the research, talk to people and question things rather [than just do it without a reason]. It [reflection] was helpful because it proved to me that I did know what I was doing and I did have the skills and knowledge to handle the situation . . . " (Dearmin, 2000, p. 163).

Attending to Self as Nurse

Nursing is a value-laden profession. When our work is consistent with our values, we find inner reward and meaning to our lives. The dissonance that comes when our work is incongruent with our values robs us of the joy of meaningful work and diminishes our emotional energy. Who we are is who we bring to practice; making sense of practice is guided by how well we attend to ourselves as person and nurse. Our actions are guided by our internal compass (Freshwater, 2008). Self-development to stay true to our internal compass helps manage the emotional work inherent in nursing. Reflective practice is a key to manage self-care, develop leadership capacity, improve responses through emotional intelligence, develop mindfulness to engage in work activities, and thus improve safety outcomes. It also supports being an authentic and caring nurse deeply rooted in one's values, finding one's voice, and having the courage to lead (Horton-Deutsch, 2016).

Engaging in Self-Care

Nurses are often challenged by attempts to balance their own personal health and wellness with their dedication, commitment, and passion in their work to improve the lives of others by engaging in practice, research, and education. Nurses have disproportionately high rates of emotional distress and depression compared to the general population (Letvak, Ruhm, & McCoy, 2012). Distress, depression, and burnout often result from the challenging work environment and culture, as well as challenges with prioritizing self-care. Distress and burnout among nurses have been associated with compassion fatigue, poor sleep quality, trouble concentrating, limitations in performing mental or interpersonal tasks, time management challenges, workplace bullying, lower productivity, absenteeism, increased turnover, and compromised quality of care provision and quality of life (Bjorvatn et al., 2012; Drury, Francis, & Chapman, 2008; Ekici & Beder, 2014; Hegney et al., 2014; Jenkins & Elliott, 2004; Sherring & Knight, 2009). In addition, research conducted over the past 20 years on nurse burnout demonstrates that *modifiable* factors associated with increased burnout include negative perceptions of support and value in the workplace, inadequate academic preparedness to meet professional challenges, inadequate coping skills, and interactions with co-workers who are experiencing significant emotional demands (Fagin et al., 1996; Hannigan, Edwards, Coyle, Fothergill, & Burnard, 2000; Sherring & Knight, 2009).

In fact, as early as 1996, Fagin and colleagues (1996) identified the need to validate ways to reduce the impact of work-related stressors on nurses and identify best strategies for delivering stress-management interventions. Workplaces are now focusing on strategies to improve quality of life among nurses through workplace wellness and mindfulness-based strategies to enhance coping and self-care. Participating in wellness activities, such as mindfulness-based stress reduction (MBSR), is associated with reduction in stress, improved coping, and better empathy among nurses and nursing students. More specifically, nurses and nursing students who participated in mindfulness courses reported improvements in well-being, relaxation, life and job satisfaction, feelings of personal accomplishment and coping skills and reductions in anxiety, stress, perceptions of time pressure, emotional exhaustion, and burnout symptoms (Bazarko, Cate, Azocar, & Kreitzer, 2013; Beddoe & Murphy, 2004; Mackenzie, Poulin, & Seidman-Carlson, 2006).

Nurses report they improve their patience, presence, and caring; develop greater ability to engage in self-care; and enhance their ability to react less and look at the big picture more when solving problems, stating, "I'm much more aware of my feelings and thoughts during stressful events," and, "I'm much clearer in my statements of my own needs" (Cohen-Katz, Wiley, Capuano, Baker, & Shapiro, 2005, p. 82). Still, we lack focused strategies on how to optimally, broadly, and sustainably translate these research findings into practice to develop a culture of wellness in healthcare settings that we know can contribute to patient outcomes (Letvak, 2013).

Developing Self-Awareness and Mindful Practice

Reflection helps develop self-awareness, an essential aspect of emotional intelligence (Freshwater, 2002; Horton-Deutsch & Sherwood, 2008; Sherwood & Horton-Deutsch, 2008). Reflection provides insights into behavior and

EMOTIONAL INTELLIGENCE

The ability to monitor our own and others' feelings and emotions, to discriminate among them, and to use this information to guide thinking and actions.

responses and contributes to self-management and self-improvement by examining relationships with self and others. It encourages the spirit of inquiry as an important link to quality care.

Horton-Deutsch and Horton (2003) cited mindfulness as the basic social process for working through difficult situations. Mindfulness allows individuals to become fully aware of perceptual experiences (O'Haver Day & Horton-Deutsch, 2004). This fully engaged yet detached stance enables mindful responses, rather than habitual behaviors that might perpetuate and intensify situations, much like the reflection required in developing emotional intelligence, empathy, and openness (Vitello-Cicciu, 2002). Through a sense of openness and curiosity about our experience, mindfulness leads to greater awareness and insight. Similarly, reflection-in-action involves paying attention to our moment-to-moment experience, including thoughts, feelings, bodily sensations, and judgments. Reflection-in-action and mindfulness help nurses develop insight into how perceptions shape actions, identify and understand other people's standpoints, and incorporate this knowledge into more deliberate and effective responses.

In essence, reflective and mindful practices serve to guide personal and professional growth, teaching one to consciously care for self while simultaneously pursuing professional goals. These two aspects of a person begin to merge. We no longer have a sense of separateness between our personal and professional lives; it becomes a way of being (Horton-Deutsch, 2016).

Cultivating the Practice of Loving-Kindness Toward Self and Others

Humanistic-altruistic values lay the foundation for caring, and Caring Science emphasizes a set of universal values including kindness, concern, and love for self and others (Watson, 2008). As nurses mature through reflective and mindful practices, they are able to cultivate an awareness and intentionality to sustain a guided vision for life and work. The practice of loving-kindness toward self and others honors the gift of being able to give and receive with a capacity to love and appreciate all of life's diversity and the individuality of each person. These emotions and experiences are the essence of what makes us human and what deepens our humanity and connection with the human spirit. This awareness connects us to our source, breath, the gift of life, and where we access energy and creativity for living and being. Through this process, we let go of the ego-self and recognize that we all belong to the universe of humanity and all living things.

Centering exercises are one way to cultivate loving-kindness and equanimity for self and others. These exercises serve as a starting point and an ongoing guide for sustaining caring-healing practices throughout our day. Table 11.1 provides a guide for setting intentionality and consciousness of caring and healing.

TABLE 11.1 Touchstones for Caring (Jean Watson © 2002)

Caring in the Beginning

- Begin the day with a silent gratitude; set your intentions to be open to give and receive all that you are here to give and receive this day; intend to bring your full self, in the day-to-day moments of this day; cultivating a loving, caring consciousness toward yourself and others who enter your path.

Caring in the Middle

- Take quiet moments to "center," to empty out, to be still with yourself before entering a patient's room or when entering a meeting; cultivate a loving-caring consciousness toward each person and each situation you encounter throughout the day; make an effort "to see" who the spirit-filled person is behind the patient/colleague.

continues

TABLE 11.1 (continued)

- Return to these loving-centered intentions again and again, throughout the day, helping yourself to remember why you are here.

- In the middle of stressful moments, remember to breathe; ask for guidance when unsure, confused, and frightened; forgive and bless each situation.

- Let go of that which you cannot control.

Caring in the End

- At the end of the day, fold these intentions into your heart; commit yourself to cultivating a loving-caring practice for yourself.

- Use whatever has presented itself to you this day as lessons to teach you to grow more deeply into your own humanity and inner wisdom.

- At the end of the day, offer gratitude for all that has entered the sacred circle of your life and work.

- Bless, release, and dedicate the day to a higher, deeper order of the great sacred circle of life.

Caring Continuing

- Create your own intentions and your own authentic practices to prepare your caritas consciousness; find your individual spiritual path toward cultivating caring consciousness and meaningful experiences in your life and work and the world.

Developing Transformational Leadership: Relating to Others

Personal development is the basis of transformative leadership. Transformative leaders influence the connection of the self with others. Reflection provides a mirror to the self by helping to confront and work to resolve actual and desired work practices. Appreciative Inquiry is a positive change process to consider how to work with others by thinking of times that have worked well, as explored in Chapter 10. To understand the work environment, leaders call upon their emotional intelligence to manage responses by considering the impact of three facets of the workplace environment: consciousness of context, self, and others, as illustrated in Figure 11.1 (Shankman & Allen, 2008).

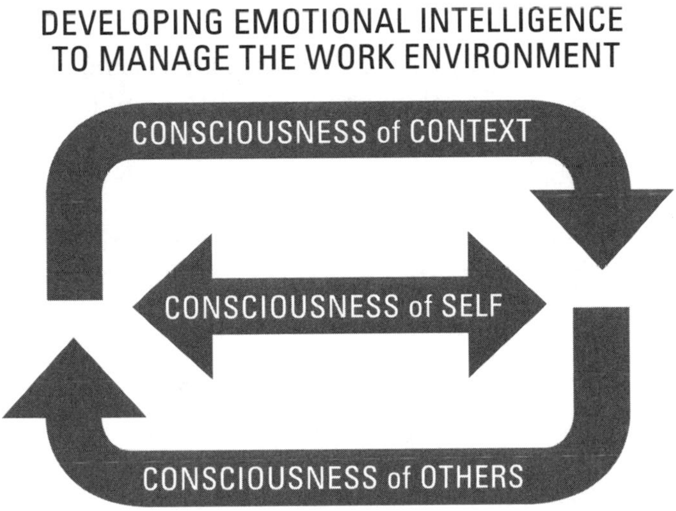

DEVELOPING EMOTIONAL INTELLIGENCE TO MANAGE THE WORK ENVIRONMENT

CONSCIOUSNESS of CONTEXT

CONSCIOUSNESS of SELF

CONSCIOUSNESS of OTHERS

FIGURE 11.1

Three Facets of Leadership to Develop Emotional Intelligence to Manage the Work Environment (Shankman & Allen, 2008).

1. **Context:** The work environment combines setting and situation. *Setting* is the structure of the organization. *Situation* is the many different forces of a particular time and place, such as individual personalities, organizational politics, and tensions or challenges within the setting. Each new context requires a different set of knowledge, skills, and attitudes to have environmental awareness.

    - **Reflection:** What are the informal traditions and values of the group? Does your style of leadership and practice fit within the culture?

2. **Self:** Self is all about the person, knowing who you are, what you stand for, your strengths and limitations, and how your answers and actions

impact others. Emotional self-perception, honest self-understanding, healthy self-esteem, emotional self-control, authenticity, flexibility, achievement, optimism, and initiative are facets of self.

- **Reflection:** What knowledge, skills, and attitudes do you bring to the organization or activity? What would others say are your strengths and weaknesses?

3. **Others:** Taking the role of others into account means awareness of those with whom you work and being attuned to them. Leadership is relationships. The facets are empathy, citizenship, inspiration, influence, coaching, change agent, conflict management, relationships, teamwork, and capitalizing on differences.

- **Reflection:** Why do members of the unit take part in activities? What is the level of innovation? Who stands out as influential or inspirational?

Bringing It Together: Professional Development Strategies

Reflection builds emotional intelligence to monitor feelings, to discriminate among emotional reactions, and to use the information to guide future responses and actions. Debriefing with colleagues after a stressful situation can help put events in perspective and build reflective capacity. By remaining open to their experiences, clinicians develop expertise when they test and refine propositions, hypotheses, and principle-based expectations in actual practice situations. Experience, therefore, can provide career and personal development (Benner, 1984). The link between reflection and confidence acknowledges the synergy among competence, confidence, experience, and reflection (Dearmin, 2000).

Reflective Narratives

Johns (1995, 2016) developed a model of structured learning to account for multiple ways of learning (Carper, 1978). He offers reflective questions as cues to guide learning based on aesthetic, personal, ethical, empirical, and reflexive ways of knowing. Nurses can use these questions along with reflective narratives such as journaling, critical incident reports, or aesthetic experiences. A model such as Johns's (see Table 11.2) can serve as a guide to multiple ways of knowing and facilitate ongoing professional development.

TABLE 11.2 Reflective Questions: Making Sense of Practice

(Adapted from Johns's [1995] Model of Structured Learning based on Carper's [1978] Ways of Knowing)

FRAMEWORK OF KNOWING	REFLECTIVE QUESTIONS
Aesthetic	What was I trying to achieve?
	Why did I respond as I did?
	What were the consequences to others and how did they feel?
Personal	How did I feel?
	How was I influenced by my internal beliefs and values?
Ethical	How did my actions match my values and beliefs?
	What influenced me to act incongruently with my beliefs and values?
Empirical	What evidence informed how I acted?
	Did I ignore evidence that should have guided my actions?
Reflexivity	How are my actions in this situation connected with previous behaviors?
	How can I handle future situations better?
	How can I anticipate the consequences on others if I change how I act in the future?
	How has this changed my ways of knowing?

Narratives encourage thinking through telling and interpreting stories. It is often how nurses think through an experience to make sense of and explain what they see in practice so they can interpret concerns, intents, and motives. Benner et al. (1996) maintain that narrative reasoning creates a deep background understanding of the patient as both a patient and a person (Benner et al.,

2010). Narrative is an important tool of reflection. It supports exploration of the context of caring, which fosters caring knowledge and skills in all situations (Barry, Gordon, & King, 2015). Telling stories of experiences helps turn experience into practical knowledge and a deeper understanding of events, which forms a basis for future meaningful responses (Levett-Jones, 2007).

Benner (1984; Benner & Wrubel, 1989) demonstrated the value of narrative as a reflective learning strategy and also as the basis for qualitative study of expert nursing practice. Qualitative analysis of practice exemplars from expert nurses illuminate the lived experience of illness and help us to understand the relationships among the person, their health, illness, and disease. Every illness has a story in how plans are interrupted, symptoms have meaning, and treatment might itself be burdensome. How nurses make sense of this has an impact on the emotional labor of nursing. As they make sense of their own way of managing this complexity, they expand leadership capacity, build professional maturity, and value the diversity of multiple perspectives.

These points are illustrated in a narrative reflection recorded by a clinical nurse specialist in which her assessment and history-taking of a patient with rheumatoid arthritis illuminated her understanding of how the disease had altered the patient's life. Demonstrating reflection-in-action in the following encounter with the patient and her daughter, the nurse, too, was transformed by what happened between them (adapted from Benner & Wrubel, 1989, pp. 9–11):

> Nurse to the patient and her daughter, noting the deformities of her hands and feet: "Rheumatoid arthritis really has not been nice to you." She then questioned the patient about how she managed dressing herself and maintaining activities of daily life.
>
> As they talked, the patient responded with tears, "No one has ever talked about it as a personal thing before; no one's ever talked to me as if this were a thing that mattered, a personal event."
>
> In reflectively retelling this encounter, transformation was evident in the nurse's observation: "Something really significant had happened between us, something that she valued and would carry away with her." The personal knowing expressed in the encounter enabled the

patient to acknowledge how the disease had altered her self-image and her way of life. The nurse's full understanding of the disease was conveyed to the patient in a personal way that allowed the mother and daughter to acknowledge the impact of the disease on their lives and on their relationship.

Reflecting-on-action, the nurse wrote, "There is a sense when you feel that you are making contact with the patient—and again, I don't know whether it is the way you talk about the illness, the way you approach the patient, the kinds of questions you ask, or the language you use—but somehow, patients know that you know what they are talking about . . . You understand what they are [experiencing]."

This exemplar illustrates the reflective process in developing tacit knowledge, how this nurse made sense of her practice to be in the privileged place of nursing through the capacity to reflect-in-action and on-action. By responding to cues from the patient, the nurse communicated her understanding of the meaning of the illness to the patient, and in that connection helped break down a wall that had isolated the patient in her crippling condition. The nurse too is transformed to bring further understanding to her own practice, reflecting on what it is that transfers between patient and caregiver. The exemplar demonstrates the value and importance of caring literacy as a way of being/knowing/evolving as a human with another in a manner that helps to affirm and sustain humanity (Watson, 2016).

REFLECTING FROM AN APPRECIATIVE APPROACH

- *What happened?*
- *How do I make sense of the situation?*
- *What was meaningful?*
- *What questions did I ask and how did I ask them in a patient-centered way?*
- *When and how did I know I had connected with the other person?*
- *How can I do it again to make it an integral part of my practice?*

Evidence links the effectiveness of reflective journals to record meaningful events in an effective way that evaluates the experience and promotes learning (Epp, 2008; Langley & Brown, 2010; Ruland & Ahern, 2007). Learning through reflective journaling helps to stimulate learning through analysis, discussion, and documentation of critical incidents. Writing can help separate oneself from the experience to be able to see it through a new lens (Freshwater, 2008). Reflective writing leads to deeper thinking, which Freshwater calls "a way of stepping forward and speaking [your] own voice" (2008, p. 228). Cranton (2006) reminds us that writing preserves one's thoughts about events that are lost in the midst of life and helps plot developmental processes, as both an assessment and evaluation that is consistent with principles of adult education. Journaling helps the learner's personal growth through increasing self-awareness for interacting with others (Freshwater, 2008). Having a systematic approach to guide the stories within the journal establishes clear aims on the purpose.

Duke (2000) wrote from the experience of becoming a reflective practitioner and how written reflection illuminated her feelings about her practice. She recorded in her journal at the end of her shift in response to caring for a patient at the end of life, "Nurse[d] a patient tired of fighting, feeling hopeless. I stayed with the patient but my heart emptied of having anything that could protect me."

Reading the journal later, she was startled by how accurately she had recorded her feelings, wondering how many times had she felt that way but not recorded it. "This was a revelation to me. I realized for the first time that the habit of debriefing myself in the car, although helpful as a coping strategy, was causing me to forget the things I was doing in practice and I was losing the opportunity to learn from them these experiences" (Duke, 2000, p. 138).

Critical incidents record snapshot views of the daily work of nurses and can provide a lens for examining opinions, personal actions, judgments, and beliefs. These narrative accounts might be similar to end-of-shift reports in their stories but add the reflective component. To record incidents, pick events in which the intervention made a difference, went unusually well, captured the essence of nursing, was particularly demanding or satisfying, or could have been handled differently (Freshwater & Esterhuizen, 2008). Some elements to include are:

- The context of where and when it happened

- What happened

- Why it was significant

- What concerns there were at the time

- What you were thinking about and feeling at the time and afterward

- What choices you made and why; if you had acted in another way, what might have happened?

Processes for developing reflection-on-action are virtually unlimited. *The Scholarship of Reflective Practice* position paper (Sherwood, Freshwater, Taylor, & Horton-Deutsch, 2005) provides an international perspective on ways to incorporate reflective learning both for self-development and for learning exercises in educational programs and gives more details on using a myriad of reflective strategies.

In addition to reflective journals, written critical incidents, narratives of work encounters, or case study analysis, learners can audiotape stories from practice as an alternative to writing and use a reflective guide as they listen to the story (Taylor, 2000). These written accounts are different from a clinical log, which is merely the recording of actions without including reflection on the experience.

"Sharing aesthetic ways of knowing helps us reach into our innermost thoughts and feelings to surface values and attitudes that are so much a part of how we respond to others."

There are multiple approaches to learning to understand the human condition, which is so much a part of both attending to self as nurse as well as making sense of practice (Sherwood, 2000). Aesthetics such as drawing, painting, montage, poetry, a literature vignette, role-playing, or other creative endeavors are all possibilities. In addition to mindfulness, reflection-in-action can include dance or other movement, meditation, singing or listening to music, or Visual Thinking Strategies as outlined in Chapter 7. Sherwood (1997) related how movies can be used as a means of examining and understanding the human condition.

By using a structured reflective format of examining the central characters, the underlying motivations, and how each stakeholder responded, we can deepen our capacity for working with and for others in our care. Some groups have used a set movie night together to build teamwork while having a focused discussion to analyze the meaning of the storyline within the context of the ethical and spiritual dimensions confronted to gain human understanding applicable in practice.

Whether we are using art, poetry, movies, or story, these narrative devices offer another language through which we can connect to another. Sharing aesthetic ways of knowing helps us reach into our innermost thoughts and feelings to surface values and attitudes that are so much a part of how we respond to others. By reflecting on the meaning found in the language of poetry, the message conveyed in a painting, or the human narrative in stories or movies, we can better appreciate how others respond to contextual and interpersonal cues. Thus, we can mindfully embrace the development of our emotional intelligence as we seek self-awareness, self-regulation, self-motivation, and empathy through various aesthetic approaches alone or collectively.

REFLECTING ON . . . THE ART OF CLAY (DEEPENING UNDERSTANDING OF SELF AS NURSE)

Purpose: *Let the self become still to engage in a personal growth strategy to focus on your self in wholeness, who you are as a nurse, to support and encourage reflection on values, attitudes, beliefs, and your state of being.*

Premise: *Aesthetic expression leads us into "inner knowing places," into our creative connection within our self, and expands our situational awareness.*

Method: Alone or with participants, sit quietly with soft, unobtrusive music in the background. Hold a piece of clay in your hands to begin to warm it to a softened state. Then work with the clay in any way you want—kneading it, opening, circling, pinching, or pounding—as you reflect inwardly on your state of being in the moment. Clear the mind of preconceived notions or barriers about creating art. Shaping the clay is about an expression of self from inside out. Using principles of reflection, go into a place within yourself where you reach beyond to transcend to your undiscovered affective dimensions that are usually crowded by your rationalities.

Reflection: *The aliveness of the clay as an organic, natural matter will be shaped into a form that might have meaning only to you, the shaper. As you come out of the shaping experience, consider what your mind is helping to bring from your soul to the surface. Share with others in the group; write your experience as a critical reflection, a poem, or other narration to explicate the changes felt from the quiet place of shaping the clay into a message of feeling.*

(adapted from Parker, 1994)

Guiding and Coaching: Developing Inquiry

In an ever-changing healthcare environment, nurses need ways to sustain themselves and remain engaged to achieve stated professional goals. Ongoing professional development through contextual learning is a reflective learning intervention. Developing the ability to think critically in practice and learn from narrative are major foundations for ongoing professional development (Forneris & Peden-McAlpine, 2006). Goodman (1984) offered a guide for planning reflective learning:

1. Reflection to achieve stated objectives: examine efficiency, effectiveness, and accountability

2. Relating principles and practice: assess implications and consequences of actions and beliefs, and underlying rationale for practice

3. Incorporating an ethical and political framework: weighing justice, valuing professional goals and practice, linking everyday practice with broader social structures

Reflective learning based on these three premises holds the possibility of helping nurses attend to their own selves as a nurse, while also wrestling with the complexities of their work to make sense of it. Taking care of oneself is fundamental to being an effective nurse.

The following sidebar provides an example of one organization's approach to creating a sustainable wellness culture to help nurses develop self-care practices for all stages of career development. Creating habits of ongoing reflective practices is the foundation for developing practice, expanding professional expertise, and encouraging attention to wholeness of mind, body, heart, and spirit.

CHERYL WOODS GISCOMBE, PHD, RN, PNMNP-BC

Director and Distinguished Associate Professor for the LeVine Wellness Program at the University of North Carolina at Chapel Hill School of Nursing

The School of Nursing is focusing on developing a wellness culture among faculty, staff, and students to both promote self-development and build a healthy work environment. The mission is to promote quality of life, workplace wellness, and overall well-being among School of Nursing students, faculty, and staff and to facilitate a sustainable culture of wellness within the School of Nursing. With the proximity of a major teaching healthcare system, the goal is to expand to include nurses from the clinical areas to model ongoing reflective practices. By modeling for learners during their academic programs, they will continue to apply wellness practices in working with clients across their careers. Nurses' commitment to caring for patients often overshadows the imperative for attention to self, contributing to stress, burnout, and compromised health. This model can be adapted in all settings to begin to transform practice habits to a culture of balancing caregiving of others with caring for self.

Objectives and Activities:

1. *Develop annual Nursing Wellness and Quality of Life institutes and continuing education seminars in collaboration with the Center for Lifelong Learning, the hospital system, and university campus.*

2. *Integrate Nursing Wellness and Quality of Life content in core courses in academic programs, particularly in courses focusing on population health, professional development, and role development courses.*

3. *Implement "Morning Mindfulness" sessions open to all nurses, students, faculty, and staff.*

4. *Collaborate with local massage therapy school to institute "Wellness Days" for students, faculty, and staff that will include low-cost chair massage sessions and other wellness activities.*

5. *Partner with University programs and initiatives, for example, health coaches and trainers from Campus Recreation programs, to provide fitness and health promoting initiatives onsite in the School of Nursing. Examples include monthly wellness workshops, demonstrations, and healthy eating socials.*

6. *Promote an ambiance of tranquility and wellness in the School through informative posters, bulletin boards, and video messaging to enhance quality of life for all.*

7. *Teach and model "wellness language" to replace "martyr language" among nurses, students, faculty, and staff. For example, replace "I only slept 4 hours last night," or "I did not use the bathroom for 4 hours," with "I make sure that I take a mobility break each day to stand or walk for 15 to 30 minutes," or "I took a nap for 10 minutes in the break room to refresh to be ready for afternoon tasks!" or "I scheduled a walking meeting to break traditional meeting habits and encourage creative thinking."*

8. *Implement semi-annual or annual wellness competitions to challenge physical fitness or other wellness activities. For example, develop competitive teams to compare steps per day, or number of stairs climbed each day.*

Final Reflections

Reflective practice is an important self-development strategy for continuing growth, making sense of our work, and applying innovative change methods. Reflection provides a systematic way of thinking about our actions and responses to change future actions and responses. Reflective practice guides our learning from experience by considering what we know, believe, and value within the context of an event. Systematic analysis through reflection contributes to sense-making to see the whole; the continuing journey helps us evaluate our contributions, leading to greater satisfaction and sense of purpose in our work. Developing reflective practice is a lifelong journey that supports and sustains career development. Reflection helps clarify how we work according to our sense of mission and purpose and as such guides us in developing the spiritual resources for managing and balancing our personal and professional lives.

References

Barry, C., Gordon, S., & King, B. (2015). *Nursing case studies in caring.* New York, NY: Springer Publishing.

Bazarko, D., Cate, R. A., Azocar, F., & Kreitzer, M. J. (2013). The impact of an innovative mindfulness-based stress reduction program on the health and well-being of nurses employed in a corporate setting. *Journal of Workplace Behavioral Health, 28*(2), 107–133.

Beddoe, A. E., & Murphy, S. O. (2004). Does mindfulness decrease stress and foster empathy among nursing students? *The Journal of Nursing Education, 43*(7), 305–312.

Benner, P. (1984). *From novice to expert: Excellence and power in clinical nursing practice.* Menlo Park, CA: Addison-Wesley.

Benner, P., Kyriakidis, P. H., & Stannard, D. (2011). *Clinical wisdom and interventions in acute and critical care: A thinking-in-action approach* (2nd ed.). New York, NY: Springer Publishing.

Benner, B., Sutphen, M., Leonard, V., & Day, L. (2010). *Educating nurses: A call for radical transformation.* San Francisco, CA: Jossey-Bass.

Benner, P., Tanner, C., & Chesla, C. (1996). *Expertise in nursing practice: Caring, clinical judgment, and ethics.* New York, NY: Springer Publishing.

Benner, P., & Wrubel, J. (1989). *The primacy of caring: Stress and coping in health and illness.* Menlo Park, CA: Addison-Wesley.

Bjorvatn, B., Dale, S., Hogstad-Erikstein, R., Fiske, E., Pallesen, S., & Waage, S. (2012). Self-reported sleep and health among Norwegian hospital nurses in intensive care units. *Nursing in Critical Care, 17*(4), 180–188.

Carper, B. A. (1978). Fundamental patterns of knowing in nursing. *Advances in Nursing Science, 1*(1), 13–23.

Cohen-Katz, J., Wiley, S., Capuano, T., Baker, D., & Shapiro, S. (2005). The effects of mindfulness-based stress reduction on nurse stress and burnout. *Holistic Nursing Practice, 18*(2), 303–308.

Cranton, P. (2006). *Understanding and promoting transformative learning: A guide for educators of adults*. San Francisco, CA: Jossey-Bass.

Day, L., & Sherwood, G. (2017a). Transforming education to transform practice: Using unfolding case studies to integrate quality and safety in subject centered classrooms. In G. Sherwood & J. Barnsteiner (Eds.), *Quality and safety in nursing: A competency approach to improving outcomes* (2nd ed.) (pp. 199–220). Hoboken, NJ: Wiley-Blackwell.

Day, L., & Sherwood, G. (2017b). Quality and safety in clinical learning environments. In G. Sherwood & J. Barnsteiner (Eds.), *Quality and safety in nursing: A competency approach to improving outcomes* (2nd ed.) (pp. 253–263). Hoboken, NJ: Wiley-Blackwell.

Dearmin, N. (2000). The legacy of reflective practice. In S. Burns & C. Bulman (Eds.), *Reflective practice in nursing: The growth of the professional practitioner* (2nd ed.) (pp. 156–172). Oxford, UK: Blackwell Science.

Drury, V., Francis, K., & Chapman, Y. (2008). Where have all the young ones gone: Implications for the nursing workforce. *OJIN: The Online Journal of Issues in Nursing, 14*(1), e1. doi:10.3912/OJIN.Vol14No1PPT03

Duke, S. (2000). The experience of becoming reflective. In S. Burns & C. Bulman (Eds.), *Reflective practice in nursing: The growth of the professional practitioner* (2nd ed.) (pp. 137–155). Oxford, UK: Blackwell Science.

Ebright, P. R., Patterson, E. S., Chalko, B. A., & Render, M. L. (2003). Understanding the complexity of registered nurse work in acute care settings. *Journal of Nursing Administration, 33*(12), 630–638.

Ekici, D., & Beder, A. (2014). The effects of workplace bullying on physicians and nurses [online]. *The Australian Journal of Advanced Nursing, 31*(4), 24–33.

Epp, S. (2008). The value of reflective journaling in undergraduate nursing education: A literature review. *International Journal of Nursing Studies, 45*(9), 1379–1388.

Fagin, L., Carson, J., Leary, J., De Villiers, N., Bartlett, H., O'Malley, P., . . . Brown, D. (1996). Stress, coping and burnout in mental health nurses: Findings from three research studies. *International Journal of Social Psychiatry, 42*(2), 102–111.

Forneris, S. G., & Peden-McAlpine, C. J. (2006). Contextual learning: A reflective learning intervention for nursing education. *International Journal of Nursing Education Scholarship, 3*(1), 1–18.

Freshwater, D. (Ed.). (2002). *Therapeutic nursing: Improving patient care through reflection*. London, UK: Sage Publications.

Freshwater, D. (2008). Reflective practice: The state of the art. In D. Freshwater, B. J. Taylor, & G. Sherwood (Eds.), *International textbook of reflective practice in nursing* (pp. 1–18). Oxford, UK: Blackwell Publishing.

Freshwater, D., & Esterhuizen, P. (2008). Reflective narratives: Developing a career pathway. In D. Freshwater, B. J Taylor, & G. Sherwood (Eds.), *International textbook of reflective practice in nursing* (pp. 223–239). Oxford, UK: Blackwell Publishing.

Goodman, J. (1984). Reflection and teaching education: A case study and theoretical analysis. *Interchange, 15*(3), 9–26.

Hannigan, B., Edwards, D., Coyle, D., Fothergill, A., & Burnard, P. (2000). Burnout in community mental health nurses: Findings from the all-Wales stress study. *Journal of Psychiatric and Mental Health Nursing, 7*(2), 127–134.

Hegney, D. G., Craigie, M., Hemsworth, D., Osseiran-Moisson, R., Aoun, S., Francis, K., & Drury, V. (2014). Compassion satisfaction, compassion fatigue, anxiety, depression and stress in registered nurses in Australia: Study 1 results. *Journal of Nursing Management, 22*(4), 506–518.

Horton-Deutsch, S. (2012). Learning through reflection and reflection on learning: Pedagogies in action. In G. Sherwood & S. Horton-Deutsch (Eds.), *Reflective organizations: On the front lines of QSEN and reflective practice implementation* (pp. 101–131). Indianapolis, IN: Sigma Theta Tau International.

Horton-Deutsch, S. (2016). Open and visionary: Remaining open to the possibilities of nursing praxis. In W. Rosa (Ed.), *Nurse leaders: Evolutionary visions of leadership* (pp. 311–322). New York, NY: Springer Publishing.

Horton-Deutsch, S., & Horton, J. (2003). Developing mindfulness: A means to overcoming conflict. *Archives of Psychiatric Nursing, 17*(4), 186–193.

Horton-Deutsch, S., & Sherwood, G. (2008). Reflection: An educational strategy to develop emotionally competent nurse leaders. *Journal of Nursing Management, 16*(8), 946–954.

Ireland, M. (2008). Assisting students to use evidence as a part of reflection on practice. *Nursing Education Perspectives, 29*(2), 90–93.

Jenkins, R., & Elliott, P. (2004). Stressors, burnout and social support: Nurses in acute mental health settings. *Journal of Advanced Nursing, 48*(6), 622–631.

Johns, C. (1995). Framing learning through reflection within Carper's fundamental ways of knowing in nursing. *Journal of Advanced Nursing, 22*(2), 226–234.

Johns, C. (2016). *Mindful leadership. A guide for the health care professions.* London, UK: Palgrave Macmillan.

Kuiper, R. A., Pesut, D. J., & Arms, T. E. (2016). *Clinical reasoning and care coordination in advanced nursing practice.* New York, NY: Springer Publishing.

Langley, M. E., & Brown, S. T. (2010). Perceptions of the use of reflective learning journals in online graduate nursing education. *Nursing Education Perspectives, 31*(1), 12–17.

Lasater, K., & Nielsen, A. (2009). A reflective journaling for clinical judgment development and evaluation. *Journal of Nursing Education, 48*(1), 40–44.

Letvak, S. (2013). We cannot ignore nurses' health anymore: A synthesis of the literature on evidence-based strategies to improve nurse health. *Nursing Administration Quarterly, 37*(4), 295–308.

Letvak, S., Ruhm, C. J., & McCoy, T. (2012). Depression in hospital-employed nurses. *Clinical Nurse Specialist, 26*(3), 177–182. doi:10.1097/NUR.0b013e3182503ef0

Levett-Jones, T. L. (2007). Facilitating reflective practice and self-assessment of competence through the use of narratives. *Nurse Education in Practice, 7*(2), 112–119.

Mackenzie, C. S., Poulin, P. A., & Seidman-Carlson, R. (2006). A brief mindfulness-based stress reduction intervention for nurses and nurse aides. *Applied Nursing Research, 19,* 105–109.

Nielsen, A., Stragnell, S., & Jester, P. (2007). Educational innovations. Guide for reflection using the clinical judgment model. *Journal of Nursing Education, 46*(11), 513–516.

O'Haver Day, P., & Horton-Deutsch, S. (2004). Utilizing mindfulness-based therapeutic interventions in psychiatric nursing practice—part II: Mindfulness-based approaches for all phases of psychotherapy. *Archives of Psychiatric Nursing, 18*(5), 170–177.

Parker, M. (1994). The healing art of clay: A workshop for remembering wholeness. In D. A. Gaut & A. Boykin (Eds.), *Caring as healing: Renewal through hope* (pp. 35–145). New York, NY: National League for Nursing Press.

Ruland, J. P., & Ahern, N. R. (2007). Transforming student perspectives through reflective writing. *Nurse Educator, 32*(2), 81–88.

Shankman, M. L., & Allen, S. J. (2008). *Emotionally intelligent leadership: A guide for college students.* San Francisco, CA: Jossey-Bass.

Sherring, S., & Knight, D. (2009). An exploration of burnout among city mental health nurses. *British Journal of Nursing, 18*(20), 1234–1240.

Sherwood, G. (1997). Developing spiritual care: The search for self. In M. S. Roach (Ed.), *Caring from the heart* (pp. 196–211). Wahmak, NJ: Paulist Press.

Sherwood, G. (2000). The power of nurse-client encounters: Interpreting spiritual themes. *Journal of Holistic Nursing, 18*(2), 159–175.

Sherwood, G. (2003). Leadership for a healthy work environment: Caring for the human spirit. *Nurse Leader, 1*(5), 36–40.

Sherwood, G., Freshwater, D., Taylor, B., & Horton-Deutsch, S. (2005). *The scholarship of reflective practice*. Position paper. Sigma Theta Tau International. Retrieved from http://www.nursingsociety.org/docs/default-source/position-papers/resource_reflective.pdf?sfvrsn=4

Sherwood, G., & Horton-Deutsch, S. (2008). Reflective practice: The route to nursing leadership. In D. Freshwater, B. Taylor, & G. Sherwood (Eds.), *International textbook of reflective practice in nursing* (pp. 137–154). Oxford, UK: Blackwell Publishing.

Tanner, C. A. (2006). Thinking like a nurse: A research-based model of clinical judgment in nursing. *Journal of Nursing Education, 45*(6), 204–211.

Taylor, B. (2000). *Reflective practice: A guide for nurses and midwives*. Buckingham, UK: Open University Press.

Vitello-Cicciu, J. M. (2002). Exploring emotional intelligence: Implications for nursing leaders. *JONA, 32*(4), 203–210.

Walton, M. K., & Barnsteiner, J. (2017). Patient-centered care. In G. Sherwood & J. Barnsteiner (Eds.), *Quality and safety in nursing: A competency approach to improving outcomes* (pp. 62–83). Hoboken, NJ: Wiley-Blackwell.

Watson, J. (2002). Intentionality and caring-healing consciousness: A practice of transpersonal nursing. *Journal of Holistic Nursing Practice, 16*(4), 12–19.

Watson, J. (2008). *Nursing: The philosophy and science of caring* (Rev. ed.). Boulder, CO: University of Colorado Press.

Watson, J. (2016). Human caring literacy. In S. Lee, P. Palmieri, & J. Watson (Eds.), *Global advances in human caring literacy* (pp. 3–11). New York, NY: Springer Publishing.

Chapter 12

Reflective Practices: Changing the Culture of Peer Evaluation

–*Sharon L. Sims, PhD, RN, FAANP*

–*Melinda M. Swenson, PhD, RN, FNP, FAANP*

As part of a reflective paradigm, a new reflective approach to evaluating educators can shift from only looking at learner satisfaction and achieving content objectives to emphasizing the interconnectedness and complementary nature of self-evaluation~peer evaluation (SE~PE). This chapter will explain ideas from Appreciative Inquiry (Cooperrider & Whitney, 2005), Shulman's Table of Learning (Shulman, 2002), Diekelmann's Concernful Practices (Diekelmann & Diekelmann, 2009), and Kelso's description of complementarity (Kelso & Engstrom, 2006).

We describe how reflective evaluation can promote a paradigm of *gathering* (welcoming and calling forth deep reflection) (Diekelmann & Diekelmann, 2009, p. 339) and *sustaining* (nurturing and retaining) nurse educators as they develop, and we explore self-evaluation~peer evaluation as a means of welcoming reflection and sustaining the teaching role, whether in academic or clinical settings. Applying a new vocabulary for looking at faculty evaluation can serve to re-form ideas about how evaluation can be used in reflective teaching and reflective learning, while also eliminating the dread often associated with evaluation of our teaching. We also suggest that SE~PE has a place in the evaluation of clinical practice. We propose that self and peer evaluation using similar approaches would foster professional growth for clinicians.

Issues With Current Approaches to Peer Evaluation

Higher education in nursing relies on self-evaluation and peer evaluation for documenting teaching effectiveness required for promotion, tenure, awards, and merit. Clinicians might benefit from a similar interactive process, particularly those who progress through a clinical ladder. Important dilemmas complicate these evaluation processes. First, few educators enjoy being evaluated using the formal, conventional criteria that focus on performance as a lecturer or seminar leader, adequacy of syllabus and course development, and the nearly exclusive use of measurable student outcomes. Few educators feel they have enough time to effectively plan and conduct an evaluation for a peer teacher because of busy classroom, clinical, and faculty responsibilities. Theoretically, educators understand that evaluation is necessary and even helpful; in practice, few like it or seek it out without encouragement. A new way of thinking about reflective evaluation can promote a new interest in evaluation and new energy in its process.

Second, most traditional systems of peer evaluation are linear, starting with a review of the educator's self-evaluation; continuing with a document review, classroom visitation, or online visitation; and followed by the evaluator's production of a document that judges the teacher's skill and effectiveness. This linearity belies the ideal integrative nature of responsive evaluation (Guba & Lincoln, 1989; Swenson, 1991). Teaching and learning are inextricably connected, and this connection is neither a polarity nor a situation of cause-and-effect.

Third, we recognize the psychometric paradox embedded in conventional thinking about teaching evaluation. As described by Shulman, "Our measurement models are psychometric but our assessment needs are often sociometric, requiring the measurement of socially-scaffolded and joint productions" (Shulman, 2008, p. 9). As teachers of nursing, we continually strive for objectivity, even in areas that are essentially subjective and reflective. Palmer (1983) addressed this embedded need for objectivity:

> "Objective" is another word central to our way of knowing. It is the ever-present adjective, continually used to modify the key nouns so there will be no mistaking what we are talking about: objective facts, objective theories, and objective reality. If a claim is not objective, it is not knowledge, but merely some species of passion or prejudice (Palmer, 1983, p. 23).

Thus, fully objective evaluation misses invisible, ineffable, reflective aspects of good teaching and sustained learning. These facets of good teaching and learning cannot be measured directly, but can be demonstrated, recognized, and assessed using more reflective techniques and approaches.

Fourth, not only is the process linear, but self-evaluation often appears subordinate and secondary to peer evaluation, privileging the power of the evaluator

Note: We illustrate the complementary nature of teaching~learning, highlighted in this chapter by the use of the tilde (~) to emphasize the back-and-forth motion between these two aspects of schooling (Kelso & Engstrom, 2006, p. xiv).

over self-reflection and review. Traditionally, self-evaluation is part of—but not equal to—the peer review. In contrast, we suggest these two evaluations exist in a relationship that cannot be reduced to before-and-after, or primary-and-secondary, but in a relationship of both~and. Kelso and Engstrom described this relationship as the "complementary nature" of apparently contradictory or separate pairs. They state:

> . . . For example, "body" and "mind" are complementary aspects of the complementary pair "body~mind." We use the tilde, not to concatenate words or as an iconic bridge between polarized aspects, but to signify that we are discussing complementary pairs. Equally, if not more important, the tilde symbolizes the dynamic nature of complementary pairs. . . . It is not only the polar complementary aspects of complementary pairs that matter but also all the stuff and all the action falling in between them (Kelso & Engstrom, 2006, p. 7).

In this view, teaching and learning are a complementary pair, and all the action involved in each takes place in the "squiggle space" (designated by the tilde) between them. As a logical extension then, self-evaluation (SE) and peer evaluation (PE) also are seen in a dynamic relationship (SE~PE) rather than a linear relationship. "All the stuff and all the action falling in between them" is the possibility that these components can be seen in a co-creative way, each informing and changing the other as they develop. This complementary view also resolves the teaching~learning paradox by privileging neither teaching nor learning and by emphasizing the nonlinear interconnectedness of these processes. The complementary view similarly illuminates the conventional polarity of evaluator and the one being evaluated and brings better balance to evaluation practices. This complementary approach, then, is aimed toward improving reflective teaching and sustaining teachers in the same reflective mode.

Fifth, conventional evaluation might work for conventional teaching, but because pedagogies evolve so quickly and in so many new directions, we are convinced that higher education needs a more responsive approach to the evaluation of teaching. In any situation where evaluation is based on predetermined, over-described criteria, it can fail to address innovative practices, new pedagogies, unconventional settings, or simulation. In extreme cases, evaluators mistakenly use instruments intended for face-to-face classroom situations to evaluate clinical, simulation, or online teaching. Similarly, self-evaluations suffer from lack of templates or instruments to focus on and promote reflection in practice and leadership.

Responsive evaluation is not a new concept. Guba and Lincoln (1989) eloquently described it nearly 30 years ago (following Stake, 1975); Parlett and Hamilton (1972) referred to "illuminative evaluation." Eisner (1991) proposed evaluation as "connoisseurship." Each of these non-conventional approaches focused on evaluation that was more reflective, more appreciative, and less centered on measurement. These thoughtful and qualitative approaches have largely been ignored in higher education, perhaps because of our reliance on rigidly objective measures, behavioral outcomes, and evidence-based/best teaching practices. Approaches to evaluation reflect normal cyclic changes in the discipline. Perhaps the time is right for a re-formed and reflective approach to SE~PE, an approach that captures the dynamic interplay—the squiggle space (Kelso & Engstrom, 2006, p. xiv) existing in the "space between" this complementary pair.

In response to these and other potential dilemmas, we propose Shulman's Table of Learning as a flexible structure and new language useful for framing an evaluation process honoring the complementary nature of SE~PE. Starting with Shulman, within an appreciative and responsive evaluation paradigm, we can re-form the evaluation of teaching.

RESPONSIVE EVALUATION

Responsive evaluation focuses on the concerns and issues of all the involved participants. It is characterized by flexibility, no structured, pre-conceived design, and is "continuously evolving and never complete." (Guba & Lincoln, 1989, p. 30)

ILLUMINATIVE EVALUATION

Illuminative evaluation concerns itself primarily with description and interpretation of findings, rather than more conventional prediction and control, focusing on the complexity of all involved participants and concerns. (Parlett & Hamilton, 1972)

The Shulman Table of Learning

Shulman proposed a Table of Learning (2002) to begin a conversation about the uses (and abuses) of educational taxonomies, specifically Bloom's taxonomies of the cognitive domain (Bloom, 1956) and of the affective domain (Krathwohl, Bloom, & Masia, 1964). Shulman maintains that taxonomies are useful as the vocabulary of a language, classification systems, protocols, checklists, and heuristics. However, he also states that taxonomy can become an end in itself and can take on theoretical claims to sequentiality and hierarchy. We see this frequently in nursing education. Critiques of course design often focus on whether objectives and outcomes are placed "high enough" in Bloom's taxonomy. If they are judged to be too low in that hierarchy, the course is seen as deficient and less stringent. This is especially true in graduate courses, as if graduate students are never in an appropriate place or time to engage in learning at the level of recall or understanding. Analysis, synthesis, and integration have come to represent the only acceptable standard of quality in graduate course syllabi.

> *"Engagement is not just a proxy or measure of learning, but a fundamental purpose of education itself."*

In contrast to Bloom and other rigidly behavioral approaches, Shulman's Table of Learning is circular, non-hierarchical, and non-theoretical. It is flexible enough to accommodate both teaching and learning. We suggest it as a conceptual scaffold for SE~PE in higher education because of its adaptability and its emphasis on complementarity.

The simplest representation of Shulman's Table of Learning presents a spiraling, continuous, and constantly responsive process. In this diagram (see Figure 12.1), we use the tilde to emphasize the complementary nature of these pairs. According to Shulman:

> Learning begins with student engagement, which in turn leads to knowledge and understanding. Once someone understands, he or she becomes capable of performance or action. Critical reflection on one's practice and understanding leads to higher-order thinking in the form of

a capacity to exercise judgment in the face of uncertainty and to create designs in the presence of constraints and unpredictability. Ultimately, the exercise of judgment makes possible the development of commitment. In commitment, we become capable of professing our understandings and our values, our faith and our love, our skepticism and our doubts, internalizing those attributes and making them integral to our identities. These commitments, in turn, make new engagements possible—and even necessary. (Shulman, 2002, p. 38)

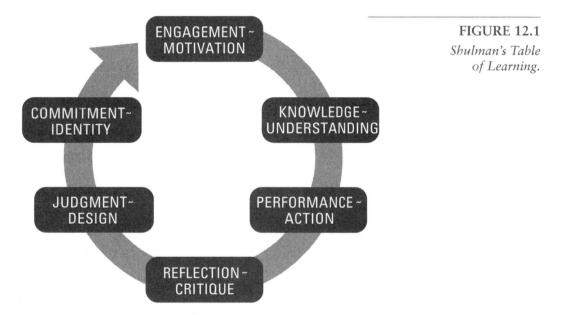

FIGURE 12.1
Shulman's Table of Learning.

Shulman describes pedagogies of engagement as approaches that have the capacity to get students actively involved with learning in new ways. This is more than getting students interested—it is finding out what opens them to learning. Shulman goes further in saying "engagement is not just a proxy or measure of learning, but a fundamental purpose of education itself" (Shulman, 2002, p. 40). Pedagogies of engagement in nursing could include service learning, practice or patient-based learning, collaborative learning, simulation, and practica.

- *Knowledge and understanding* move the student beyond memorizing content, always with an eye toward engaging the students in the practice world. It allows them to be in a different relationship with discipline-specific content, to talk about the ideas of others without plagiarizing.

- *Performance and action* are perhaps the most recognizable elements for nurse educators. We see this as putting knowledge and understanding into action in a clinical arena. Shulman describes practice as the "pivot point of education."

- *Critical reflection* is the honest critique of one's own practice (nursing or teaching nursing) or the practices of others. Through reflection, we make decisions on what to keep doing and what to stop doing.

- *Judgment and design* almost always take place in environments filled with uncertainty and ambiguity. This certainly describes the world of nursing practice. When students exercise judgment and design, they can invent new approaches to meet the needs of particular patients in particular situations.

- *Commitment and identity* arise when students see the relationship between and among their judgments in practice, their professional values, and the values and attributes of nursing. They see who they are as nurses, and this commitment leads to new engagements.

Given its inherent plasticity and adaptability, we can imagine using the Table of Learning for various evaluation situations. In this sense, we propose that the Table of Learning is also a Table of Teaching~Learning. Specifically, the Table of Learning could become a template for SE~PE of teaching, using the complementary aspects in the Table as the foundation for appreciative questions to uncover the immeasurable but crucial aspects of teaching effectiveness. In SE~PE, appreciative interviews and appreciative writing are the means for collecting data for review and critique, in addition to course materials, publications, and student evaluations. Table 12.1 describes and elaborates on the complementary pairs in the Table of Learning. An Appreciative Inquiry approach, added to Shulman's ideas, helps to generate questions, narratives, and innovative ideas for faculty development.

TABLE 12.1 Guidelines for Complementary Pairs in Table of Learning

GUIDE FOR, DIALOGUE, PLANNING, AND REVIEW DISCUSSION	TEACHER'S ENACTMENT OF THE COMPLEMENTARY PAIRS	EXAMPLES THAT MIGHT BE ASSESSED BY REVIEWER AND TEACHER OR QUESTIONS THAT MIGHT STIMULATE
Engagement~ Motivation	Finds out what drives student learning and captures students' interest Adopts approaches to get students actively involved with learning	What actions or activities foster engagement~motivation? For example, Service Learning, PBL (Problem-Practice-Project-Patient-Based Learning), Collaborative Learning, Simulation, Field Work
Knowledge~ Understanding	Encourages going beyond memorizing content Models ways to state ideas learned from others (texts, clinical resources) to establish a form of ownership of the content	Uses motivation and engagement with the real world to enhance engagement with the world of the mind—books, experts, resources What opportunities are created for students to listen attentively and to put ideas into their own words in public? Encourages students to build on ideas/statements of others in an accountable/ethical way
Performance~ Action	Facilitates and demonstrates practices that allow putting knowledge and understanding into action	Evidence of balance between coaching~directing during clinical practice or simulation How is reflective listening evident in teaching/clinical practice? Develops assessment techniques that maintain fairness and equity

continues

TABLE 12.1 (continued)

GUIDE FOR, DIALOGUE, PLANNING, AND REVIEW DISCUSSION	TEACHER'S ENACTMENT OF THE COMPLEMENTARY PAIRS	EXAMPLES THAT MIGHT BE ASSESSED BY REVIEWER AND TEACHER OR QUESTIONS THAT MIGHT STIMULATE
Reflection~Critique	Reflects on one's own nursing practice, on one's own practice of teaching nursing Critiques one's own work and the work of others Considers stopping some action or practice to make space for innovative practices	How is reflective practice modeled for students? Provides specific and appreciative feedback on student learning Provides specificity and openness in syllabus and grading practices
Judgment~Design	Makes judgments in the face of uncertainty in the real world Creates new approaches, innovation, and invention to meet particular situations and constraints	Goes beyond teaching and assessing for understanding to encourage flexibility and innovation Creates situations for uncertainty to emerge in safe ways and is prepared to deal with whatever comes up
Commitment~Identity	Understands and articulates clearly the values inherent in nursing Enhances learners' opportunities for moving inward (reflection) and connecting outward (with patients and peers)	Points out when students start to think and act like a nurse, clinically and pedagogically How is ethical awareness modeled in teaching~learning? Shows and promotes moral courage, advocating for patients and for students
Engagement~Motivation	Guides students into new engagements and finding new motivations	Continues with cycles in Table of Learning

Adding Appreciative Approaches

In our teaching practice, we enact evaluation using ideas from Appreciative Inquiry (Cooperrider & Whitney, 2005; Cooperrider, Whitney, & Stavros, 2003; Whitney & Trosten-Bloom, 2003). *Appreciative Inquiry* (AI), expressed simplistically, is a process for individual and group development that uses narratives to identify what is best in the history of the person or group and what aspects of that past should be preserved and amplified. The determination of "what works" and "what we want more of" leads to the generation of innovative ideas for future development, grounded in the best of the past and situated in the present.

The AI process includes four phases: initiating, inquiring, imagining, and innovating (Reed, 2007). In the initiating phase, the stakeholders learn about AI processes and determine the focus for the project (peer evaluation, in this case). They also develop a structure for the project, including a timeline for completion. The inquiry phase includes the interviews and discussion that provide the co-created data for the evaluation. Imagining, the third phase, brings the data together, and participants identify ideas and themes relevant to the project. The innovation phase returns these ideas to practice.

We suggest integrating these AI process steps into all aspects of SE~PE. Table 12.2 summarizes the proposed process for integrating the complementary nature of the evaluative pairs, the Table of Learning, and the appreciative approach.

TABLE 12.2 Self-Evaluation~Peer Evaluation Process

Design Conference (Initiating and Inquiring)

Teacher and evaluator have an appreciative conversation about how the teacher enacts the six elements of the Table of Learning (TOL). Questions to explore: What actions worked to foster student engagement and motivation, knowledge and understanding, performance and action, reflection and critique, judgment and design, and commitment and identity? What would the teacher like more of? What evidence can the evaluator expect to see in the class observation or the student assignments that reflect each element?

continues

TABLE 12.2 (continued)

Are all six elements appropriate for the kind, degree, and level of courses taught by this teacher? Teacher and evaluator decide what kind and how many class observations will be useful.

Based on this conversation, the teacher prepares a self-evaluation, addressing the TOL elements and identifying themes of success across all the elements.

Based on this conversation, the evaluator prepares a template of what to look for in the class observation.

Class Observation (Inquiring)

Evaluator visits class or other setting (for example, Internet, clinical site, or simulation/lab) as negotiated with teacher and makes observations focused on the preconference discussion of what works.

Review syllabus for clarity and transparency, level and purpose of assignments, teacher feedback, grading rubrics, online interactions, and review of student evaluation data.

Ideas Conference (Imagining and Innovating)

Teacher and evaluator meet to co-construct the report. Both contribute notes on how the class or learning situation went, including judgment on whether elements were evident in the situation.

Ideas for how to do more of what works for each element and how to integrate them more effectively are also co-developed.

Self-evaluation, observation, and final report merge into one document that becomes the basis for imagining future possibilities and planning the teacher's continued development.

Enacting SE~PE

We have used SE~PE in evaluating teachers of undergraduate and graduate nursing courses, including online, clinical, and face-to-face didactic courses. One of the first things we discovered is that not all of the Table of Learning elements are predominant in every course. Depending on the subject of the course and its placement in a particular curriculum, some of the elements are more foregrounded than others. We offer three examples in the following sections to demonstrate our process of enacting SE~PE.

Exemplar #1: Online Course: Design Conference Determines Process

The teacher in a graduate online pharmacology course noticed that Engagement~Motivation and Knowledge~Understanding were stronger foci in the course than other aspects. For most students, this course was their introduction to advanced pharmacology and prescribing, and they were not yet fully engaged in their clinical work. Opportunities for practicing Judgment~Design were thus limited for them. Though all the elements were touched on, Engagement~Motivation and Knowledge~Understanding were most important. It was enlightening for both teacher and peer evaluator to unpack each element in relation to the course content and outcomes as we progressed through the inquiry phase to see how, where, and in what degree they were enacted in the course. In addition, this initial dialogue/conversation was very helpful in focusing the work of the evaluation for both teacher and evaluator. The teacher used the dialogue to begin her self-evaluation, and the evaluator used it to organize and focus her investigation of the course and course materials. In the words of the teacher:

> The process was orderly, conversations were not rushed, and the outcome incredibly helpful. My course is a better class because of it. I am a better and more reflective teacher because of it. I was encouraged to reflect on the development process, as well as the possible changes to strengthen the experience for both faculty and students. I implemented every suggestion and the course is a better course, and I am enjoying teaching it even more, because of that. The process has helped me to understand better how the course information is received (what I intended to communicate vs. what I actually communicated) and the clarity of the instructions I had given. Ultimately, the process strengthened the course.

This teacher noticed that she enjoyed teaching her course even more following this reflective process—it opened a possibility for her that she could grow and sustain her enthusiasm for the work and her commitment to the faculty role. It also served as affirmation that she was on the right path.

Exemplar #2: Graduate Clinical Course: Design Conference and Observation of Online Teaching

In reviewing a graduate course in a psych-mental health program, the initial dialogue regarding the online syllabus revealed that Reflection~Critique was the main emphasis. This course occurred near the end of the program, and students were immersed in their clinical practice as clinical nurse specialists (CNSs). Learning to reflect on that practice was the most crucial part of the course. All of the elements were present in some degree or another, but Reflection~Critique was the core.

As the teacher and evaluator began this dialogue, the teacher clearly saw that how she enacted reflection in her own teaching was at least as important as how she created reflective assignments for the students. This teacher said:

> . . . What I found to be different from previous peer reviews is that this process went beyond instructional feedback (i.e., just change this teaching strategy or learning activity) to something deeper—it asked me to question who I am as a teacher, what are my values, and how will I convey this to/with students. It got at the heart of who I am as a teacher and asked me to reflect on who I am and how I want to be. I found it much more transformative, empowering, and humbling. At the same time, it has led to more confidence—an opportunity to recognize and balance the complementary pairs of humility~confidence, transformation~change, openness~structure, and others. For example, we chose to explore the nature of feedback. This process gave me the opportunity to think about what feedback means to me, the ways I like to receive feedback from others, and how I might translate this to the way I give and receive feedback to/from

students. When we had this deeper conversation about feedback, it went beyond what instructional feedback I give to students to how I approach and present feedback as well as how I remain open to feedback from students.

This is a remarkable story in many respects, but one of the most important points it illustrates is the power of reflective dialogue to create a space into which gathering and sustaining can emerge. This teacher opens up to her own practices of reflection as she considers how she makes that same opportunity available for her students, and she begins a process that allows teacher and students to shape each others' views and actions as reflective practitioners. She gathers the practices, and in the process of reflection, she discovers ways to sustain herself as a teacher. The peer evaluator, in looking over course documents (online), found that same emphasis on reflection and feedback in the syllabus and assignments.

Exemplar #3: Undergraduate Capstone Course Illustrates an Ideas Conference

We also used the model with an undergraduate capstone course—a combination of online and clinical work. This course places senior students with individual preceptors, and the faculty role is assisting students with an evidence-based inquiry project that meets a unit need, working with preceptors to guide the students' clinical experience, and working with students to reflect on their own experiences.

The evaluator was invited to meet with the teacher, a new preceptor, and the student. During this conversation (and after the initial inquiry conversation with the evaluator), the teacher articulated how she wanted to emphasize reflection as a major part of the experience. She invited the preceptor and student to participate with her in this endeavor. In this way, she gathered (welcomed) both student and new preceptor into a dialogue that encouraged growth for all three. Conversation with the evaluator at semester's end revealed that she was better able to engage in reflection and that she could re-frame student critique of the course from more than one point of view. She could reflect on her own experience differently. She noted that the usual checklist for evaluating courses and faculty seemed very narrow to her after her experience with SE~PE. She articulated many new ideas about changes she wanted to make in her teaching and how she would build on these ideas for future possibilities for her own development.

The Ideas Conference and Reports

The final report represents writing as reflection-in-action and is co-created by the teacher and peer reviewer. The teacher begins by creating a reflective introduction about his or her teaching, including his or her philosophy of teaching~learning, general approach to students, and specifically, the aims for the particular course. The reviewer responds by adding a reflection on this introduction, supporting or challenging the ideas presented as useful ways of thinking about teaching.

Following this introduction, the dialogue continues as the teacher presents the relevant complementary pairs from the Table of Learning and describes how he or she tried to enact each one. The reviewer follows by discussing how the evidence from the course illustrates success or reveals places where more could be done. The final section of the dialogue contains both self and peer reviewer ideas for future work—innovations, places where the enactment of the elements was less clear, and ideas for extending the successful strategies. This mirroring dialogue engages both teacher and evaluator in new ways. It gathers their ideas into a place of co-creating a template for continued growth and success. It sustains the conversation about teaching~learning and creates a path for ongoing reflection.

SE~PE Application to Clinical Nursing Practice

The process of peer review in clinical practice is not evident in the literature. Clinical performance critique, based on a measurement model of skills and competence, is almost entirely driven by the need for supervisory evaluation

(Meretoja & Leno-Kilpi, 2001; O'Connor, Pearce, Smith, Voegeli, & Walton, 2001; Watson, Stimpson, Topping, & Porock, 2002). We note that there are no current articles on the topic of peer evaluation of clinicians. We propose that the SE~PE model outlined in this chapter could be effective in developing a mindful, interactive, and non-hierarchical evaluation, aimed at development of reflective nursing practices that are not easily measured: therapeutic presence, compassion, mindfulness, resilience, and professional insight.

In all SE~PE encounters, listening must be a central focus of reflective evaluation so that *interior insights* are privileged equally with behavioral observation (Swenson, & Sims, 2003). Nurses working together on a team have long been committed to listening to personal stories of providing care and to helping and supporting one another. A natural extension of this mutual support can be SE~PE. We propose that self-evaluation and peer evaluation, in listening pairs, can enhance nursing care by supporting and encouraging observed and reported best practices.

Final Reflections

The SE~PE process reveals the complementary nature of teaching~learning for the teacher. We are "always already" teaching and learning—the movement between this pair is constant and fluid. We have used the process with different teachers, both graduate and undergraduate, teaching clinical, didactic, and online courses. The same principles translate to application for educators in clinical settings, whether working with new graduates in transition to practice programs or providing other forms of instruction for clinically based learners, or for educators in lifelong learning programs teaching continuing education courses. The SE~PE model shows much promise in changing from the current culture of measurement-exclusive evaluation to one that fosters reflection. We can use the model to construct a world in which we gather creative possibilities for teaching~learning and sustain each other in the challenging work of educating the next generations of nurses.

References

Bloom, B. S. (1956). *The taxonomy of educational objectives: Cognitive domain*. New York, NY: David McKay.

Cooperrider, D. L., & Whitney, D. (2005). *Appreciative Inquiry: A positive revolution in change*. San Francisco, CA: Berrett-Koehler Publishers, Inc.

Cooperrider, D. L., Whitney, D., & Stavros, J. M. (2003). *Appreciative Inquiry handbook*. San Francisco, CA: Berrett-Koehler Publishers, Inc.

Diekelmann, N., & Diekelmann, J. (2009). *Schooling learning teaching: Toward narrative pedagogy*. Bloomington, IN: iUniverse, Inc.

Eisner, E. W. (1991). *The enlightened eye: Qualitative inquiry and the enhancement of educational practice*. New York, NY: Macmillan.

Guba, E. G., & Lincoln, Y. S. (1989). *Fourth generation evaluation*. Thousand Oaks, CA: Sage Publications.

Kelso, J. A. S., & Engstrom, D. A. (2006). *The complementary nature*. Cambridge, MA: MIT Press.

Krathwohl, D. R., Bloom, B. S., & Masia, B. B. (1964). *Taxonomy of educational objectives, book 2: Affective domain*. New York, NY: David McKay.

Meretoja, R., & Leno-Kilpi, H. (2001). Instruments for evaluating nurse competence. *JONA, 31*(7–8), 346–352.

O'Connor, S. E., Pearce, J., Smith, R. L., Voegeli, D., & Walton, P. (2001). An evaluation of the clinical performance of newly qualified nurses: A competency based assessment. *Nurse Education Today, 21*(7), 559–568.

Palmer, P. J. (1983). *To know as we are known: Education as a spiritual journey*. San Francisco, CA: Harper.

Parlett, M., & Hamilton, D. (1972). *Evaluation as illumination: A new approach to the study of innovatory programs*. Edinburgh, UK: University of Edinburgh Centre for Research in the Educational Sciences.

Reed, J. (2007). *Appreciative Inquiry: Research for change*. Thousand Oaks, CA: Sage Publications.

Shulman, L. S. (2000). From Minsk to Pinsk: Why a scholarship of teaching and learning? *JoSTL, 1*(1), 48–53.

Shulman, L. S. (2002). Making differences: A table of learning. *Change, 34*(6), 36–44.

Shulman, L. S. (2008). When coaching and testing collide. Retrieved from http://archive. carnegiefoundation.org/perspectives/when-coaching-and-testing-collide

Stake, R. E. (Ed.). (1975). *Evaluating the arts in education: A responsive approach.* Columbus, OH: Merrill.

Swenson, M. M. (1991). Using fourth-generation evaluation in nursing. *Evaluation & the Health Professions, 14*(3), 78–87.

Swenson, M. M., & Sims, S. L. (2003). Listening to learn: Narrative strategies and interpretive practices in clinical education. In N. L. Diekelmann (Ed.), *Teaching the practitioners of care: New pedagogies for the health professions* (154–193). Madison, WI: University of Wisconsin Press.

Watson, R., Stimpson, A., Topping, A., & Porock, D. (2002). Clinical competence assessment in nursing: A systematic review of the literature. *Journal of Advanced Nursing, 39*(5), 421–431.

Whitney, D., & Trosten-Bloom, A. (2003). *The power of Appreciative Inquiry: A practical guide to positive change.* San Francisco, CA: Berrett-Koehler Publishers, Inc.

Chapter 13

Reflective Ways of Working Together: Using Liberating Structures

–Melinda M. Swenson, PhD, RN, FNP, FAANP
–Sharon L. Sims, PhD, RN, FAANP
–Keith McCandless, MMHS
–With Learning Activity by Dawn Vanderhoef, PhD, DNP, PMHNP-BC,
FAANP

This chapter explores working together in groups, from small to large. We base our discussion on the principle that groups of any size reflect relationships that can be complex, confusing, and sometimes counterproductive. Secondly, we challenge traditional approaches to group interaction with approaches derived from complexity theory, in which we demonstrate how Liberating Structures can create new and more effective ways of working together. Groups and organizations have been studied through many lenses to understand how they develop, manage change, improve processes, and generally just get better (however that might be defined). Systems theory, cultural theory, group process, political theory, and change theory (among others) have been applied in nursing. Each approach has made valuable contributions to the work, and each has strengths and limitations. Through the discussions in this chapter, we propose Liberating Structures as another way of understanding the work of groups.

Beyond Tradition: Complexity Science Advances Organizational Relationships

The application of complexity science to the study of organizations is a fairly recent addition to this panoply of perspectives and is most relevant to this discussion of new and more reflective ways of working with each other. According to Lindberg, Nash, and Lindberg (2008), "Complexity science is not a single theory, but rather an interdisciplinary field that recognizes multiple theoretical frameworks. Complexity science examines [complex adaptive] systems comprised of multiple and diverse interacting agents . . ." (p. 32). Lindberg et al. continue their discussion of complexity science:

> Complex situations display properties of uniqueness, and thus must be approached and understood individually. A high degree of uncertainty is inherent in complex problems and situations, and outcomes are not predictable. Solutions cannot be assured through application of known formulas. Likewise, expertise and experience are helpful, but do not always ensure successful resolution. Complex problems call for unique solutions (p. 27).

Traditional approaches to organizational life have been critiqued for their mechanistic, linear view of the world, as discussed by Westley, Zimmerman, and Patton:

> Traditional methods of seeing the world compare its working to a machine. We say "things are working like clockwork" or "like a well-oiled machine," and people are seen as "human resources" who use management "tools." By using a machine metaphor, often unconsciously,

we ignore the living aspects of our world and our work. Complexity science embraces life as it is; unpredictable, emergent, evolving, and adaptable—not the least bit machine-like. And though it implies that even though we cannot control the world the way we can control a machine, we are not powerless, either. Using insights about how the world is changed, we can become active participants in shaping those changes (Westley et al., 2006, p. 7).

When complexity is the interpretive lens for organizational life, the relationships in that organization become the most important focus. Complexity science teaches different ways of examining groups and organizations—simply put, the more complex the organization, the less effective linear and hierarchical leadership and communication will be. Westley et al. (2006) describe the elements of working from a complexity stance:

> Questions are key. In complex situations there are no final answers. But certain key questions illuminate the issues of social innovation.
>
> Tensions and ambiguities are revealed through questioning. Social innovation both reveals and creates tensions. Once understood these tensions can then be engaged—not simply managed—in the interests of amplifying the desired change.
>
> Relationships are key to understanding and engaging with the complex dynamics of social innovation. For social innovations to succeed, everyone involved plays a role. As systems

COMPLEXITY SCIENCE

Complexity science is based on a view of systems that includes highly interrelated and rapidly adaptable parts. Each element in these complex adaptable systems affects the behavior of all other elements, and small changes can lead to large effects.

shift, everyone—funders, policy makers, social innovators, volunteers, evaluators—is affected. It is what happens between people, organizations, communities and parts of systems that matter—"in the between" of relationships.

A certain mindset is crucial—framed by inquiry not certitude, one that embraces paradoxes and tolerates multiple perspectives (Westley et al., 2006, pp. 21–22).

Beneath all of the theoretical language lives a deceptively simple premise:

> . . . If it is change we are after, and when we see the patterns and our role in their creation, we can make different choices in how we participate in a conversation . . . In complexity terms, this introduction of diversity into a pattern of interacting may represent the small change that triggers an entirely new pattern of relating or meaning. This emergence happens through a self-organizing process we can influence but not control. This self-organization is happening all around us and we are active players (Lindberg et al., 2008, p. 42).

Using Liberating Structures to Change the Way We Interact and Reflect

Non-hierarchical methodologies based in complexity science offer new ways to work in organizations that can "unleash" the power of everyone to think and act in new ways. Lipmanowicz and McCandless developed Liberating Structures (LS) to provide access to the benefits of complexity science without the associated theoretical burden (Lipmanowicz & McCandless, 2013). Ordinary people can take advantage of complexity principles in eminently practical ways. We use LS to act our way into new thinking, rather than thinking our way into action. This way of "unlearning" old habits and biases improves engagement in nursing education and practice.

Liberating Structures are a collection of methods designed for easy use by anyone to shift the patterns of interaction and "unleash the collective wisdom and creativity of nearly everyone in an organization" (Lipmanowicz & McCandless, 2010, p. 7). Business and healthcare organizations around the world have used LS with widespread effect. Because LS were created from field experience, they operate at the ground level of people's daily experience of their work. "The way we see organizing and leading has shifted profoundly. We have acted our way into new thinking. Our attention is no longer focused on overcoming resistance to change, buy-in strategies, expert training programs, best practices, visionary planning, or charismatic leadership. Many complicated control-heavy practices have faded away" (K. McCandless, personal communication, January 10, 2012).

The list of Liberating Structures in Figure 13.1 is itself a reflection of adaptability and emergence—new ones are being invented all the time and old ones are modified as they are used. "The basic idea is that Liberating Structures are combinations of freedom and control—they provide minimal structures or rules to maximize engagement by all. They are easy to learn and use and need not be implemented perfectly to produce results and change the pattern of interactions. Many of them create conversational spaces for people to self-organize and discover latent innovations that remain hidden when too many decisions and controls are imposed from the top. They make it easy for people at all levels to speak up, participate, and contribute" (Lipmanowicz & McCandless, 2010, p. 10). They are intended to allow groups to create solutions through "informal social networks and decentralized communities-of-practice" (p. 6). LS structures work in large and small groups, over a few minutes or whole days.

Figure 13.2 illustrates two possibilities for organizational/group behavior: One pattern is centered on control, whereas the other is focused on letting go. Control-centric cultures create a cycle of dependence, whereas cultures focused on letting go foster cycles of self-organization. Control tends toward a focus on tasks and alignment, whereas letting go tends toward a focus on engaging people. When control is ascendant, the culture fosters negative behaviors, such as aggression, forced "buy-in," secrecy, burnout, not taking responsibility, blame and mistrust, and caution. Dependency feeds back to the creation of ever more control. When letting go is predominant, the culture engages in interdependent work and shared accountability. Some commonly experienced behaviors in that kind of system include listening, asking for help, removing barriers to innovation, taking more responsibility, seeking full participation by all, information sharing, and risking action. Liberating Structures can be the catalyst for moving from control to letting go.

FIGURE 13.1

Liberating Structures Menu (Lipmanowicz & McCandless, 2013, p. 68).

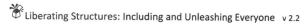 Liberating Structures: Including and Unleashing Everyone v 2.2

 Impromptu Networking
Rapidly share challenges and expectations, building new connections

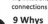 **9 Whys**
Make the purpose of your work together clear

What, So What, Now What?
Together, look back on progress to-date and decide what adjustments are needed

 TRIZ
Stop counterproductive activities & behaviors to make space for innovation

 Appreciative Interviews
Discover & build on the root causes of success

 1-2-4-All
Engage everyone simultaneously in generating questions/ideas/suggestions

 User Experience Fishbowl
Share know-how gained from experience with a larger community

 15% Solutions
Discover & focus on what each person has the freedom and resources to do now

 25-To-10 Crowd Sourcing
Rapidly generate & sift a group's most powerful actionable ideas

 Troika Consulting
Get practical and imaginative help from colleagues immediately

 Conversation Café
Engage everyone in making sense of profound challenges

 Min Specs
Specify only the absolute "Must do's" & "Must not do's" for achieving a purpose

 Wise Crowds
Tap the wisdom of the whole group in rapid cycles

 Wicked Questions
Articulate the paradoxical challenges that a group must confront to succeed

 Drawing Together
Reveal insights & paths forward through non-verbal expression

 Improv Prototyping
Develop effective solutions to chronic challenges while having serious fun

 Agreement-Certainty Matrix
Sort challenges into simple, complicated, complex and chaotic domains

 Shift & Share
Spread good ideas and make informal connections with innovators

 Heard, Seen, Respected
Practice deeper listening and empathy with colleagues

 Social Network Webbing
Map informal connections & decide how to strengthen the network to achieve a purpose

 Design StoryBoards
Define step-by-step elements for bringing projects to productive endpoints

 Open Space
Liberate inherent action and leadership in large groups

Discovery & Action Dialogue
Discover, spark & unleash local solutions to chronic problems

Integrated~Autonomy
Move from either-or to robust both-and solutions

Generative Relationships
Reveal relationship patterns that create surprising value or dysfunctions

Critical Uncertainties
Develop strategies for operating in a range of plausible yet unpredictable futures

Purpose-To-Practice
Define the five elements that are essential for a resilient & enduring initiative

Ecocycle Planning
Analyze the full portfolio of activities & relationships to identify obstacles and opportunities for progress

 Panarchy
Understand how embedded systems interact, evolve, spread innovation, and transform

What I Need From You
Surface essential needs across functions and accept or reject requests for support

Celebrity Interview
Reconnect the experience of leaders and experts with people closest to the challenges at hand

Helping Heuristics
Practice progressive methods for helping others, receiving help, and asking for help

 Simple Ethnography
Observe & record actual behavior of users in the field

 Keith McCandless & Henri Lipmanowicz www.liberatingstructures.com

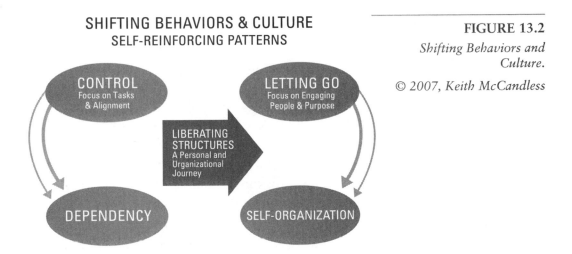

FIGURE 13.2

Shifting Behaviors and Culture.

© 2007, Keith McCandless

Liberating Structures can be scaled up or down, depending on the size of the group and the nature of the work to be done. This approach works in teacher-learner dyads, in classrooms, in governance groups such as committees and task forces, or in entire institutions.

Liberating Structures: Reflecting-in-Action and Reflecting-on-Action

Reflection is integral to Liberating Structures but emerges later in the process. The idea behind acting our way into thinking is that we can use LS to quickly make changes in our patterns of interaction, leading to reflection. Sometimes when the initial changes are small, we might take some time to realize what has happened: Reflection takes time to develop. Changing the ways we interact with each other is about changing our culture, which is about changing our habits and behaviors. Reflection is the means by which we notice how (and how much) our relationships have changed. This conversation about LS in groups shows up in the What, So What, Now What Cycle, which provides a useful template for reflection-on-action.

- *What?* What stands out in the stories we have shared? What do you notice?

- *So What?* Is there a pattern underneath the stories? Does it make a difference?

- *Now What?* What action can help us move forward? Who else should be here?

The conversations often involve telling, hearing, and thinking about stories, great and small. From a reflective perspective, engaging in conversations in this manner cues us to reflect on our thoughts and whether our responses within the experience were effective. Johns (2006) calls this dialogue between the retelling of the story (text) and other sources of knowing *theoretical framing*, helping us to uncover the relevance and validity to inform our practice. By conversing in a manner that involves sharing our own stories and incorporating relevant literature, we further inform and frame our ideas, and insights emerge.

Using Liberating Structures in a School of Nursing

The remainder of this chapter provides examples of using Liberating Structures in a school of nursing. They were very useful in informing our reflective practices and advancing our complex work, and could be used in multiple settings.

Story: Using a Conversation Café to Move From Small Talk to BIG Talk

We found an emerging need to take our everyday conversations to a higher level, as part of our efforts to determine a new vision, mission, and core values for the School of Nursing. The Conversation Café model (originating in Seattle soon after September 11, 2001) seemed to be a good fit. Conversation Cafés are open, hosted conversations where people gather to make sense of their world. At a Conversation Café, there is nothing to join, no agenda—just a simple process that helps to shift participants from small talk to BIG talk, focusing on conversations that matter.

The approach we present is derived from both Conversation Café the website, www.conversationcafe.org, and from our own experiences participating in various forms and modifications of the approach. The website includes an introductory video and print resources to help start a Conversation Café. Principles of the model include inclusivity and diversity (everyone can participate; in our case, this meant faculty, staff, and students); a designated host or hosts (but not a permanent host; anyone can host and all are invited to try); and open access to the conversation, in keeping with very few "rules," including the following:

- **What is said cannot be owned by anyone:** Clarify that what is said in the Conversation Café must be considered to be in the public domain. No one at the table or outside the conversation can claim exclusive ownership of the ideas that emerge.

- **Commercial-free [and agenda-free] zones:** No one can attend primarily to promote or impose a particular agenda, point of view, outcome, or solution.

- **No committees:** No political networking, committee formation, or action groups allowed.

- **Continuing to push our edges:** Encourage people to become hosts in a wide variety of settings on their own topics.

- **Empowering hosts:** Provide clear information to all hosts and participants about the mechanics of hosting Conversation Cafés and the open, inquisitive spirit of hosting.

As we worked with the Conversation Café idea, we proposed questions for conversation that we thought would interest a broad range of participants. We set up a café atmosphere in the conference room, with checkered tablecloths, tea, cookies, and a comfortable arrangement of chairs around a single table. We used a "talking stick" to keep the conversation focused on one person at a time and to enable everyone to have ample time to talk and be heard. We encouraged "deep listening" during which the person talking was encouraged to say as much as he or she wanted without comment or questions from anyone else. Everyone had a chance to respond once to the question, then to respond again, in turn, after all had spoken (or "passed") once.

> *"Creative conversation happens in a generative space that lies between. Notions of leading or following dissolve. A keen attentiveness and responsiveness among participants takes over. The process evokes a fine attunement to each other and what is happening in the moment."* –Keith McCandless

Our proposed conversations were stimulated by questions related to the newly developed core values for the school: respect, responsibility, trust, and dialogue. Each Conversation Café experience asked participants to tell about a time when a core value was clearly demonstrated by them or someone else. On the second round, each person could enlarge or clarify what they or another participant had said.

The discussion on each core value enabled participants to identify when the value had been clearly demonstrated, what behavior and language were used, and what feelings were evoked when the value was evident (or absent). Faculty members and staff members were able to have a conversation on the same plane, with no worry about repercussion or retaliation. The group felt safe and assured of the confidentiality of the discussions.

Conversation Cafés in our school took about 90 minutes. We scheduled some at the end of the school day and others at midday to enable participation by different people with differing schedules. For 2 years, we had a conversation about twice a semester, with different people attending.

Story: 1-2-4-All: A Way to Get Started

We used the Liberating Structure called "1-2-4-All" to start a different kind of conversation about our graduate nursing programs. We invited all faculty, staff, and students interested in looking at the relationships between and among our graduate nursing programs—in particular, our MSN and DNP programs. The impetus for the meeting focused on our first 2 years of implementing our new post-master's DNP, during which the disconnects between the master's and doctoral programs became visible. Prerequisite courses for the DNP were not part of our MSN program; DNP students could not obtain additional specialty preparation as part of their DNP program plan; and movement from the MSN to the DNP was not seamless in any way.

The 1-2-4-All structure is a rapid cycle conversation that begins with self-reflection on the question at hand. After this individual reflection, participants share their thoughts with one other person. The "duets" then share with another group of two, and finally, the groups of four share their conversations with the whole group (All). The themes from the "All" conversation generate next steps for the group. The initial conversation cycles (1-2-4) are designed to be short, perhaps 5 minutes for each cycle. The rapid cycles allow for jointly shaping solutions and insights in-the-moment (Lipmanowicz & McCandless, 2010). The whole-group conversation allows for broadening and deepening the themes from the rapid cycles.

The appreciative question we posed for our 1-2-4 cycle was, "What opportunities do you see for making the relationship between our graduate programs seamless?" The rapid cycle conversations were productive and positive and set the stage for an appreciative conversation by the whole group. The rapid cycle applies a type of reflection-in-action approach. The themes that emerged from this conversation focused mainly on tailoring student programs, increasing flexibility, facilitating easy transition from the master's program into a doctoral program, improving administrative and infrastructure processes, and nurturing connections among faculty and students.

The group did not focus on the details of courses and administrative process ("magnifying glass" level); rather, we kept our thinking at a higher level of abstraction ("satellite" level, as discussed at www.ThePrimes.com). This process enabled us to plan our next steps at a more conceptual level. After the meeting, we constructed a "word cloud" to summarize our thoughts and lead to an open and creative future.

After much discussion about what we would need to give up to create our preferred vision for graduate programs, we created an online project site where people could share their best ideas for moving the work forward. We continually strive to create open-space work groups and encourage innovation.

Story: TRIZ: Turning It Upside Down

We used the LS called TRIZ during a department meeting. Our aim was to discover what we might do to make our work environment more welcoming. The TRIZ process is about creative destruction and making a space for something new to emerge. It allows participants to recognize and amplify the dysfunctional parts of a system and then choose to eliminate them.

We started with a question: What would a totally reliable system for making us all miserable at work look like? What is the most terrible result we could imagine? Faculty and staff members worked in groups of four, using a rapid cycle process to answer these questions. It was challenging at first, because we were not used to thinking ridiculous thoughts about our department. We encouraged participants to let their minds go wild in this imagining and to have fun.

When the groups debriefed, several elements of a totally terrible workplace were generated. First, everyone must keep their doors shut at all times. No one was allowed to talk to anyone else in person. If two people encountered each other in the halls, they were not allowed to greet one another, nor have any conversation. Everyone would be required to eat lunch in their own office, and always alone. The secretaries would make sure they never got work done on time, and they would make as many mistakes as possible. The best result would be that the faculty member would eventually stop giving secretaries work—they would just do it themselves, behind their closed doors. We would never acknowledge any elements of our lives away from school—no birthdays would be noted, no flowers or cards sent if someone was hospitalized, no congratulations on significant life achievements. In short, the perfectly terrible system we designed would ensure that all of us would work in total isolation, with no humane or supportive interactions whatsoever.

The next step was to reflect on how this terrible system was similar to what we were already doing, and what actions we could take to stop doing things that lead to isolation and unhappiness. When we reflected on this TRIZ process, we realized we were already doing things to isolate socially from one another, by eating lunch alone in our offices and using electronic communication almost to the exclusion of face-to-face conversation. Our decision was that we would stop eating alone and/or skipping lunch and would instead reserve a conference room every day at noon for an hour and eat lunch together as often as possible. When we were able to stop something (isolating ourselves), it made room for something new to happen. It is this kind of small difference that encourages us to change our habits of interaction, which in turn changes a culture of isolation into one of sustaining human connection.

Story: Clearness Committees to Enable Discernment

We added Clearness Committees to our personal repertoire of reflective practices after learning about the use of these committees during our participation in a "Courage to Lead" workshop. The idea arises out of the Quaker tradition and is aimed at the protection of individual integrity in decision-making (discernment) while drawing on the resources of a supportive community. We used Clearness Committees with a new faculty member working through a decision on her career path, with doctoral students striving to determine their research focus, and with a faculty member considering retirement options.

Discernment is the concept describing differentiation between and among various choices or directions. The process aims at enabling the individuals to listen to themselves, to their "inner teacher" when faced with dilemmas or difficult choices. The Clearness Committee does not purport to give advice or make suggestions; instead, the committee helps to remove pre-judgments and other interferences so that individuals can hear their own inner voices.

Palmer (2004) describes these guidelines regarding how to best use a Clearness Committee:

1. The "focus person" chooses the members of the Clearness Committee, usually three to six trustworthy people who are diverse in gender and background.

2. We applied the "What/So What/Now What" Liberating Structure to the Clearness Committee. The focus person writes about the issue: What is the issue, what are the background issues, and what are our beginning speculations on approaches to the problem or dilemma. Members of the committee read this statement before the meeting.

3. The committee and the focus person meet together in a quiet and private place. Each member keeps notes during the meeting (or the session could be tape recorded). The focus person receives the notes at the end of the session. We planned sessions of approximately 1 to 2 hours. When the time is agreed upon, the session continues until the end, without any attempt to stop earlier.

4. We start with silence and a few contemplative moments. Then members of the committee start by asking honest, open questions of the focus person. These questions must be questions that no one but the focus person could possibly answer. Only the focus person can speak the answer, and only the focus person can really have access to the "truth" of the situation. Questions might be, "What have you thought about this issue up until now?" or "Have you ever faced a decision like this before?"

5. Questions might solicit ever deeper, more thoughtful responses from the focus person. The person might choose not to answer.

6. Questions and deep listening must not be rushed; it must be gentle, quiet, calm, and humane. The group might have long periods of silence.

7. All members of the committee remain totally engaged with the focus person and the issues at hand. The committee must be completely present in the moment, without distraction.

8. In the last few minutes of the meeting, members might read back some of the issues and discussion recorded. The focus person might respond and reflect, or not. Each member of the committee has a few minutes to comment on strengths of the focus person that emerged, celebrating the ability of the group and the person to open themselves up to the discernment process. All notes from the meeting are a gift to the focus person.

9. The committee does not fix the person, nor does it seek to solve any problems. If the focus person wants, he or she can discuss the "Now What" of the discernment process.

The beauty and utility of LS lie in the idea that new structures always are emerging, changing, and being re-invented. The use of LS is site-specific, depending on the people, places, problems, and issues involved. LS are fundamentally malleable and responsive to evolving circumstances. LS developers constantly rethink how to restructure and revise. For example, a few of the newest LS include the ideas described in the following sections.

Positive Gossip

The purpose of positive gossip is to reverse destructive patterns of negative gossip in a group or organization. Face to face in pairs, people are asked to say something positive about colleagues' actions or contributions. The pairs then debrief in groups of four, then engage in subsequent rounds of positive gossip with others in the larger group.

The nature of gossip is self-reinforcing. If the polarity of the gossip can be changed from negative to positive, the possibility exists that risk-taking and innovation will increase. Positive gossip can interrupt organizational malaise and discontent, replacing negativity with optimism and productivity (McCandless & Lipmanowicz, n.d.).

Talking with Pixies

The purpose of "Talking with Pixies" is to examine beliefs, ideas, and assumptions that limit one's progress. The central idea is that we all have lots of mental chatter about competing goals or commitments. This chatter can stifle progress, unless there is a path to examining what lies beneath—unchallenged assumptions or logic.

This LS starts with a group of three people—two to play the "pixies" and one listener who presents a personal or professional challenge. The pixies ask several questions aimed at illuminating why the goal is important, what actions have been taken that prevent the goal from being reached, and what will happen if the goal is not achieved. The pixies then chatter energetically about these things. One represents taking a safer course of action, maintaining the status quo, and the other represents the benefits of moving into different behaviors that stop undermining achievement. The pixies neither talk to each other nor offer advice to the listener; they are the listener's "inner voices." The roles switch so that each person in the group can be the listener. In contrast to the traditional Clearness Committee, the pixies may suggest consequences if the listener's assumptions are wrong. Once the process is complete, each person considers what actions they could take now and chooses one that could be started immediately.

Using Liberating Structures

Responding to increasing complexity, universities, colleges, and individual departments use Liberating Structures all over the United States and the world. Older linear models are no longer as effective or efficient. A recent survey of institutions of higher learning (Harris, Lilly, Semura, & Johnston, 2016) revealed that 90% of the schools who used this approach agree LS produce positive results by engaging groups, focusing on everyday solutions for big and small projects, suggesting design strategies, and transforming decision-making. The six most-used structures were 1-2-4-All (93%), What, So What, Now What (55%), TRIZ (52%), 25/10 Crowd Sourcing (51%), Impromptu Networking (35%), and Trioka Consulting (35%) (Harris et al., 2016).

Harris reports (personal communication, August 26, 2016) that the use of Liberating Structures can trigger a "healthy virus" effect. People who have been in LS sessions may try various structures in other situations, including small meetings, classrooms, and informal conversations. When positive outcomes emerge, more people become interested, and the move toward liberation grows exponentially. These are situations where the phenomenon can quickly spread throughout an organization, a school, or a community.

In addition to higher education settings, LS have been used for leadership and professional development, clinical practice, adult education, and with students in a wide variety of fields (Harris et al., 2016). Professions represented included communications, medical center administration, prevention science, public service, professional education, rhetoric and writing studies, social justice, and teaching/learning programs. Users of Liberating Structures learned the techniques in formal training workshops (83%), from knowledgeable colleagues (42%), or taught themselves using the website (www.liberatingstructures.com) and the book by Lipmanowicz and McCandless (13%) (Lipmanowicz & McCandless, 2013). Much of the diffusion of LS is informal, colleague to colleague and friend to friend.

DEVELOPING A PERSONAL NURSING PHILOSOPHY STATEMENT USING LIBERATING STRUCTURES: STORY BOARDS TO GUIDE THE PROCESS, BY DAWN VANDERHOEF, PHD, DNP, PMHNP-BC, FAANP

With graduation, advanced practice registered nurses (APRNs) enter the workforce within complex healthcare systems. Patients too are complex and increasingly present with more comorbid health conditions. APRNs must learn to navigate healthcare systems simultaneous with transitioning to practice as an advanced practice nurse. Many APRNs are introduced to reflective practice in

continues

continued

their academic studies; however, little is known about how APRNs engage as reflective practitioners aware of their personal philosophy of nursing and how this conceptualization guides their professional practice and development.

The ability to "know thy self" when working with systems and patients and as a member of the healthcare team is important. Articulation of a personal nursing philosophy grounds a new APRN. The ability to state one's beliefs, assumptions, and values about nursing in a succinct philosophy statement demonstrates a level of self-awareness. Holistic expression of one's beliefs, assumptions, and values incorporates the art and science, or theory and practice, of nursing (Marchuk, 2014).

Self-reflection, clinical experiences, and self-identity as an APRN validate the ability to seamlessly connect theory and practice (Johns, 2009, p. 82). Nursing philosophy development promotes critical thinking and self-reflection (Hernandez, 2009). Using one's experiences to make sense of and express a personal philosophy is productive and purposeful. As Dewey states, one learns through an arc, connecting present with previous experiences (Nelson, 2012).

Engaging students in group work further facilitates development of critical thinking and self-reflection (Hernandez, 2009). The ability to embrace reflection as a skill in the journey of lifelong learning is important. Throughout an APRN's career, individual beliefs, assumptions, and values will change; having the skills to revisit and revise a personal philosophy of nursing embraces and encourages ongoing reflection, critical analysis, and growth.

APRN students in their final semester have the theoretical knowledge and clinical experience to develop a personal nursing philosophy statement. The purpose of the nursing philosophy statement group assignment is to promote reflection and critical thinking. The process learned in this exercise can be replicated in other situations to promote reflective lifelong learning. Creating a classroom environment that encourages APRN students to engage as members of a team facilitates communication, sharing of ideas, and participation. The use of Liberating Structures (LS) design story boards facilitates group discussion in a safe environment, which lends to creative and innovative thinking (McCandless & Lipmanowicz, n.d.). Developing a philosophy of nursing statement in a group setting is risk-taking, and using an LS process promotes success.

The following exemplar uses an adaptation of the LS story board to facilitate a group classroom experience for APRN students to develop a personal philosophy of nursing statement.

LS Story Board Learning Activity

(Pre-class reading: Hernandez, C. A. (2009). Student articulation of a nursing philosophical statement: An assignment to enhance critical thinking skills and promote learning. Journal of Nursing Education, 48(6), pp. 343–349.)

- *Students and faculty engage in a 30-minute class discussion about the Hernandez (2009) article focusing on development of a personal nursing philosophy statement and ongoing refinement; definition of beliefs, assumptions, and values about APRN practice and how these terms guide the development of a nursing philosophy. Nursing's four metaparadigm concepts (nursing, person, health, and environment) help frame the discussion.*

- *Students are divided into groups of six and provided three poster boards taped to the wall, each with one of the following headings: Beliefs, Values, and Assumptions. The LS story board process is explained. Each student is provided a unique color of sticky notes such as yellow, blue, orange, etc.*

- *Each group is allowed 10 minutes to individually write keywords or phrases that come to mind when thinking about nursing beliefs. Each keyword or phrase is written on a separate sticky note and then posted on the poster board titled "Assumptions." Each student group selects a spokesperson to lead a 10-minute discussion of the statements on the poster board, and the group begins to create themes. A group member clusters sticky notes based on the identified themes and creates headings.*

- *Each student group repeats the process of writing keywords and phrases about assumptions, grouping the posted notes and developing themes (20 minutes), and then follows the same process for values (20 minutes).*

- *Groups are allowed 20 minutes to discuss the themes in each of the three areas—beliefs, assumptions, and values—and identify two or three key themes for each heading. Guided by the key themes, the group develops a philosophy of nursing statement.*

- *Each group has 10 minutes to describe to the class their process using the "what, so what, now what" reflective approach (see Liberatingstructures. com). A group spokesperson then reads the newly developed philosophy of nursing statement.*

- *Students take a picture of the poster board to guide an out-of-class reflection assignment.*

- *Students submit a written reflection about the process of developing a group nursing philosophy statement based on the group process and present their own nursing philosophy statement.*

Final Reflections

This chapter offered some practical, grounded ideas for ways to help complex groups, large and small, to enact reflective thinking by doing. These are ideas-in-practice to promote reflection-in-action and reflection-on-action. The next chapter presents more theoretical approaches to complexity through the use of integral theory, which both transcends and includes the perspectives presented in this chapter. The combination of Liberating Structures and integral theory has the potential to lead to even more productive and fulfilling reflective practices for nursing.

References

Harris, D., Lilly, C., Semura, J., & Johnston, R. (August 19, 2016). *LS: Scaling up across higher education.* Presentation at NCCI, Montreal, Quebec, Canada.

Hernandez, C. A. (2009). Student articulation of a nursing philosophical statement: An assignment to enhance critical thinking skills and promote learning. *Journal of Nursing Education, 48*(6), 343–348.

Johns, C. (2006). *Engaging reflection in practice: A narrative approach.* Oxford, UK: Blackwell.

Johns, C. (2009). *Becoming a reflective practitioner.* Ames, IA: John Wiley & Sons.

Lindberg, C., Nash, S., & Lindberg, C. (2008). *On the edge: Nursing in the age of complexity.* Bordentown, NJ: PlexusPress.

Lipmanowicz, H., & McCandless, K. (2010). Liberating Structures: Innovating by including and unleashing everyone. *E&Y Performance, 2*(3), 6–20.

Lipmanowicz, H., & McCandless, K. (2013). *The surprising power of Liberating Structures: Simple rules to unleash a culture of innovation.* Seattle, WA: Liberating Structures Press.

Marchuk, A. (2014). A personal nursing philosophy in practice. *Journal of Neonatal Nursing, 20,* 266–273.

McCandless, K., & Lipmanowicz, H. (n.d.). Liberating Structures. Retrieved from http://www.liberatingstructures.com/

Nelson, S. (2012). The lost path to emancipating practice: Towards a history of reflective practice in nursing. *Nursing Philosophy, 13*, 202–213.

Palmer, P. (2004). *A hidden wholeness: The journey toward an undivided life.* San Francisco, CA: John Wiley & Sons.

Westlcy, F., Zimmerman, B., & Patton, M. Q. (2006). *Getting to maybe: How the world is changed.* Toronto, Canada: Vintage Canada

Part V

Future Directions in Reflective Practice

Chapter 14

An Introduction to Integral Philosophy and Theory: Implications for Quality and Safety

–Daniel J. Pesut, PhD, RN, FAAN

The first four sections of this book have described the overall framework for reflective practice, presented applications with a variety of objectives, and illustrated ways for practice improvements and self-development. This chapter introduces readers to integral philosophy and theory to further advance our capacity for reflective thinking and acting. *Integral theory* is a comprehensive framework that supports multiple perspectives and enables practitioners to become more aware of their personal experiences through analysis, consideration, reflection, and understanding of any situation.

Integral theory is an emerging paradigm offering a useful framework that transcends and includes other theoretical orientations. Initially, integral theory might seem complex; however, with mindful effort, practitioners can gain understanding and appreciate the comprehensive value of integral theory. The philosophy, principles, and concepts of integral theory can offer an awareness of new units of analysis and methods that support inquiry, reflection, and good science. Integral understanding enhances self-management in regard to others and the contexts in which we live and work. Thus, it is an expanded application of reflective practices.

Consideration of quality and safety issues through integral philosophy pushes one to the learning edge of sense-making and results in new ways of perceiving. Use of an integral lens supports analyzing, evaluating, and understanding personal experiences, relationships with others, as well as the behavior of self and others that is embedded in systems and the collective cultures in which we live and work. Reflecting on the Quality and Safety Competencies (knowledge, skills, and attitudes; see www.qsen.org) through an integral lens provides a comprehensive way to navigate the territories related to self, relationships with other, behaviors, and systems dynamics. Learning more about integral methodological pluralism opens a way to study quality and safety through eight zones of inquiry, thus contributing to the evidence, knowledge base, and science of quality and safety. Finally, given the complexities of the environments in which clinicians practice, integral philosophy, theory, and methods all support teaching and learning into the future.

Learning at the Integral Edge: What Is Integral?

Wilber (2000, 2001, 2005, 2007) is a philosopher-scientist-practitioner who has advanced an integrally informed approach to being and doing in the world. *Integral* means comprehensive, balanced, whole, and complete. Dossey (2008) has proposed an integral theory of holistic nursing, and Jarrin (2006) goes further to suggest that integral theory can be used as a unifying meta-theory for nursing. Dacher (2006) has written about the need for an integral approach to health and human flourishing, and Watson (2008) asserts that while nursing practice has tended to locate itself professionally with the right side of the quadrant, much of the evolving work in the academic world leans toward the left side of the quadrant. Integral theory allows for all ways of knowing and is consistent with a comprehensive approach for Caring Science.

An excellent overview and introduction to integral theory, written by Esbjorn-Hargens (n.d.), can be found at the Integral Life website. Bhaskar, Esbjorn-Hargens, Hedlund, and Hartwig (2016) argue that there is a deep need for integrative metatheories to help impact and influence understanding and insight into the complex, wicked methodological challenges of the twenty-first century.

According to Forman (2010), integral philosophy involves attention to the following principles:

- What is real and important depends on one's perspective.

- Everyone is at least partially right about what they argue is real and important.

- By bringing together these partial perspectives, we can construct a more complete and useful set of truths.

From an integral philosophy, a person's perspective depends on five central things:

- The way the person gains knowledge (the person's primary perspective, tools, or discipline)

- The person's level of identity development

- The person's level of development in other key domains or lines

- The person's particular state at any given time

- The person's personality style or "type" (cultural and gender style)

The integral viewpoint is often relayed using the acronym AQAL:

- All

- Quadrants

- All

- Levels, lines, states, and types

Experience Through an Integral Lens: Four Dimensions of Awareness

AQAL represents the four major overarching perspectives, which are:

- Subjective-individual

- Objective-individual

- Subjective-collective

- Objective-collective

Given the AQAL model posits, you have four major overarching perspectives or dimensions of awareness. The quadrants refer to four dimensions of a person's being in the world. This is portrayed in Figure 14.1 and can be described as follows:

1. The first dimension is your individual interior—your thoughts, feelings, intentions, and psychology. Basically, this is the "I" of you.

2. The second quadrant refers to your *collective interior*—your relationships, culture, and meaning that you share with others. This quadrant is often referred to as the "we" space.

3. The third quadrant is your *individual exterior*—your physical body and behaviors and actions. This is referred to as the "it" space.

4. Finally, the fourth quadrant is your *collective exterior*—the environment and social systems and structures in which you operate. This is referred to as the "its" space.

These four quadrants represent four perspectives of awareness.

Stop for a moment and tune inward into awareness of your sense of self. This "I" space is composed of thoughts, ideas, opinions, motivations, values, beliefs, and a sense of identity, purpose, mission, and vision. All of these exist within the interior of your personal consciousness. All of these things are invisible to those around you—they are only available to you. You might study these aspects of your own experience through the use of journaling, prayer, self-inquiry, mindfulness practices, meditation, reflection, or phenomenology. What you know about yourself depends on your sincerity of expression, truthfulness, honesty, integrity, and your willingness to acknowledge your biases and identify your assumptions and experiences. Self-knowledge influences how you see the world and thus begins the sense-making of practice, work, and relationships with others.

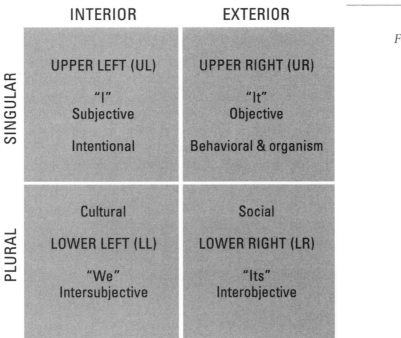

FIGURE 14.1

Four Quadrants of the AQAL Model.

Next, stop for moment and think about a relationship you are in—imagine being together with another person. Chances are you can recognize that by being with this person you share emotions, communicate with them, share feelings, and participate in the ups and downs of relating. The feeling and awareness of the "we" you get from this relationship is different from the awareness of "I." What you know about the "we" is often derived from resonance and mutual understanding, empathy, collective reflection, storytelling, and dialogue and/or debate.

"Integral philosophy and theory challenges us to be aware of being aware of the four dimensions in an intentional way. Such awareness sharpens our intention and attention and provides us with alternative ways to investigate phenomena while appreciating and valuing multiple perspectives in the pursuit of learning, inquiry, and knowledge."

The "it" space is the perspective or dimension of objectifying people and things and sensing behaviors. This is the dimension of individual exteriors. This is the dimension of body and brain—you can see it, hear it, touch it, taste it, and smell it. The focus on the exterior individual nature of something gives it a "thingness" sense. The dimension of it can be studied through observations and measures from the outside in—controlled conditions, representative samples, empirical measures, fieldwork observations, surveys, documentation, and examinations. It is often described in third-person descriptions and supported with statistics and charts. Physical behavior and the things you do with the body are a part of the "it" dimension, because others can see and observe these behaviors and actions.

Now consider the "its" dimension. The "its" dimension involves the social and political systems in which you live and work. It includes the environment, ecology of the planet, social systems of schools, and government. It encompasses policies and procedures that regulate your work and family life, as well as the legal system in which you participate. "Its" awareness includes experiences with multiple interacting systems that focus on function, sustainability, and the ecology of the planet and local environment where you live and work.

Integral philosophy supports people who aspire to integral life practices (Wilber, Patten, Leonard, & Morelli, 2008); individuals who recognize these four different dimensions of awareness are arising at the same time. The simultaneous arising is described as the four dimensions of being "tetra-arising." None of the dimensions exist separately, yet we often segregate and discuss them one at a time, as if one dimension does not influence the other dimensions. Integral philosophy and theory challenges us to be aware of being aware of the four dimensions in an intentional way. Such awareness sharpens our intention and attention and provides us with alternative ways to investigate phenomena while appreciating and valuing multiple perspectives in the pursuit of learning, inquiry, and knowledge. In this way, we expand our reflective capacity.

The AQAL framework has several other elements. The notion of four quadrants combines two of the most fundamental integral distinctions: the interiors and exteriors of an individual and collective. The other elements of the AQAL framework are levels, lines, states, and types.

Levels are ways to describe developmental structures that evolve over time. For example, as an individual grows and matures, he or she evolves and develops through a series of developmental stages. People often mature and evolve from an egocentric view of the world to an ethnocentric, and then to a world-centric stage of development.

Lines are specific areas of growth and development. Lines or streams of development are similar to the ideas of multiple intelligences. Important lines of development and life questions include the following:

- Cognitive: What am I aware of?
- Self: Who am I?
- Values: What is significant to me?
- Moral: What should I do?

TETRA-ARISING

Tetra-arising integral is about quadratic or four-quadrant thinking, because at any moment in time, experiences can be considered from one or more of the four quadrants—I, We, It, and Its.

- Interpersonal: How should we interact?

- Spiritual: What is of ultimate concern?

- Needs: What do I need?

- Kinesthetic: How should I physically do this?

- Emotional: How do I feel about this?

- Aesthetic: What is attractive to me?

Lines of development can arise in any of the four quadrants. Some lines of development in the "I" quadrant include such things as cognitive awareness, emotional access, interpersonal skills, psychosexual expression, moral capacity, spiritual experience, and self-identity dynamics. Lines of development in the "we" quadrant include such things as worldviews, intersubjective dynamics, linguistic meaning, cultural values, background cultural contexts, philosophical positions, and religious understandings. Lines of development in the "it" quadrant include organic structures, neuronal systems, neurotransmitters, brainwave patterns, skeletal-muscular growth, nutritional intake, and kinesthetic capacity. Examples of the lines of development in the "its" quadrant include forces of production, geopolitical structures, ecosystems, written legal codes, architectural styles, grammatical systems, and evolutionary paths.

From an integral perspective, *states* matter. *States* in the integral framework are temporary, changing levels of awareness. Consider how you personally transition every day from dreaming to sleeping to waking states. An individual can also alter his or her states through meditating or exercising. Some people have psychic state experiences, whereas others alter their states through the use of chemicals or substances. So in the "I" quadrant, there are phenomenal states, natural states, and altered states. In the "we" quadrant, there are group states, intersubjective states, and religious states. In the "it" quadrant, there are brain states, hormonal states, and behavioral states. In the "its" quadrant, there are weather states, economic states, and ecological states.

Finally, another basic building block in the integral model is the notion of *types*. These are categories of differences, such as masculine or feminine, cultural types, or personality types like Myers-Briggs personality definitions that become influential as one thinks about integral paths of growth and development through time. In the "I" quadrant, you can reference personality and gender types. In the "we" quadrant, you can reference types of religious and kinship systems. In the "it" quadrant, you can reference blood types and body types. In the "its" quadrant, types include biome types and regime types.

Dr. Alan Watkins (2014, 2016) has proposed that taking an integral perspective can lead to vertical development and enlightened leadership. There are 10 dimensions to enlightened leadership: physical intelligence, physical management, emotional intelligence, emotional literacy, emotional self-management, emotional resilience, self-motivation, optimistic outlook, social intuition empathy and rapport, and social intelligence. Watkins argues that a person's energy can be measured by paying attention to the physiology of the body, especially one's heart rate variability. From an integral perspective, there is power to heart rate variability and coherence.

Consider the HeartMath Institute paradigm and research that focuses on personal development by unifying heart, breath, and mind through mindful evocation of a calming positive heart image. This practice raises awareness to a deeper heart and breath connection through biofeedback, leading to increased awareness of emotions, greater order and mind coherence, and energy to a more positive conscious presence (Edwards, 2015). HeartMath techniques support the development of an integral consciousness that illuminates wisdom and skillful compassion through the practice of inner work that radiates to outer work of service in the world. The embodiment of integral philosophy requires noticing and valuing every kind of intelligence, including that of the heart (Wilber et al., 2008).

The integral framework contains more complexities that are beyond the scope of this chapter. Interested readers are directed to the reference list and resources noted at the end of this chapter to learn more about the background and development of integral philosophy and theory. The AQAL model provides a framework for most of life. Personal development and evolution within the context of the AQAL framework is about harmonizing development across all four quadrants to reach higher levels of development and awareness, based on a reflective stance.

An Integral Circle of Awareness

A person can use the AQAL model to assess any situation. For example, differing situations challenge us individually, so *interior considerations* and *interpersonal* communications pose challenges to us in terms of evaluating possible *actions to take*. And the influence of our actions has a reciprocal relationship, affecting *systems* in which we operate. Visualizing the challenges in teamwork communication, an essential aspect of quality and safety, within these considerations of the four quadrants is easy. Forman and Ross (2013) suggest that the upper left quadrant relates to purpose and personal thoughts and beliefs, emotions, motivations, satisfaction, desires, attitudes, and values. The lower left quadrant is the space of guiding principles, organizational ethos, language, priorities, styles, and taboos. The upper right is about individual behaviors, actions, stress responses, and a person's health, physical skills, and appearance. The lower right is about processes, whether administrative, financial, legal, or reporting structures and communication channels. Meaning-making must take place through the perspective of these four quadrants.

REFLECTING ON . . . SIZING UP ANY SITUATION

A person is able to size up any situation by using the following questions (Wilber et al., 2008):

- *Interior considerations: What do I think, feel, or value about _____? (Focus on "I," interior individual.)*

- *Communication: How can I take the greatest amount of people into consideration at the deepest levels? (Focus on "we," the collective interior of relationships and relating.)*

- *Evaluate possible actions: What creative action can I take regarding _____? (Focus on "it," the exterior individual behavior and actions.)*

- *Interconnections: How do the larger systems in which I live affect my range of choices? How will my choices affect these systems? (Focus on "its," the collective exterior systems.)*

Imagine that the four quadrants represent a complete circle. To have an integral perspective means that you pay attention to all four quadrants and all

360 degrees of the circle. To limit your attention or awareness to only one of the quadrants means that you are only attending to 90 degrees of what is tetra-arising or possible at any given moment. Quality and safety mindfulness requires 360 degrees of awareness. If you attend only to what is going on in your personal interior without attending to the impact that relationships, behavior, and systems have on you, then you will not be able to offer mindfulness of the entire circle. (This concept is displayed in Figure 14.2.)

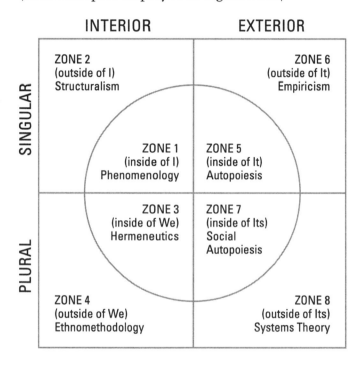

FIGURE 14.2

The Eight Zones and Methodologies of Integral Methodological Pluralism (IMP) (Esbjorn-Hargens, 2006).

Evolving Quality and Safety Science Through an Integral Lens

The QSEN competencies are organized around knowledge, skills, and attitudes associated with six main areas of concern. As described in the tables in Appendix B, the competencies are:

1. *Patient-centered care:* Recognize the patient or designee as the source of control and full partner in providing compassionate and

coordinated care based on respect for the patient's preferences, values, and needs.

2. *Teamwork and collaboration:* Function effectively within nursing and interprofessional teams, fostering open communication, mutual respect, and shared decision-making to achieve quality patient care.

3. *Evidence-based practice:* Integrate best current evidence with clinical expertise and patient/family preferences and values for delivery of optimal healthcare.

4. *Quality improvement:* Use data to monitor the outcomes of care processes and use improvement methods to design and test changes to continuously improve the quality and safety of healthcare systems.

5. *Safety:* Minimize risk of harm to patients and providers through both system effectiveness and individual performance.

6. *Informatics:* Use information and technology to communicate, manage knowledge, mitigate error, and support decision-making.

REFLECTING ON . . . AN INTEGRAL EXERCISE

Challenge yourself with this integral exercise. Create a two-by-two table in a blank document based on the four integral quadrants. Label them accordingly: the upper left quadrant would be "I," interior individual dimensions of self; the lower left quadrant would represent the interior collective, or the "we" of an interpersonal space; the upper right quadrant would be the "it" space, or the exterior individual zone; and the lower right quadrant represents the social systems, or the "its" space. As you review the knowledge, skills, and attitudes associated with all the QSEN prelicensure and graduate level competencies, in which quadrant do you place each of the skills and/or attitudes from an integral perspective? After you do this exercise, what sense do you make of the areas that need most attention in terms of your development of mindfulness and reflection? What insights do you gain about the collective interiors of teamwork and patient family relationships? What behaviors and actions do you need to master? Finally, how do the systems in which you work influence you and your integral quadratic thinking about quality and safety?

HEART-FOCUSED BREATHING™ TECHNIQUE

Heart-Focused Breathing is a self-regulation strategy designed to reduce the intensity of a stress reaction and to establish a calm, alert state. To practice Heart-Focused Breathing, begin by taking 5 minutes to simply focus your attention in the area of the heart and imagine your breath flowing in and out of your heart. Breathe a little slower and deeper than usual, and try practicing with your eyes open so that you can learn to do it on the go. (HeartMath, 2014)

HeartMath techniques such as Heart-Focused Breathing support the development of the dimensions and skills associated with Watkins Enlightened Leadership Model. Heart-Focused Breathing leads to measurable physiological changes, shifting heart rhythms to a more coherent state and drawing attention away from an issue, which further calms our thoughts and stabilizes our emotions. By creating an inner pause, we become aware that we have a choice of how to respond to a situation (HeartMath, 2014).

Final Reflections

In many ways, this entire text is nudging all of us toward a more integral way of teaching and learning. The purpose of the book is to help us make sense of our work while using inquiry-based reflective practices. As we engage in mindful examination of ourselves within the context of our environment, self, and others, we expand our emotional intelligence in ways that increase our capacity for change and transformation. Integral theory helps us move toward a higher level of self-awareness by applying the four-quadrant thinking and analysis. As we integrate the principles of integral thinking into habits of the mind, we are freer to be in the world, respond to the challenges we confront daily, and bring a holistic perspective to our work and self-development. Who we are is who we bring to work. Thus, integral-based self-development changes our work presence and potentiates our focus on doing our work well. Quality and safety are based on doing the right thing for all those around us, whether working with patients, learners, or co-workers. We can experience a renewed focus that will change patient outcomes, improve learner achievement, and increase our own satisfaction with our work. Enlightened leadership practices and managing the energy of our physiology (and especially heart math practices) are ways to self-regulate and master our leadership, which contributes to the health of patients, teams, and organizations in which we practice. The next two chapters will further enhance our views of applying integral theory to advance our capacity for reflection and commitments to action.

References

Bhaskar, R., Esbjorn-Hargens, S., Hedlund, N., & Hartwig, M. (Eds.). (2016). *Metatheory for the 21st century*. New York, NY: Routledge.

Dacher, E. (2006). *Integral health: The path to human flourishing*. Laguna Beach, CA: Basic Health.

Dossey, B. (2008). A theory of integral nursing. *Advances in Nursing Science, 31*(1), E52–E73.

Edwards, S. D. (2015). HeartMath: A positive psychology paradigm for promoting psychophysiological and global coherence. *Journal of Psychology in Africa, 25*(4), 367–374.

Esbjorn-Hargens, S. (n.d.). *An overview of integral theory: An all-inclusive framework for the 21st century*. Integral Life Institute. Retrieved from http://integrallife.com. (Also available as Integral Life Institute, Resource Paper No. 1, March 2, 2009.)

Esbjorn-Hargens, S., Reams, J., & Gunnlaugson, O. (2009). The emergence and characteristics of integral education: An introduction. In S. Esbjorn-Hargens, J. Reams, & O. Gunnlaugson (Eds.), *Integral education: New directions for higher learning* (pp. 1–16). Albany, NY: State University of New York (SUNY) Press.

Forman, M. (2010). *A guide to integral psychotherapy: Complexity, integration, and spirituality in practice*. Albany, NY: State University of New York (SUNY) Press.

Forman, J., & Ross, L. (2013). *Integral leadership: The next half step*. Albany, NY: State University of New York (SUNY) Press.

HeartMath. (2014). *HeartMath certified trainer leader's guide*. Boulder Creek, CA: Institute of HeartMath.

Jarrin, O. F. (2006). An integral philosophy and definition of nursing: Implications for a unifying meta-theory of nursing. *School of Nursing Scholarly Works*. Paper 46. Retrieved from http://digitalcommons.uconn.edu/son_articles/46

Sullivan, D. T., Hirst, D., & Cronenwett, L. (2009). Assessing quality and safety competencies of graduating prelicensure nursing students. *Nursing Outlook*, *57*(6), 323–331.

Watkins, A. (2014). *Coherence: The secret science of brilliant leadership*. London, UK: Kogan Page Publishers.

Watkins, A. (2016). *4D leadership: Competitive advantage through vertical leadership development*. London, UK: Kogan Page Publishers.

Watson, J. (2008). *Nursing: The philosophy and science of caring* (Rev. ed.). Boulder, CO: University Press of Colorado.

Wilber, K. (2000). *Integral psychology: Consciousness, spirit, psychology, therapy*. Boston, MA: Shambhala Publications.

Wilber, K. (2001). *A theory of everything*. Boston, MA: Shambhala Publications.

Wilber, K. (2002). *The many ways we touch: Three principles helpful for an integrative approach*. Unpublished manuscript.

Wilber, K. (2005). Introduction to integral theory and practice: IOS Basic and the AQAL map. *AQAL: Journal of Integral Theory and Practice*, *1*(1), 1–36.

Wilber, K. (2007). *The integral vision*. Boston, MA: Shambhala Publications.

Wilber, K., Patten, T., Leonard, A., & Morelli, M. (2008). *Integral life practice: A 21st century blueprint for physical health, emotional balance, mental clarity, and spiritual awakening*. Boston, MA: Integral Books.

Chapter 15

Reflecting as a Team: Issues to Consider in Interprofessional Practice

–Daniel J. Pesut, PhD, RN, FAAN
–Gwen D. Sherwood, PhD, RN, FAAN, ANEF
–Sara Horton-Deutsch, PhD, RN, FAAN, ANEF

The purpose of this chapter is to put forward ways that interprofessional health professions practice can be transformed through the use of integral theory, methods of research, action inquiry, and principles of reflection. *Integral theory* is a common framework and model to support perspective-taking, dialogue, understanding, and reflection among healthcare providers. Development of integral consciousness combined with the cooperative and action inquiry methods are proposed as skillful means to enhance interprofessionality. The models and methods described in this chapter suggest that interprofessional reflection, teamwork in practice, and transformation of health professions education and practice can be accelerated with the adoption of integral perspectives and methods of inquiry that support transformational learning.

Transformational Learning

According to Merriam (2004), transformational learning requires a level of cognitive development that supports content, process, and premise reflection in adults. Mezirow (1991) differentiated among these three types of reflection on experience and determined that only premise reflection can lead to transformative learning. *Content reflection* is thinking about the actual experience itself; *process reflection* is thinking about how to handle the experience; and *premise reflection* involves examining long-held, socially constructed assumptions, beliefs, and values about the experience or problem. Premise reflection, or critical reflection of assumptions, is about assumptions we hold regarding the self (narrative), the cultural systems in which we live (systemic), our workplace (organizational), our ethical decision-making (moral-ethical), or feelings and dispositions (Mezirow, 2000, 2003). According to Mezirow (1991), the transformation process "always involves critical reflection upon the distorted premises sustaining our structure of expectation" (1991, p. 167). The ideas and strategies proposed in this chapter are intended to stimulate inquiry and action related to team reflection in interprofessional health practices and promote critical premise reflection.

An Integral Approach to Transformation of Interprofessional Practice

Wilber (2007) is a philosopher-scientist-practitioner who has advanced an integrally informed approach to being and doing in the world. *Integrally informed* is a phrase that denotes a consciousness, approach, or product informed by integral theory (Rentschler, 2006). Integral theory, as discussed in Chapter 14, is synonymous with the acronym AQAL, which stands for:

- **All**
- Quadrants
- **All**
- Levels, lines, states, and types

See Figure 15.1. For a general overview of these topics, consult Wilber's "Introduction to Integral Theory and Practice: IOS Basic and the AQAL Map" (2005), *A Theory of Everything* (2001), and *Integral Psychology* (2000).

According to Wilber, the six main components of a human experience made explicit through an integral model are:

1. The four quadrants of interior and exterior, individual and collective

2. Consciousness and its *waves* and *levels*

3. *Lines* of development

4. Normal and altered *states* of consciousness

5. *Styles* or *types* of personality

6. The concepts of *ego, self,* or *self-system*

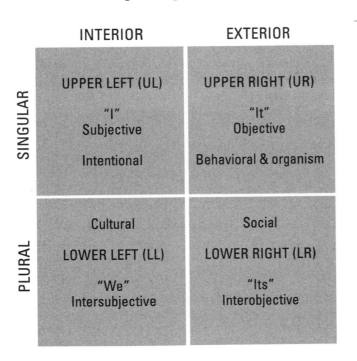

FIGURE 15.1
AQAL Model.

Forman (2010) writes, "The integral model represents a constructive response to overspecialization and positions itself as a kind of 'next step' in intellectual dialogue and practical application" (p. 11). Integral philosophy involves attention to the following principles:

- What is real and important depends on one's perspective.

- Everyone is at least partially right about what they argue is real and important.

- By bringing together these partial perspectives, we can construct a more complete and useful set of truths.

- A person's perspective depends on five central things:

  1. The way the person gains knowledge (the person's primary perspective, tools, or discipline).

  2. The person's level of identity development.

  3. The person's level of development in other key domains or lines.

  4. The person's particular state at any given time.

  5. The person's personality style or "type" (including cultural and gender style).

"As nurses, we can inform ourselves and appreciate the theories and standards of our partners in healthcare; recognize and acknowledge where our work complements and interfaces; and question from various perspectives how we can draw upon all of these sources to create an integrated whole."

Koller (2006) explains the core premise of an integral science is that every scientific discipline has some partial yet important truth to tell us, and to exclude the stories that emerge from any given discipline will create unfortunate gaps in our overall understanding. To that end, one of the key functions of integral science is to organize the various scientific disciplines relative to each other in such a way that we can honor their respective achievements in their areas of inquiry without over-exaggerating their importance.

To be integral involves adoption of three integrative principles. These principles are nonexclusion, enfoldment, and enactment (Wilber, 2001). *Nonexclusion* requires the acceptance of truth claims that go by the validity tests for their own paradigms in respective fields. Some examples of truth claims include truthfulness and sincerity, justness, objective truth, and functional fit. *Enfoldment* requires sets of practices that are more inclusive, holistic, and comprehensive than others, such as ensuring continuity of care in nursing. *Enactment* requires various types of inquiry that reveal and disclose different phenomena depending on the "I," "we," "it," and "its" quadrants and associated levels, lines, states, and types of the inquirer.

As nurses, we can inform ourselves and appreciate the theories and standards of our partners in healthcare; recognize and acknowledge where our work complements and interfaces; and question from various perspectives how we can draw upon all of these sources to create an integrated whole.

Esbjorn-Hargens (2006a) and Esbjorn-Hargens, Reams, and Gunnlaugson (2010) write that integral theory informs an integral approach to education and is committed to all of the following:

- The best components of conventional and alternative approaches to curriculum, pedagogy, evaluation, and methods of inquiry

- The engagement of transformative practices among teacher, student/practitioners, and classroom

- Inclusion of subjective experience, objective behavior, intersubjective culture, and interobjective systems

- Attention to the depth, dimensions, and developmental levels of students/practitioners as the four dimensions of the integral framework are explored

- Attention to the interaction and complexity of relationships between and among students'/practitioners' developmental lines and levels

- Attention to the variety of ordinary and non-ordinary types of experiential knowing

- Attention, use, and understanding of typologies and narrative styles (first-, second-, and third-person)

Rentschler (2006, p. 1) defines AQAL as a "comprehensive approach to reality that attempts to explain how time-tested methods and experiences fit together in a coherent fashion." Short (2010) suggests that the five elements of the AQAL model (quadrants, levels, lines, states, and types) provide a meta-theory to advance clinical practice. George (2006) uses Wilber's AQAL model in his medical practices and observes, " . . . the fact remains, medical schools today have no comprehensive model for understanding how various treatments fit together or how and when they should be used" (2006, p. 50). George also notes:

> Treating patients with an AQAL perspective, which includes awareness of quadrants, levels, lines, states, and types, greatly improves the quality of the doctor-patient relationship. High-quality relationships correlate with better compliance and improved outcomes. The most important aspect of an Integral medical practice is the practitioner's commitment to ongoing self-development of Integral consciousness (George, 2006, p. 69).

Quality, Safety, and Integral Methodological Pluralism: Eight Zones of Inquiry

Integral theory is committed to three strands of good science: instrumental injunction, direct apprehension, and communal confirmation or rejection. As explained by Esbjorn-Hargens & Wilber (2006):

> Instrumental injunction refers to an actual practice, an exemplar, a paradigm, an experiment, or an ordinance. It is always of the form, "If you want to know this, do this." Direct apprehension refers to an immediate experience of the domain brought forth by the injunction: that is, a direct experience or apprehension of data (even if those

data are mediated, at the moment of experience they are immediately apprehended) . . . Communal confirmation or rejection is a checking of the results, the data, the evidence, with others who have completed the injunction and apprehensive strands adequately. Thus all kinds of science are in fact empirical in the broadest sense of experiential. This is a much broader definition of science than the narrow definition of sensory experience usually associated with it (p. 534).

Given the nature of perspectives in the AQAL theory, it follows that eight fundamental methodologies can be applied to examine perspectives of experiences, cultures, behaviors, and systems (see Figure 15.2). The methodologies relate to the dimensions defined by the AQAL model and relate to subjective individual and intersubjective interiors and objective and interobjective individual exteriors. As explained by Esbjorn-Hargens and Wilber (2006):

The eight methodological families are *Phenomenology,* which directly explores experiences (the insides of individual interiors); *Structuralism,* which explores formal patterns of direct experience (the outsides of individual interiors); *Autopoiesis Theory,* which explores self-regulating behaviors (the insides of individual exteriors); *Empiricism,* which explores observable behaviors (the outsides of individual exteriors); *Social Autopoiesis Theory,* which explores self-regulating dynamics in systems (the insides of collective interiors); *Systems Theory,* which explores the functional fits of parts within an observable whole (the outside of collective exteriors); *Hermeneutics,* which explores intersubjective understanding (the insides of collective interiors); and *Ethnomethodology,* which explores formal patterns of mutual understanding (the outsides of collective interiors) (p. 530).

From an integral perspective, you can use a number of methods to explore and gather evidence from each of the quadrants. Because each method has its own set of validity claims in terms of scientific integrity, you have ways and means to develop a more integrally informed body of evidence about quality and safety from an integral view. In addition, each of the four quadrants provides guidance about teaching and learning practices that can be useful for developing lines of inquiry and pedagogy in that particular dimension.

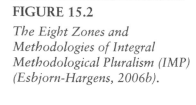

FIGURE 15.2

The Eight Zones and Methodologies of Integral Methodological Pluralism (IMP) (Esbjorn-Hargens, 2006b).

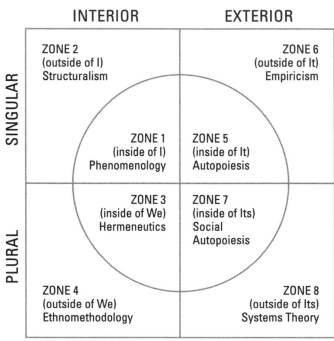

For example, to study self and consciousness, the interior-individual experiences (which are subjective), you are likely to use methods from Zone 1 (Phenomenology) or Zone 2 (Structuralism).

Potential methods of study include self-inquiry, phenomenology, reflection, prayer, journaling, shadow work, and mindfulness practices. The validity claims associated with different scientific approaches invite truthfulness, honesty, authentic expression, sincerity, integrity, the identification of assumptions, and acknowledgment of bias. Structuralism invites the use of psychometric measures, developmental tests, video recordings, notice of speech and behavioral patterns, and interviews. These methods require attention to the validity issues of established developmental models, psychological tests, descriptions with analysis, and triangulation. Educational practices that support teaching and learning in this particular quadrant involve contemplative inquiry, critical reflection, and experiential knowing.

To study the interior-collective of culture and worldview, you can focus inquiry on the feeling of "we"—Zone 3 (Hermeneutics)—or the structure of "we"—Zone 4 (Ethnomethodology). Methods of study might include interviews; role-playing; small group work; storytelling; interpretive analysis; textual analysis; collective reflection; focus groups and ethno methodologies, such as use of participant observer; Appreciative Inquiry; cultural anthropological techniques; coaching; mentoring; forms of structural analysis; cross-cultural comparisons; observation of group dynamics; documented observations; and member checks. Educational teaching-learning practices and methods or ways of knowing culture might include ethical participation, perspectival embrace, and connection encounters.

To examine the exterior-individual phenomena of behaviors or the objective, you can look to Autopoiesis (Zone 5) and/or Empiricism (Zone 6). Methods of study in these two zones include surveys, documentation, exams, fieldwork observations, third-person description, charts, statistics, case studies, gap analysis, as well as traditional approaches to empiricism that include repeatable controlled conditions that employ empirical, logical, measurable tools and metrics that involve use of multiple senses and representative samples. Educational teaching-learning practices and ways of knowing in this quadrant would include competency-based evaluations that examine skillful action, practical application, and empirical observation.

To study social systems and the environments or the interobjective collective exteriors of systems, the validity issues of the focus of inquiry shift to Social Autopoiesis (Zone 7) or communication between organisms and Systems Theory (Zone 8), the study of networks and exchanges. Methods of study in these two zones include statistical analysis, network mapping, scientific studies, library research of previous studies, monitoring, and evaluation. Validity issues in these zones revolve around issues of functional fit, repeatability, control of conditions, and the logical empirical metrics associated with system dynamics and direct experience with the system. Educational teaching-learning practices in these zones include knowing educational systems and understanding global dynamism, social sustainability, and the adaptive cycle of ecological flourishing. From a Caring Science perspective, nurses must attend to the social-community, visible norms, collective behaviors of a group, village, nation-state. From this broader and deeper aspect of tending to basic needs, nursing is simultaneously touching upon all quadrants of integral theory (Watson, 2008).

Enacting Integral Education

Esbjorn-Hargens, Reams, and Gunnlaugson (2010) suggest that the following foci, commitments, and elements help to enact integral education and research:

- Exploring multiple perspectives
- Including first-, second-, and third-person methodologies of learning and teaching
- Weaving together the domains of self, culture, and nature
- Combining critical thinking with experiential feeling
- Including the insights from constructive-developmental psychology
- Engaging regular personal practices of transformation
- Including multiple ways of knowing
- Recognizing various types of teachers and learners
- Encouraging "shadow work" within learners and teachers
- Honoring other approaches to education

Dossey (2008) has proposed an integral theory of nursing based on holistic care, and Jarrin (2006) suggests integral theory can be used as a unifying meta-theory for nursing. Watson (2008) sees the integral model as providing a Caring Science context for grasping the totality of a broader disciplinary focus for providing views of the body and thus basic nursing care. The model supports all ways of knowing—an integration of the inherent with the transcendent-transpersonal, the sacred with the ordinary (Watson, 2005). Similarly, Dacher (2006) has written about the need for an integral approach to health and human flourishing.

Goddard (2006) suggests that integral theory supports a comprehensive approach to healthcare management issues, such as quality improvement efforts; accreditation processes and procedures; and issues of patient safety, compliance, and team-building. Integral theory, when combined with methods of inquiry and reflection, has the potential to support more effective teamwork in healthcare contexts. The nature of interdisciplinary and interprofessional practice is complex and deserves critical examination to develop explanatory models. Though the term *interdisciplinary* has some very specific notions, we are going to use *interdisciplinary* and *interprofessional* as equivalent in the following discussion.

The Nature and Definition of Interprofessionality

In her book, *Interdisciplinarity, History, Theory and Practice,* Klein writes that:

> Interdisciplinarity has been variously defined in this century as methodology, a concept, a process, a way of thinking, a philosophy, and a reflexive ideology. It has been linked with attempts to expose the dangers of fragmentation, to reestablish old connections, to explore emerging relations, and to create new subjects adequate to handle our practical and conceptual needs. Cutting across all of these theories is one recurring idea, interdisciplinarity is a means of solving problems and answering questions that cannot be satisfactorily addressed using single methods or approaches. Whether the context is a short range instrumentality or a long range reconceptualization of epistemology, the concept represents an important attempt to define and establish common ground (Klein, 1990, p. 196).

Lattuca (2001) cites a definition of *interdisciplinary* offered by the Centre for Educational Research and Innovation:

> Interdisciplinary—an adjective describing the interaction among two or more different disciplines. This interaction may range from simple communication of ideas to the mutual integration of organizing

concepts, methodologies, procedures, epistemology, terminology, data and organization of research and education in a fairly large field. An interdisciplinary group consists of persons trained in different fields of knowledge (disciplines) with different concepts, methods and data and terms organized into a common effort on a common problem with continuous intercommunication among the participants from the different disciplines (Organization for Economic Cooperation and Development [OECD], 1972, pp. 25–26).

Most recently, the term *interprofessionality* has been defined by the Interprofessional Education Collaborative Expert Panel (2011) in the following way:

The processes by which professionals reflect on and develop ways of practicing that provides an integrated and cohesive answer to the needs of the client/family/population . . . It involves continuous interaction and knowledge sharing between professionals, organized to solve or explore a variety of education and care issues all while seeking to optimize the patient's participation . . . Interprofessionality requires a paradigm shift, since interprofessional practice has unique characteristics in terms of values, codes of conduct, and ways of working. These characteristics must be elucidated (p. 14).

Klein suggests five tasks important to interdisciplinary futures:

- Compiling narratives to understand how interdisciplinary work is actually done by individuals and teams, including the work done within projects, organizations, institutions, conferences, and journals

- Conducting empirical studies of current interdisciplinary research, teaching, and practice to broaden the database on which general observations are drawn and theories constructed

- Writing histories of particular fields, problem areas, and patterns of relations among disciplines, to understand the "local" nature of interdisciplinarity

- Disclosing the "concealed reality" of interdisciplinarity to have more accurate knowledge of both its nature and consequence

- Exploring the connections among creativity, problem-solving, and the interdisciplinary process (Klein, 1990, p. 196)

The Demand of Interprofessionality

Stein notes that the demands of interdisciplinary/interprofessional work require attention to two main issues: 1) the complexity of thinking and collaboration; and 2) the epistemological structure of interdisciplinary validity claims that relate to level of analysis issues and perspectives issues (Stein, 2007). He advises that meta-disciplinary reflection requires attention to developmental lines of expertise. Reflecting together in an interprofessional team requires members to transcend and include their unique disciplinary perspectives and rise to a meta-disciplinary frame for sense-making, meaning-making, and actionable inquiry.

Multiple pre-disciplinary engagements build on a foundation of general education. Pre-disciplinary knowledge leads to professional grounding in disciplinary knowledge, which leads to expertise. After disciplinary expertise is achieved, we gain evolution and awareness of the emergence of other disciplinary perspectives. This emergence fosters a meta-disciplinary reflection that transcends and includes attention to multidisciplinary, cross-disciplinary, interprofessional, and trans-disciplinary perspectives that frame and facilitate epistemological reflections about education, practice, and research goals. For this reflection to take place, members of an interprofessional team need to acknowledge some of the issues related to group life, their own developmental status, and types of narrative styles.

The Nature of Group Life: Implications for Interprofessionality

Interprofessional group life contains some inherent paradoxes and invisible dynamics. Smith and Berg (1997), in their classic work *Paradoxes of Group Life,* note that an invisible aspect of group life is its inherently paradoxical nature. The coordination dynamics of group life revolve around several complementary pairs and paradoxical tensions. Consider the tensions between the individual~group, self~other, conscious~unconscious processes, dependency~independence, stuckness~movement, framing~reframing, participation~control, disclosure~non-disclosure, fear~courage, isolation~intimacy, belonging~not belonging, splitting, and issues of introjection~projection.

Making this invisible dynamic visible is a significant contribution that explains group conflict, paralysis, and dynamics. Clustered under the three essential group concepts of belonging, Smith and Berg (1997) identify and explain paradoxical tensions related to identity: involvement, individuality, and boundaries. Under the concept of *engaging*, they discuss the tensions and issues associated with the dynamics of disclosure, trust, intimacy, and regression. The issue of *peaking* in group life is discussed in terms of the dynamics of individual versus collective voice, authority, dependency, creativity, and courage.

> *"How is it that we can make the invisible visible in interprofessional work and reflect on the paradoxes and dynamics that bind us to move forward more intentionally with different ways of relating and practicing?"*

Because group life is permeated with contradictory thoughts, actions, and emotions, any group spends considerable time trying to negotiate and unravel these contradictory forces that often result in the creation of a paralyzing circular process that leads to conflict, enmeshment, and paralysis. These authors suggest the dynamic that is responsible for the paralysis and difficulty in group life is a "self-referential bind" (Smith & Berg, 1997). Framing and reframing these contradictory perspectives in different ways leads groups to growth and developmental insights that evolve the group beyond intractable, paralytic dynamics. Reframing changes the meaning, content, or context of a situation so people develop new insights about intentions and actions. They write, "When a social entity uses itself as a mirror through which it judges what it is like, it often only sees those parts of itself that confirm what it wants to know, that is, that it will enable it to remain as it wants to be. Systems that are self-referential create binds for themselves that are difficult to get out of" (Smith & Berg, 1997, p. 48).

One way to overcome self-referential binds is to embrace a greater number of perspectives. Integral theory helps us understand and value perspective-taking, because given an integral perspective, we can take at least eight perspectives: dynamics arising from self and consciousness, culture and worldview, brain and organism, and social systems and environment along developmental lines.

Both academic and clinical organizations have exhibited the paradox when trying to initiate interprofessional education and practice. Bound by traditional silos, processes, and educational models, both faculty and clinicians sometimes experience inertia as they engage in circular conversation around what they know to be a desired future state of education and practice, but they are unable to reconcile existing differences across the professions. In the end, they conclude that interprofessional is beyond their reach, or they settle on low-level activities rather than immersion in interprofessionalism.

The bind that groups create is the paradox that emerges as a result of projections and introjections, and groups engage in splitting and fractionation around issues of identity (we/they) and issues related to logical errors. *Projections* are defined as taking something from the inside and mapping it to the outside. *Introjections* are the mapping of outside/external onto the individual. Projections and introjections are forms of displacement, where some dynamic that belongs in one place is moved to another. When the projection~introjection dynamic is co-mingled with sub-group formation in a group, role-taking and collective splitting result in social interactive processes that are paradoxical and paralyzing. Different frames create conflicts that appear to be irresolvable and foster double-bind situations that elicit multiple contradictions and meanings. Providing models and methods to help professionals recognize and respond to multiple perspectives and differences in frames and framing enables professionals to transcend their disciplinary perspective, supersede conflict, and move toward more appreciative and respectful interprofessional engagement and cooperation.

How is it that we can make the invisible visible in interprofessional work and reflect on the paradoxes and dynamics that bind us to move forward more intentionally with different ways of relating and practicing? Perhaps understanding dynamics with an integral perspective that embraces different narrative styles and developmental action logics is a way forward. Application and use of integral theory that promotes first-, second-, and third-person perspectives and single-, double-, and triple-loop learning provides the framework for future thinking.

Torbert (2004) suggests that cooperative collaborative inquiry (interprofessional practice) is an explicit, shared reflection about an organization's mission and the open interpersonal relationships among people in the organization that includes support, confrontation, exploration of value differences, and the performance of the organization and the people in the organization. Such collaborative inquiry includes and is not limited to creative resolution of paradoxes and the polarities of inquiry~productivity, freedom~control, quality~quantity, and interactive development of self and others. Such collaborative practice requires attention to structuring interactions in a four-frame way.

The structure for speaking and communicating in all four territories of experience is as follows (Torbert, 1991, p. 233):

- *A frame:* The assumptions that bound the conversation, the "name of the game," the purpose of speaking

- *An advocacy:* A particular goal to be achieved, an abstract assertion about perception or action

- *An illustration:* A concrete example, a colorful story

- *An inquiry:* An invitation to respond, an effort to determine the effects of one's action (one's speaking), or others' perspectives on the matter

Such a structured approach to dialogue and discovery supports collaborative-cooperative inquiry and reflection.

Heron (2006) defines cooperative inquiry as a participative research method that " . . . involves two or more people researching a topic through their own experience of it, using a series of cycles in which they move between this experience and reflecting together on it. Each person is a co-subject in the experience phases and co-researcher in the reflection phases" (Heron, 2006, p. 116). Heron suggests there is a four-fold circuit of knowing that involves the embodied feeling of experiential knowing—translating experiential knowing into a form of presentational knowing, expressing the patterns of felt experience into some graphic, moving, musical, verbal art form that leads to the creation of propositions or expressed statements that describe the experiences, which is then translated into some practical knowledge or skill. Similarly, a Caring Science orientation includes the arts and humanities beyond the conventional empirical knowing of human healing and health. A Caring Science epistemology as an ethic grounded in human relationships and caring encompasses human-to-human dialogue and asks us to consider meaningful and expanded forms of authentic data (Watson, Porter O'Grady, Horton-Deutsch, & Malloch, 2017).

Consider the nature of an interprofessional case conference in a hospital or clinic. Each clinician comes to the conference with experience of the patient encounter. As they begin to present and represent the issues in various ways—diagrams, drawings, lab data, and results of tests and markers—they explain how specifically this data is related and then develop propositions or hypotheses about how data is related. They look for patterns and try to engage in sense-making about what practically can be done in the situation given the constellation of facts, experiences, feelings, intuitions, and knowledge at hand.

Heron (2006) suggests that the person initiating a cooperative inquiry needs to do three things to integrate the cognitive, emotional, and interpersonal aspects of cooperative learning inquiry:

- Initiate group members into the methodology of the inquiry so the group can make it their own.

- Support and facilitate the emergence of participative decision-making and authentic collaboration so that inquiry is truly cooperative.

- Create a climate where emotional states can be identified so that distress and tension aroused by inquiry can be processed.

Such guidelines are essential to support interprofessionality and reflection as a team. Such actions also require a highly evolved professional self.

REFLECTING ON . . . QUESTIONS TO STIMULATE META-DISCIPLINARY REFLECTION

- *Professionally, what are you open to believe or open to doubt about a post-disciplinary, post-metaphysical, integral science perspective?*

- *How does your discipline currently define, frame, study, and reference the nature of science? Is the discipline open to consider distinctions between narrow science and broad science?*

- *To what degree do you agree that good science consists of instrumental injunctions, direct apprehension, and communal confirmation or rejection?*

- *What evidence and validity claims (truthfulness, truth, justness, and functional fit) are most valued, given your disciplinary foci and perspectives? How does this apply in implementing interprofessional education and practice?*

- *Specifically, how can your discipline apply the integral theory principles of non-exclusion (acceptance of truth claims that pass the validity tests for their own paradigms in respective fields), enfoldment (sets of practices that are more inclusive, holistic, and comprehensive than others), and enactment (various types of inquiry disclose different phenomena depending on the quadrants, levels, lines, states, and types of the inquirer) in a disciplinary or multidisciplinary context? What factors limit implementation of interprofessionalism?*

- *How does the discipline currently account for phenomena in the four dimensions of experience outlined by the AQAL theory—"I" (subjectivity), "we" (intersubjectivity), "it" (objectivity), and "its" (interobjectivity)? Examine how the phenomena are both drivers and inhibitors to promote interprofessional teamwork.*

- *Given that the AQAL model suggests eight fundamental perspectives and eight fundamental methodologies (Phenomenology, Structuralism, Autopoiesis Theory, Empiricism, Social Autopoiesis Theory, Systems Theory, Hermeneutics, and Ethnomethodology), how might you use this information and knowledge to consider disciplinary and multidisciplinary phenomena of concern and practice? How might this explain conflicts that emerge in curricular discussions or decisions about professional practice models?*

- *How might an integral perspective influence teaching, learning, research, and professional socialization in your discipline and in efforts to reach across disciplines?*

- *From a disciplinary and multidisciplinary perspective, what are the advantages and disadvantages of integral methodological pluralism?*

- *Given your disciplinary perspectives, how does the AQAL model support the process of meta-disciplinary reflection?*

Interprofessional Practice, Team Reflection, and the Development of a Self-Authoring Mind

Psychologist Robert Kegan (1994) notes that personal and professional transformation takes place as we realize the complexity of subject-object relationships. As people grow and develop, they realize differences between self and other—the "me" and "not me." They evolve from self-consciousness to "self-other" consciousness. Developmentally, they progress to yet another level of consciousness that Kegan calls the "we" or "socialized mind." Most people's growth and development become arrested at this third level of consciousness. Kegan and Lahey (2016) have begun to document the contributions of organizations that focus deliberately on the development of people in the organization.

With experience, and as people learn the hidden curriculum of daily life, they grow into fourth order consciousness. People know they have developed fourth order consciousness if they have what Kegan (1994) calls a "self-authoring mind." A self-authoring mind is less rule-bound, understands competing commitments, and can manage paradoxes in service of personal growth and development. Self-authoring minds exercise critical, creative, and systems thinking and take responsibility for self. Self-authoring individuals view work, school, parenting, therapy, intimate relationships, and citizenship differently than those who operate at the third level of socialized mind. Kegan suggests that the fourth order consciousness manifests at work in the following ways (Kegan, 1994, p. 302). People begin to:

- Be the inventor or owner of their own work and distinguish work from job

- Be self-initiating, self-correcting, and self-evaluating rather than dependent on others to frame the problems, initiate adjustments, or determine whether things are going acceptably well

- Be guided by their own visions at work rather than be without vision or captive of the authority's agenda

- Take responsibility for what happens to themselves at work externally and internally (rather than seeing present internal circumstances and future external possibilities as caused by someone else)

- Be accomplished masters of their own particular work roles, jobs, or careers (rather than have an apprentice or imitating relationship to what others do)

- Conceive of the organization from "outside in" as a whole and see their relation to the whole, see the relation of the parts to the whole rather than see the rest of the organization and its parts only from the perspective of their own part, from the "inside out"

"Kegan argues that professional growth and development in a postmodern society might in fact require another level—a 'fifth order of consciousness,' or 'self-transforming mind'."

Fourth order consciousness that operates in educational settings requires people to (Kegan, 1994, p. 303):

- Exercise critical, creative, and systems thinking

- Examine self, culture, and milieu to understand what they feel from what they should feel, what they value from what they should value, and what they want from what they should want

- Be self-directed learners (take initiative; set their own goals and standards; use experts, institutions, and other resources to pursue these goals; take responsibility for their direction and productivity in learning)

- See themselves as co-creators of the culture (rather than shaped by the culture)

- Read actively (rather than receptively) with their own purpose in mind

- Write to themselves and bring their teachers into their self-reflection (rather than write mainly to teachers and for teachers)

- Take charge of the concepts/theories of a course or discipline, marshaling on behalf of their independently chosen topic its internal procedures for formulating and validating knowledge

Kegan argues that professional growth and development in a postmodern society might in fact require another level—a "fifth order of consciousness," or "self-transforming mind." At this level, people integrate polarities and contradictions in their own behavior as they develop and appreciate integral perspectives and engage in the really hard work of psychological and spiritual integration. Perhaps this level of consciousness is what interprofessional health practitioners should strive to develop as they engage the complexities and challenges of working with each other.

Final Reflections

This chapter described and discussed reflective strategies to support transformational learning among members of an interprofessional healthcare team. Integral theory was proposed as an organizing framework that promotes multiple perspectives and forms of inquiry. Appreciating and valuing disciplinary perspectives supports group interaction and cohesion. To be a part of a group and embrace interprofessionality requires personal insight into one's own developmental action logics and the principles and practices of action and cooperative inquiry. The professional evolution of self, striving to develop a self-authoring or self-transforming mind in the context of interprofessional healthcare teams, is one path toward a future that helps put the pieces of the puzzle together in order to accomplish the patient quality and safety goals identified throughout the book.

References

Dacher, E. S. (2006). *Integral health: The path to human flourishing.* Laguna Beach, CA: Basic Health.

Dossey, B. (2008). A theory of integral nursing. *Advances in Nursing Science, 31*(1), E52–E73.

Esbjorn-Hargens, S. (2006a). Integral education by design: How integral theory informs teaching, learning, and curriculum in a graduate preprogram. *ReVision, 28*(3), 21–29.

Esbjorn-Hargens, S. (2006b). Integral research: A multi-method approach to investigating phenomena. *Constructivism in the Human Sciences, 11*(2), 79–107.

Esbjorn-Hargens, S., Reams, J., & Gunnlaugson, O. (Eds.). (2010). *Integral education: New directions for higher learning.* Albany, NY: State University of New York (SUNY) Press.

Esbjorn-Hargens, S., & Wilber, K. (2006). Toward a comprehensive integration of science and religion: A post-metaphysical approach. In P. Clayton & Z. Simpson (Eds.), *The Oxford handbook of religion and science* (pp. 523–546). Oxford, UK: Oxford University Press.

Forman, M. (2010). *A guide to integral psychotherapy: Complexity, integration, and spirituality in practice.* Albany, NY: State University of New York (SUNY) Press.

George, L. (2006). Diagnostics in integral medicine. *AQAL Journal of Integral Theory and Practice, 1*(2), 60–72.

Goddard, T. (2006). Integral health care management: An introduction. *AQAL Journal of Integral Theory and Practice, 1*(1), 449–458.

Heron, J. (2006). *The complete facilitators handbook.* London, UK: Kogan Page Limited.

Interprofessional Education Collaborative Expert Panel. (2011). Core competencies for interprofessional collaborative practice: Report of an expert panel. Washington, DC: Interprofessional Education Collaborative.

Jarrin, O. F. (2006). An integral philosophy and definition of nursing: Implications for a unifying meta-theory of nursing. *School of Nursing Scholarly Works*. Paper 46. Retrieved from http://digitalcommons.uconn.edu/son_articles/46

Kegan, R. (1994). *In over our heads: The mental demands of modern life*. Cambridge, MA: Harvard University Press.

Kegan, R., & Lahey, L. L. (2016). *An everyone culture: Becoming a deliberately developmental organization*. Watertown, MA: Harvard Business Review Press.

Klein, J. (1990). *Interdisciplinarity: History, theory, and practice*. Detroit, MI: Wayne State University Press.

Koller, C. (2006). An introduction to integral science. *AQAL Journal of Integral Theory and Practice, 1*(2), 237–259.

Lattuca, L. (2001). *Creating interdisciplinarity: Interdisciplinary research and teaching among college and university faculty*. Nashville, TN: Vanderbilt University Press.

Merriam, S. (2004). The role of cognitive development in Mezirow's transformational learning theory. *Adult Education Quarterly, 55*(1), 60–68.

Mezirow, J. (1991). Interdisciplinarity: Problems of teaching and research in universities. Organization for Economic Cooperation and Development (OECD). (1972). Washington, DC: OECD.

Mezirow, J. (2000). Learning to think like an adult: Core concepts of transformation theory. In J. Mezirow & Associates (Eds.), *Learning as transformation* (pp. 3–34). San Francisco, CA: Jossey-Bass.

Mezirow, J. (2003). Transformative learning as discourse. *Journal of Transformative Education, 1*(1), 58–63.

Rentschler, M. (2006). AQAL glossary. *AQAL Journal of Integral Theory and Practice, 1*(3), 1–40.

Short, B. (2010). Introduction to integral psychiatry. *Journal of Integral Theory and Practice, V1. 2*, 105.

Smith, K., & Berg, D. (1997). *Paradoxes of group life: Understanding conflicts, paralysis, and movement in group dynamics*. San Francisco, CA: Jossey-Bass.

Stein, Z. (2007). Modeling the demands of interdisciplinarity: Toward a framework for evaluating interdisciplinary endeavors. *Integral Review, 4*(2), 91–107.

Torbert, B. (2004). *Action inquiry: The secret of timely and transforming leadership*. San Francisco, CA: Berrett-Koehler Publishers.

Torbert, W. R. (1991). *The power of balance: Transforming self, society, and scientific inquiry*. Newbury Park, CA: Sage Publications.

Watson, J. (2005). *Caring Science as sacred science*. Philadelphia, PA: F. A. Davis.

Watson, J. (2008). *Nursing: The philosophy and science of caring* (Rev. ed.). Boulder, CO: University of Colorado Press.

Watson, J., Porter O'Grady, T., Horton-Deutsch, S., & Malloch, K. (2017). Quantum caring leadership: An evolving model for nursing and healthcare leadership. (Submitted for publication.)

Wilber, K. (2000). *Integral psychology: Consciousness, spirit, psychology, therapy*. Boston, MA: Shambhala Publications.

Wilber, K. (2001). *A theory of everything*. Boston, MA: Shambhala Publications.

Wilber, K. (2005). Introduction to integral theory and practice: IOS Basic and the AQAL map. *AQAL: Journal of Integral Theory and Practice, 1*(1), 1–36.

Wilber, K. (2007). *The integral vision*. Boston, MA: Shambhala Publications.

Chapter 16

Emancipatory Nursing Praxis: Becoming a Social Justice Ally

–*Robin R. Walter, PhD, RN, CNE*

Nurses and other healthcare professionals are being called to understand and thoughtfully address professional values and beliefs in culturally and bureaucratically complex healthcare systems (Ray & Turkel, 2014) and underserved community settings. Social justice and human rights issues are being brought forth globally, calling for nurses to help address inequities and eradicate barriers to sustainability identified in the Sustainable Development Goals (SDGs) (United Nations, 2016).

Emancipatory nursing praxis (ENP) is professional practice directed by and toward social justice goals and outcomes through reflection, action, and transformation. This form of reflective practice supports and grounds nurses with the sense of self needed to enact real and meaningful contributions toward the realization of a sustainable world (Rosa & Horton-Deutsch, 2017).

Social Justice in Nursing

Social justice is a professional expectation of nurses nationally and globally, as described in the educational mandates of the American Association of Colleges of Nursing (AACN), the professional codes of the American Nurses Association (ANA), and the International Council of Nurses (ICN).

Buettner-Schmidt and Lobo (2011) define the concept of *social justice* for nursing as the "full participation in society and the balancing of benefits and burdens by all citizens, resulting in a just ordering of society" (p. 948). Social justice is primarily concerned with identifying and redressing systems of oppression. These systems operate on individual, organizational, and societal levels to subjugate certain individuals or groups and privilege others, based solely on actual or perceived membership in various social groups, e.g., race, sexual orientation, religion, class, socioeconomic status, gender, and physical ability. Consequently, some group members (e.g., white, heterosexual, upper-class, male) socially benefit from unearned privilege. These privileges are referred to as "unearned" because they are not socially bestowed as the result of hard work, talent, virtue, or accomplishment. Instead, they are the consequence of inequitable social systems that confer dominance to some groups and subordination to all others. Nurse engagement in social justice requires expanding the professional nursing role to include the role of social justice ally.

As social justice allies, nurses function as members of a privileged, dominant social group working *with* those from an oppressed group to remedy the systemic denial of privilege and power based solely on social group membership. Functioning as an ally requires an ongoing commitment to listening to—and learning from—oppressed groups, for it is the members of the oppressed group who will ultimately decide what does (and does not) constitute an effective ally.

Emancipatory nursing praxis offers nurses a substantive theoretical framework for developing the role of social justice ally across all areas of nursing education and practice. Key to this process is engaging in critical, reflexive dialogue. This chapter explores how reflection and reflexive dialogue are used to facilitate the transformational learning needed for nurses to become social justice allies.

Emancipatory Nursing Praxis: Overview of the Theory

Emancipatory nursing praxis (ENP) is a hermeneutic-dialectic, relational learning process comprised of four conceptual processes and two contextual categories. The four conceptual processes are becoming, awakening, engaging, and transforming. The two contextual categories are relational and reflexive.

In learning to become social justice allies, nurses move dynamically through processes of "becoming" and "awakening" that help them to recognize the unearned privileges that unjustly (and invisibly) advantage them over others. The processes of "engaging" and "transforming" offer additional learning experiences through critical, reflective dialogue with others. Nurses learn to engage with clients in more authentic and emancipatory ways and, ultimately, to leverage their privilege to identify and challenge oppressive systems. Although the process of becoming an ally is not linear, it is presented sequentially here for purposes of clarity.

The major driving force in ENP occurs within the context of reflexivity. Reflective practices are initially introspective and intrapersonal but evolve to a type of reflexivity that is firmly grounded in the social process of conversation: specifically, dialogue. The reflexivity that occurs as part of this dialogical process initially allows nurses to identify and deconstruct the personal beliefs, assumptions, and behaviors that inhibit their ability to work with an individual or group in an emancipatory way.

Reflexive dialogue also allows for a collaborative reconstruction of these attitudes and beliefs that generate new meaning-in-action (praxis). As will be demonstrated, these collaborative deconstruction-reconstruction reflexive processes create a powerful sense of individual and professional agency in nurse-allies, even in the most disempowering contexts of their nursing practice. These reflexive processes are explained next and include illustrative comments from the nurse-allies who participated in a study that explored how nurses came to know, understand, and engage in social justice. This dissertation research was international in scope and used a constructivist grounded theory methodology to develop a middle-range theory of social justice in nursing (Walter, 2014; Walter, 2016).

Becoming

Becoming is a process that reflects an individual's earliest memories and perceptions of social injustice or unfair social situations. Becoming is a largely unconscious, initial exploration of perceptions and ways of being in the world. Intrapersonal characteristics and socio-environmental factors work in concert to provide a basic awareness that "something is not right" or "something needs to be done." Nurses in the becoming process may intrapersonally feel a moral obligation to those they see as less fortunate, or a desire to make a difference:

> I had a very strong feeling of the need to do something to make a better world for everybody. When I was 14, I worked in a migrant camp watching children while their parents worked . . . I was only vaguely aware of the differences between them and us, primarily in an economic sense. My understanding of privilege was limited to a very vague idea of the haves and the have-nots (Walter, 2014, p. 108).

Socio-environmental factors—parental and familial role modeling, faith-based experiences, direct or indirect experiences of marginalization or stigmatization, and sensitizing social and educational experiences—also influence the process of becoming:

> People in my family would never straight out make slurs or say anything that was straight out racist, but I always felt like something was there. My dad, on the street, being like, "Don't bring me home someone that looks like that." Totally writing people off because of what they look like or where they were at in life. There was this fear and there was this criticism . . . I remember crying at the dinner table . . . I just felt so upset and didn't know what to do with it. I think that's when I started . . . the Band-Aid kind of solutions, like, oh, I can give someone a dollar (p. 112).

Reflective practices in becoming—if they occur at all—tend to be intrapersonal, retrospective, and largely descriptive. As a nurse educator, this is often the level of reflection I see in students' written submissions following community service or service learning experiences. Their perceptions are typically limited to recounting details of the experience—where they were, who they talked to, and what they did. Students may express pity/compassion for the clients, gratefulness for their own good fortune, or a sense of helplessness, but an awareness of the problems' root (social) causes, and one's place in those processes, is neither evident nor emergent in their writing. It is important, however, that exposure to individuals and groups experiencing oppression, marginalization, or stigmatization is a critical component of learning to become an ally.

As stated earlier, the cognitive processing that occurs in "becoming" is largely unconscious, so it is not surprising that description is the reflective product. Becoming is also ongoing. Even experienced nurse-allies will seek out—or serendipitously encounter—different ways of being in the world, time and again. Clarity, in terms of recognizing one's place in the larger, structural forces that give rise to these social injustices, will develop as a function of the next learning process in ENP: Awakening.

Awakening

Awakening is the ENP learning process through which nurses come to identify or recognize their role or place in the larger, societal-structural forces that impact the health and well-being of others. Awakening is marked by a change in how the nurse sees himself or herself in relation to others (see Figure 16.1). This new awareness happens along several dimensions. One dimension is when formerly held beliefs, attitudes, and assumptions are compared to alternative beliefs, attitudes, and assumptions regarding the same situation. This comparison can help nurses to position themselves contextually within larger social systems and to begin to identify intersecting sources of privilege and oppression in their own lives:

> It took me sort of a long time to recognize my role . . . in the sense that I carry a lot of privilege. I come from an upper middle class background, so I have class privilege. I have the social conditioning it takes to get jobs, apply for nursing school . . . and then I have white privilege. My white skin makes me able to never have to think twice about whether people are going to judge me by my skin color. I used to think that, "Oh, I can save poor people!" and I didn't really understand that there is . . . a "sticky place" where it becomes this "White Savior" sort of thing. Since then I've been working pretty hard to avoid that (Walter, 2014, p. 118).

FIGURE 16.1.

Relationship of the Processes and Sub-Processes of ENP (Walter, 2014).

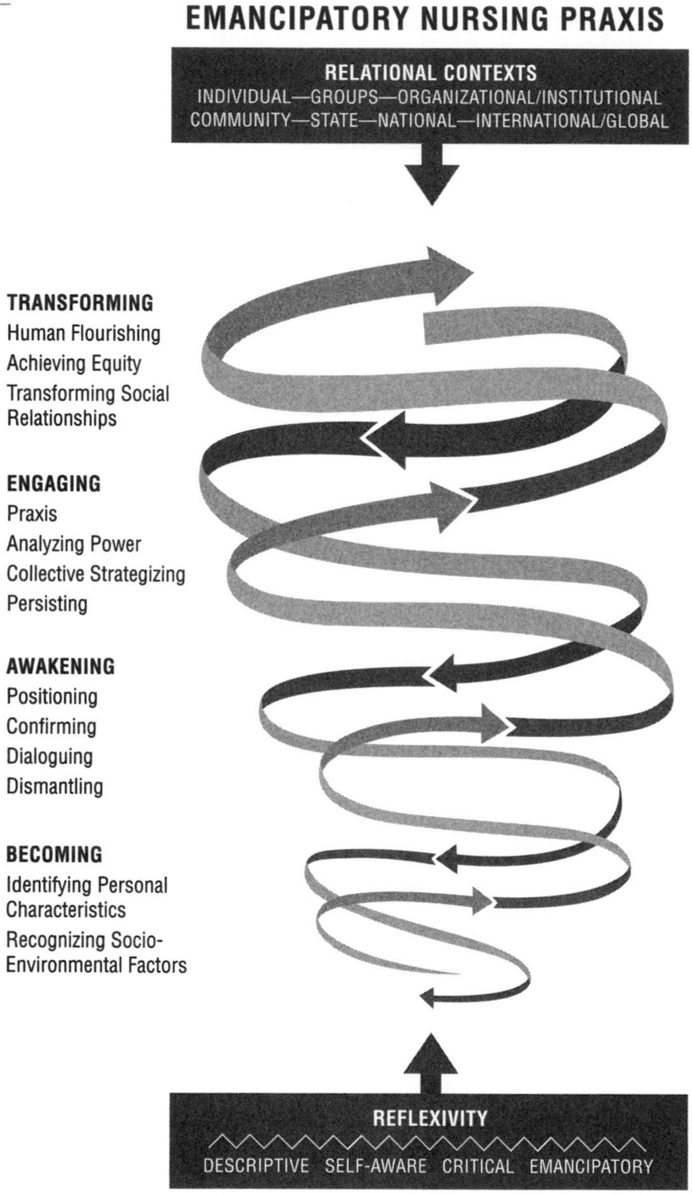

EMANCIPATORY NURSING PRAXIS

RELATIONAL CONTEXTS
INDIVIDUAL—GROUPS—ORGANIZATIONAL/INSTITUTIONAL
COMMUNITY—STATE—NATIONAL—INTERNATIONAL/GLOBAL

TRANSFORMING
Human Flourishing
Achieving Equity
Transforming Social
Relationships

ENGAGING
Praxis
Analyzing Power
Collective Strategizing
Persisting

AWAKENING
Positioning
Confirming
Dialoguing
Dismantling

BECOMING
Identifying Personal
Characteristics
Recognizing Socio-
Environmental Factors

REFLEXIVITY
DESCRIPTIVE   SELF-AWARE   CRITICAL   EMANCIPATORY

Another key dimension of awakening involves dismantling—and ultimately discarding—culturally conditioned attitudes, perceptions, and assumptions that limit one's ability to live authentically. Heidegger (1962) described living authentically as not succumbing to the actions or beliefs of predominance without considering what is true for oneself. Multiple examples of dismantled concepts/ideas emerged from the original ENP study data (Walter, 2014). Nurse-allies dismantled their socially conditioned understanding of gender, race/ethnicity, sexuality, cultural competence, noncompliance, and teaching patients/clients to "cope with" or "adapt to" socially created, unjust circumstances (rather than seek liberation from them) (see Table 16.1).

Table 16.1 Dismantling Socially Conditioned Concepts (adapted from Walter, 2016)

CONCEPT	DISMANTLING
Gender	I think your (demographic) form only has like male or female checkboxes. I didn't want to fill it out. (Consider) just putting, like—"Other"—or "How do you identify?"
Race	We're still taught pretty routinely that race is a risk factor for this (diabetes), but it's never qualified any further. Race is a social construct . . . (In) nursing . . . race is presented as a biological risk factor. It's not a biological risk factor so much as an economic-social-political determinant of health, but that is never unpacked. So it's very possible to go through nursing school and just leave feeling that black people are genetically predisposed to all the poverty diseases.
Teaching clients to cope/adapt	We have to teach people how to manage their situation and have good health, but at the same time—if we really want to advocate for our patients—it's not just about advocating that they can get free medicine, it's about advocating so that they don't need free medicine . . . that they have the opportunity everyone else has, and they can manage their own healthcare at the same level that we do—that's what real advocacy does. It doesn't help people adapt to the status quo—when the status quo is bad and unhealthy.

continues

Table 16.1 (continued)

CONCEPT	DISMANTLING
Nonadherence/ Noncompliance	I worked as a research nurse for a while, and I had all these papers coming up "noncompliant with medication." And I mean it's almost like a naughty child isn't it, not doing what they're told? It's not a very nice term . . . it's paternalistic . . . and it relieves the medical doctor or the nurse of responsibility if you say that they're noncompliant.
Cultural Competence	You go through (a course) that covers, like, 12 cultures in a semester. You can't do that without reducing it to stereotypical factoids. You're not going to be competent. As soon as you start using the words "Latino culture," then you're already missing the point. First of all—there is no "Latino culture" . . . are we talking about Mexican, Central American, Peruvian—are we talking about urban, northern Mexico, or rural Mexico—are we talking about Chiapas, which is an indigenous culture? You're not going to be competent. You just need to check your assumptions.

It is during "awakening" where self-awareness and dialogue emerge as pivotal forces in ally development. Reflection that is self-aware is marked by heightened intrapersonal awareness of feelings, emotions, and biases. Self-awareness, however, often stops short of contextualizing these perceptions within the larger social context and may leave developing nurse-allies feeling overwhelmed. Critical, reflective dialogue with others serves to mediate these disempowering attitudes and facilitates the initial process of deconstructing (dismantling) socially conditioned beliefs that perpetuate systems of oppression. For example, through dialogue, nurses can process experiences that confirm or challenge their new worldview and learn how to handle pressure from others to return to former beliefs and behaviors:

> I'm taking this Bible class that's a requirement, and there was a march on campus—it was called Human Beings Are Not Illegal, something like that. It was in support of immigrants, and against deportations, and so forth. And so the professor of the class brought up this march, and he wanted to see what the students thought of it, and whether some had

participated. He brought up this Bible verse about how we're supposed to respect authority, and pay our taxes . . . And, I think he was bringing it up in order to say that these protests are not good. He was being very careful, but . . . if we're discriminated against or put upon— we're supposed to endure that—persecution is part of the Christian life—and that's a big sign of how good a Christian you are. But, then I was saying to him that I don't think there's really a problem here. I know I have friends who are here illegally, and who are under a lot of stress every day . . . I feel like we can be biblically consistent by supporting a good life for them . . . exercise your obligation to help your neighbor. And I think that a protest like this . . . helps other people to have a life that's humane and—and—isn't unbearably stressful (Walter, 2014, p. 126).

The introduction of critical, reflexive dialogue in "awakening" will dominate the reflexive activities in the next ENP process, "engaging" in social justice.

REFLECTIVE QUESTIONS

- *Within the healthcare delivery system, where are positions of power?*
- *What power dimensions are part of being a patient in the hospital?*
- *How do issues of social justice impact nurse-patient relationships and caring?*

Engaging

Engaging is composed of the actions and interactions involved in doing social justice work as allies. Engaging is a dynamic, evolving process in which nurses actively explore and cultivate the role of ally with the expressed intent of advancing specific transformative goals (these goals are explicated in the fourth conceptual category, transforming). A fundamental process of engaging in social justice is the identification and analysis of sources and balances of power. Social justice allies must identify the stakeholders in a given unjust situation—those who benefit from the status quo and those who do not:

> You can get an enormous amount of attention and support for social justice in (organizations)—as long as it reinforces the larger hierarchy

and doesn't do anything to undermine that . . . in the sense that you are not asking for an inordinate amount of funding or any sacrifices up the chain. It's great to be helping people below you as long as everyone above you does not have to sacrifice anything and as long as it's clear that you are *helping* the people below . . . not that you are *empowering* the people below. As long as the work you are doing in the name of social justice is reinforcing the hierarchy, then it's really great, very positive. But when anything that happens to flip that, it gets much more contentious in a hurry (Walter, 2014, p. 131).

Identifying sources of power (and power imbalance) facilitates the ally's ability to engage in collective strategizing. This is also a critical, dialogic process of assessing, coalescing support, and planning the actions/interactions that will be required to move toward one or more social justice goals. Social justice engagement is collaborative-action driven, largely by members from the oppressed or marginalized groups with whom the nurse-allies are affiliated. The role of the ally is to leverage his or her position of social advantage in ways that are not only beneficial to the oppressed group, but that also seek to dismantle the system of oppression that created the inequity in the first place.

Nurses should be aware that engaging in social justice is not without risk. Participants in the original ENP study spoke of overcoming and integrating several dimensions of risk as they engaged as allies. The risks they experienced ranged from minimal to significant and crossed personal, professional, social, and financial boundaries (see Table 16.2).

Table 16.2 Risks Identified with Ally Behavior (adapted from Walter, 2016)

RISK	EXEMPLAR
Personal	There's been a huge PR campaign by the coal companies in North Queensland, Bulk Ports, the owner of the port since basically 2007 when we started making our concerns known. They're in direct opposition to us... they labeled us as extreme green radicals and bong-smoking hippies. And people, they fall for it... I was abused by a taxi driver. He told me that I was a traitor to Bowen... he told me to get out of his taxi and get out of Bowen.

RISK	EXEMPLAR
Career	The consequences for engaging in social justice, I've found, are essentially career-ending ones. I've been told that the work I do does not bring in the money and does not contribute in the same way to the rankings of the university. And because of that, as long as I engage in this work, my possibility of career progression is very small.
Financial	If you're working with the poor, you are usually not making a lot of money. Somewhere in the Jesuit literature, it asks, "Who are you going to align yourself with?" Are you going to align yourself with the poor or the rich? And if you align yourself with the rich, well, what comes with that? Power, maybe fame, money—which are all good things. But if you choose to align yourself with the poor, you're probably going to be treated like the poor are treated... I think that's a real risk... oftentimes you'll be categorized as being in the same boat.
Professional	I can't imagine it [social justice] not being a part of nursing for me, but I also can't imagine having daily battles with other nurses who might not feel this way . . . the idea of framing things within social justice terms is a source of conflict... Trying to find other nurses who are interested in social justice—it's definitely an oasis.

PRAXIS

Praxis was described by Paulo Freire as simultaneous "reflection and action upon the world in order to transform it" (1970, p. 33). In ENP, praxis involves paying attention to the ways in which our beliefs, assumptions, and behaviors foster or inhibit the ability to work with an individual or group in an emancipatory way. Stated another way, praxis fully integrates reflection with specific courses of action; the "praxis" in emancipatory nursing praxis is fundamentally relational.

The more that we are attuned to listening to the voice of the people who receive our services or need our support or our help, and the more that we can make sure that we're attending to those voices, the better we are in terms of social justice.

Transforming

Transforming reflects the motivation for learning to become a social justice ally. It is often experienced as an expansion of consciousness that fundamentally reconditions our thoughts, feelings, and actions. Three goal-directed processes include human flourishing, achieving equity, and transforming social relationships. The initial nurse participants did not articulate a singular definition of what might constitute *human flourishing* other than to intimate that it was a condition of wellness and quality of life deserved by all people.

Achieving *equity*, the second subcategory of transforming, encompasses more than access to healthcare. It extends to all basic human necessities (education, housing, food security, employment, transportation), as well as full connectedness, belonging, and participating in society. Nurses learning to become allies see these conditions as foundational to human flourishing, conditions that should be met prior to conception/birth. No individual should have to "fight" for equity once in the world, but should, instead, be conceived and born into it. The third subcategory of transforming addresses an ally's commitment to transforming social relationships. This encompasses more than simply adopting a new belief or a different way of thinking about others. *Transforming social relationships* constitutes the unfolding reality of learning how to engage authentically, in critical reflective dialogue, for the purpose of dismantling systems of oppression.

Reflexive Contextual Conditions

Nurses learning to become allies move dynamically through the process of emancipatory nursing praxis via four dimensions of reflection: descriptive, self-aware, critical, and emancipatory. Descriptive reflection—first seen in becoming—is a straightforward, retrospective accounting of events wherein emotive reactions are objectively reported, if at all. Reflection that is self-aware emerges in awakening, as a heightened awareness of personal feelings, emotions, and biases, but stops short of contextualizing these attitudes within the larger social context. Critical and emancipatory reflection characterizes the processes of engaging and transforming. This level of reflection promotes praxis, the ability to envision and take action toward possibilities of individual and collective self-determination.

Significantly, critical reflection in ENP does not occur as an intrapersonal, self-reflective process. It occurs as a social process through reflective dialogue. Brockbank and McGill (2006) argue that "while intrapersonal reflection is effective and may offer opportunities for deep learning . . . it is ultimately not enough to promote transformational learning" (p. 53). They posit that self-reflection, while important in professional development, is limited to individual insight, and critically examining oneself is inherently difficult. Critical reflection on one's own assumptions in a collaborative manner through dialogue transforms not only the quality of the conversation, but also the thinking that lies beneath it (Isaacs, 1999). Critical reflective dialogue with others initiates a process of deconstruction. *Deconstruction* helps developing allies to make explicit the implicit assumptions that keep them from authentically engaging in emancipatory nursing praxis.

Emancipatory reflection also promotes praxis and the ability to envision and take action toward the possibilities of individual and collective self-determination. Emancipatory reflection always occurs in dialogue with others and initiates processes of reconstruction. *Reconstruction* involves the collaborative creation of new meaning-in-action from the attitudes, beliefs, and assumptions deconstructed in critically reflective dialogue. In this way, dialogue becomes more than a communication tool for change; it is "the very medium within which change occurs" (Ford & Ford, 1995, p. 542). Emancipatory nursing praxis facilitates social change through a "recursive process of social construction in which new realities are created . . . sustained, and modified via processes of communication" (p. 542).

Killian provides an exemplar of how dialogic critical reflection progressed to emancipatory reflection across multiple relational contexts. He comments on a liberation encounter that occurred on an individual level, and his experience demonstrated how reflection can be used to evaluate not only the individual impact, but also the impact at organizational and national levels. He states:

We worked with a woman who was about 28 years of age, and she had Down's syndrome, and she was living at home without any parents. She was attending a day service for people with intellectual disabilities. She was the Secretary for our Board, and we had another person who was the shadow secretary who supported her in her role. She wanted to speak at a conference in the United Kingdom. She'd never traveled to the UK, had never spoken in front of a group of people, but she wanted to do this. So, we arranged for funds so that she could go . . . and she was going to speak about her experience as a Board member of an intellectual disability rights group. So we spent hours, six or seven hours, working with her . . . so that the words that went on the slides were her words and that the words that went on the script were her words. So, this is tremendously empowering for her . . . She went back to her service, and on one of the days she was practicing her words, and there was one line in all of this. It's important to know that she was identified with (our) group, not with her service, and . . . in no place was her day service named. The line in her script that raised problems was that she said, "In my center I feel treated like a kid, but I'm not a kid. I'm an adult and I want to be treated as an adult." And they said, "You can't say that." And the advocate—she was working with me—and who worked in that service as well, challenged this and said, "She wants to say it," and they said, "No, you can't say it and if you want to say that you must make a formal complaint to the Rights Review Committee person, who of course, was (an employee) of the service. So, they weren't really independent. And of course, that was striking fear into the person to try and keep her quiet (Walter, 2014, pp. 148–159).

Killian and the advocate engaged critically in reflective dialogue: "We sat down and we talked and she said, 'Should we change this?' I said, 'If we change her words and get her to change her words, what role have we played? We've become essentially—We censored her. Are we going to stand by and do that?' And we said, 'no.' She went to the conference and she spoke the words and it was hugely positive and she was very positively received."

This individual act of liberation, however, had repercussions for the person at the organizational level. Killian's critical reflection evolved into emancipatory reflection through dialogue with the client:

> She came back, and they eventually started working to get her out of the service because . . . she was asking questions. And she was saying, "I want more than I have now." And they said, "Well, you can't go to that (Board) meeting anymore because . . . you're supposed to be with us. We're responsible for you and it's too much risk." And they said she couldn't use the trolley, but she used the trolley every weekend to go into the city from her home. They said, "It's not safe." They brought up the safety legislation and said she couldn't go (Walter, 2014, p. 150).

Emancipatory reflexivity promoted praxis. The board changed its meetings to the weekend, so the secretary could participate without increasing the tension in her relationship with the day service. Killian continued:

> And they then started working on her parents, who were elderly, to say to them that they could not guarantee that the service would be available to her if she wasn't fully availing of it and doing what they wanted. And so, she had to leave the group (Walter, 2014, p. 150).

Killian's continued emancipatory reflection through dialogue ultimately changed the relational context in which he would take further action:

> We got close to what would be social justice [the Board member's right to freedom of speech], but then we found ourselves up against a bigger force of social injustice, veiled in an intellectual disability service. It really was a structure that maintained a societal status quo. And those types of things are the things that have to be challenged. That's the level at which we're trying to—that's where we're trying to bring our action at this point . . . I'm of the belief that many of these things happen not only at that place but they happen in other places as well and that we need to be raising questions at a national level, at a political level (Walter, 2014, p. 151).

The relational conditions provided the actual and potential contexts of liberation, and Killian's critical reflexivity exemplified the transformative learning that was taking place. This hermeneutic-dialectic, ethical, and relational-dialogic process was characterized by his reflective-actions with others, intended to liberate individuals and groups from socially determined oppression, marginalization, or stigmatization that negatively impacted health and well-being. Freire defined *liberation* as "praxis: the action and reflection of men and women upon their world in order to transform it" (1979, p. 70). The phrase "in order to transform it" explicitly reflects the teleological nature of the participants' experiences of emancipatory nursing praxis: changing the social conditions that sustained disadvantage for some and privilege for others.

Using a Pedagogy of Intersectional Privilege to Develop Nurses as Social Justice Allies

As stated earlier, ENP is a transformational learning theory of ally role development in nursing that is primarily informed by multiple, intersectional identities of privilege. Therefore, a pedagogy of intersectional privilege is proposed as the educational model for nurse educators seeking to develop students as social justice allies (Case, 2013; McIntosh, 2012). This model is philosophically congruent with ENP and offers nursing faculty the unique opportunity to make unearned privilege visible and to help students deconstruct and reconstruct essentialist beliefs that perpetuate health inequities and disparities (see Table 16.3).

Table 16.3 Key Elements of Intersectional Privilege Pedagogy (adapted from Case, 2013)

ELEMENT	EXAMPLE
Privilege	Provide a definition of privilege (unearned social advantage); extend learning outcomes to include the identification of privileged social identities and how privilege operates to maintain oppression; focus on the invisibility of privilege and the consequences of that

ELEMENT	EXAMPLE
	invisibility across all social groups (e.g., if privileged voices and experiences are used to deny the existence of privilege or oppression, then there is a need for further student engagement in critical, reflexive dialogue).
Intersectionality	Teach privilege across a wide spectrum of privilege systems (white, male, able-bodied, heterosexual, Christian, citizenship, etc.); frame learning about privilege through the lens of intersectionality theory.
Reflexive Dialogue	Include opportunities for faculty and student reflection and discussion on their own privileged identities and how these identities shape their own lives, attitudes, perceptions, and behaviors.
Experience	Provide opportunities for student learning outside the classroom that promotes identifying personally held assumptions and deconstructing and reconstructing belief systems that maintain privilege and oppression.

In order for learning about privilege to take place, it is important to consider several psychological barriers that may prevent students from accepting or absorbing this new information. Wise and Case (2013) identified these barriers as: 1) the need to avoid being judged as deliberately trying to harm others; 2) feeling complicit in the suffering of others; 3) the fear of losing one's privileged status; and 4) feeling hopeless and helpless to change the status quo.

Faculty may observe students engaging in defensive behaviors, such as focusing on personal experiences of marginalization or oppression, rather than exploring the unearned benefits of their privileged social identities. Students may also fail to acknowledge interpretations of course materials from alternate perspectives, or they may engage in avoidant or disruptive behaviors when certain topics are covered (e.g., class absences, unexpected changes in the level of in-class participation, texting during class, or engaging in side conversations during class) (Bishop, 2015; Case & Cole, 2013). Students may be in denial that any form of oppression exists, or if they do acknowledge some aspects, they "tend to think it can be dealt with quickly and easily by education and good intentions, and . . . certainly do not see themselves as perpetrators" (Bishop, 2015, p. 88).

An intentional focus on intersectionality may prevent many forms of student defensiveness. Intersectionality serves to validate students in their own experiences by recognizing that each individual is a complex mix of more- and less-privileged identities (Wise & Case, 2013, p. 24). It also allows for an exploration of the exceptions-to-the-rules that students often cite to discredit the role of privilege in maintaining oppression. For example, students may cite accomplished black individuals (e.g., former President Obama, Oprah Winfrey, Condoleezza Rice) to dismiss the advantages accorded to whites relative to people of color. Intersectionality allows for a deeper exploration of how the very nature of an exception may, instead, function to prove the rule. Finally, intersectionality facilitates the instructor's ability to "draw parallels between privilege systems that may be less threatening for students to explore" (p. 23). A comparison of the privilege accorded an able-bodied, attractive professional paves the way for communicating the importance of all aspects of social identity, including the more emotionally charged ones associated with race, gender, religion, social class, and sexuality.

The Interplay of Experiential Learning and Critical Reflective Dialogue

Kolb (1984) defines *experiential learning* as knowledge that is generated from reflection on personal experiences. Privilege-focused learning activities such as readings, formal written assignments, projects, service learning, and in-class activities allow students to think critically about the relationship between privilege and oppression. Williams and Melchiori (2013) found that when experiential learning is combined with structured reflection, students are more effective in identifying and challenging socially conferred privilege. What is interesting about their teaching methods is that many of these seemingly passive, receptive learning activities are never stand-alone. They are always performed in concert with face-to-face feedback and collaborative student reflection with faculty.

Their approach to service learning as a strategy for examining social class privilege is particularly resonant with ENP's focus on the deconstructive and reconstructive aspects of critical, reflective dialogue. First, they identify a common student assumption that service learning is a type of charity endeavor: "Students may think they are serving people who are unable to help themselves" (Williams & Melchiori, 2013, p. 176).

Viewing service learning as this type of helping activity diminishes the reciprocal power that can be possible between the students and community members (Weah, Simmons, & Hall, 2000). Once this assumption is laid bare, faculty are able to help students deconstruct their service learning experiences and question the privileged discourses that reinforce oppression based on social class. Community partners and their constituents are positioned as co-educators and equal stakeholders in the students' service learning experience. They are involved in "creating the service learning assignments . . . and provide input on the students' final grades" (Williams & Melchiori, 2013, p. 176). They devote multiple class sessions to reflective dialogue with students during the service learning experience. These ongoing, collaborative, dialogic reflections help students to reconstruct their experiences by acknowledging their social class privilege and consciously deciding to use it to ameliorate disadvantage rather than maintain oppressive structures and social interactions.

Nurses as Social Justice Allies: The Caring Mandate for a Global Society

Jean Watson, after acknowledging a deeply embedded—yet subjugated—social justice model of caring in nursing, once asked, "At a time when there are those of us who are longing to respond, can we find hope from within our midst?" (Watson, 2008, p. 59). Emancipatory nursing praxis offers evidence that social justice engagement continues to emerge and evolve as a profoundly caring and transformational force within the profession of nursing. Nurses around the globe are reclaiming the profession's sacred social mission as they commit to the emancipatory practices defining their roles as social justice allies. They ascribe to what Flaskerund and Nyamathi refer to as the "new paradigm that recognizes societal factors as primary pathogenic forces in . . . major health problems" (2002, p. 139). They courageously examine and dismantle their witting and unwitting roles in perpetuating systems of oppression. They stand with, rather than stand-in for, the marginalized, who are often oppressively blamed for their own circumstances.

This recommitment to our social mandate is happening at a time in history when health disparities, inequities, and atrocities against human rights and the environment continue despite international mandates seeking to redress them. The lack of uniform progress in achieving the United Nations' Millennium Development Goals (MDG, 2001–2015) has been met with a renewed call to action in the 2015–2030 Sustainable Development Goals (SDG). The 17 SDGs and 169 benchmark targets build on the MDGs and seek to complete what was not achieved: environmental sustainability; food and water security; gender equality; the empowerment of women, girls, and vulnerable/marginalized populations worldwide; and a "resolve to free the human race from the tyranny of poverty" (United Nations [UN], 2015, p. 1).

These are social, economic, and environmental expectations for all countries, not just resource-poor, developing nations. As nurses, we are called professionally and ethically to identify and redress social injustice—locally and globally. We must expand our professional role as advocates to include the role of social justice ally:

> We are running out of time. Each new generation of nursing students we produce as novice nurses entering the health care arena *without* an analysis of power and structure . . . and the intersection of gender, class, and sexuality (among other domains of life) with health, perpetuates the strength of ineffective systems and structures of healthcare delivery . . . and leads to increased constraints on individual agency and (global) sustainability (Kagan, 2014, p. 323).

Final Reflections

This chapter highlighted the importance of critical and emancipatory reflection in nursing's emerging professional role as social justice ally. Allies engage in social justice from positions of privilege, and as we have discussed, privilege intersects with oppression to create complex social identities for each of us. It is fitting, therefore, to close this chapter with a quote and an invitation to reflect on your own social identity and the myriad ways it may prepare you to become an ally. The quote is by Adrienne Rich (1986, p. 199):

"When those who have the power to name and to socially construct reality choose not to see you or hear you, whether you are dark-skinned, old, disabled, female, or speak with a different accent or dialect than theirs, when someone with the authority of a teacher, say, describes the world and you are not in it, there is a moment of psychic disequilibrium, as if you looked into a mirror and saw nothing."

In closing, realize that becoming a social justice ally will raise many more questions than it will answer. Integrating social justice into professional nursing practice requires concerted effort, ongoing reflection, and mindfulness of how privilege impacts your thoughts, beliefs, and actions that—knowingly and unknowingly—perpetuate the oppression of others. Becoming a social justice ally is a lifelong process of authentic collaboration of the "privileged" with the "other," toward the ultimate goal of emancipation for both.

REFLECTIVE QUESTIONS

- *How are you socially privileged given your gender, nationality, race, religious affiliation (or non-affiliation), able-bodiedness, cognitive ability, sexual preference, or body type? (Feel free to explore other areas of privilege that may not be identified here.)*

- *Explore the dimensions of your social identity where you have experienced the exclusion referred to in Rich's "moment of psychic disequilibrium."*

- *Reflect on your practice setting. Who is not being heard or represented? How does your reflection on your own privilege and oppression inform a new way of seeing this situation?*

References

American Association of Colleges of Nursing. (2006). *The essentials of doctoral education for advanced nursing practice.* Washington, DC: Author.

American Association of Colleges of Nursing. (2008). *The essentials of baccalaureate education for professional nursing practice.* Washington, DC: Author.

American Association of Colleges of Nursing. (2011). *The essentials of master's education in nursing.* Washington, DC: Author.

American Nurses Association. (2010a). *Code of ethics for nurses.* Washington, DC: American Nurses Publishing.

American Nurses Association. (2010b). *Nursing: Scope and standards of practice.* Washington, DC: American Nurses Publishing.

American Nurses Association. (2010c). *Nursing's social policy statement.* Washington, DC: American Nurses Publishing.

Bishop, A. (2015). *Becoming an ally: Breaking the cycle of oppression* (3rd ed.). Black Point, Nova Scotia, Canada: Fernwood Publishing.

Brockbank, A., & McGill, I. (2006). *Facilitating reflective learning through mentoring and coaching.* Philadelphia, PA: Kogan Page.

Buettner-Schmidt, K., & Lobo, M. L. (2011). Social justice: A concept analysis. *Journal of Advanced Nursing, 68*(4), 948–958.

Case, K. A. (Ed.). (2013). *Deconstructing privilege: Teaching and learning as allies in the classroom.* New York, NY: Routledge.

Case, K. A., & Cole, E. R. (2013). Deconstructing privilege when students resist: The journey back into the community of engaged learners. In K. A. Case (Ed.), *Deconstructing privilege: Teaching and learning as allies in the classroom* (pp. 34–48). New York, NY: Routledge.

Flaskerund, J., & Nyamathi, A. (2002). New paradigm for health disparities needed. *Nursing Research, 51*(3), 139–140.

Ford, J. D., & Ford, L. W. (1995). The role of conversation is producing intentional change in organizations. *Academy of Management Review, 20*(3), 541–570.

Freire, P. (1970). *Pedagogy of the oppressed.* New York, NY: Continuum International Publishing Group.

Heidegger, M. (1962). *Being and time*. Oxford, UK: Blackwell Publishers, Ltd.

International Council of Nurses. (2012). *The ICN code of ethics for nurses*. Geneva, Switzerland: Author.

Isaacs, W. (1999). *Dialogue and the art of thinking together*. New York, NY: Doubleday.

Kagan, P. (2014). Afterword. In P. Kagan, M. Smith, & P. Chinn (Eds.), *Philosophies and practices of emancipatory nursing: Social justice as praxis* (pp. 323–326). New York, NY: Routledge.

Kolb, D. A. (1984). *Experiential learning: Experience as the source of learning and development*. Englewood Cliffs, NJ: Prentice Hall.

McIntosh, P. (2012). Reflections and future directions for privilege studies. *Journal of Social Issues, 68*(1), 194–206.

Ray, M. A., & Turkel, M. C. (2014). Caring as emancipatory nursing praxis: The theory of relational caring complexity. *Advances in Nursing Science, 37*(2), 132–146.

Rich, A. (1986). Invisibility in academe. In A. Rich (Ed.), *Blood, bread, and poetry: Selected prose 1979–1985* (pp. 198–201). New York, NY: W.W. Norton & Company.

Rosa, W., & Horton-Deutsch, S. (2017, in press). The importance of reflective practice in creating the world that we want. In W. Rosa (Ed.), *Global nursing global health: Our contributions to sustainable development*. New York, NY: Springer.

United Nations (UN). (2015). The Millennium Development Goals report 2015. Retrieved from http://www.un.org/millenniumgoals/reports.shtml

United Nations (UN). (2016). Sustainable Development Goals: 17 goals to transform our world. Retrieved from http://www.un.org/sustainabledevelopment/sustainable-development-goals/

Walter, R.W. (2014). *A grounded theory study of the critical factors influencing nurse professionals' perceptions of their role in social justice* (Doctoral dissertation). Retrieved from ProQuest Dissertations and Theses Global. (Order No. 1836057479.)

Walter, R. (2016). Emancipatory nursing praxis: A theory of social justice in nursing. *Advances in Nursing Science*. Advance online publication. doi:10.1097/ANS.0000000000000157

Watson, J. (2008). Social justice and human caring: A model of Caring Science as a hopeful paradigm for moral justice for humanity. *Creative Nursing, 14*(2), 54–61.

Weah, W., Simmons, V. C., & Hall, M. (2000). Service learning and multicultural/multiethnic perspectives. *Phi Delta Kappan, 81*(9), 673–676.

Williams, W. R., & Melchiori, K. J. (2013). Class action: Using experiential learning to raise awareness of social class privilege. In K. A. Case (Ed.), *Deconstructing privilege: Teaching and learning as allies in the classroom* (pp. 169–187). New York, NY: Routledge.

Wise, T., & Case, K. A. (2013). Pedagogy for the privileged: Addressing inequality and injustice without shame or blame. In K. A. Case (Ed.), *Deconstructing privilege: Teaching and learning as allies in the classroom* (pp. 17–33). New York, NY: Routledge.

Part VI
Appendices

Appendix A
For Further Reflection: Useful Websites

Part I: The Transformation of Nursing Education Through Reflective Practice

- American Association of Colleges of Nursing, essential curricular components for baccalaureate, masters, and doctor of nursing practice programs: www.aacn.nche.edu

- The Center for Compassion and Altruism Research and Education: http://ccare.stanford.edu/education/about-compassion-cultivation-training-cct/

- Emotional Intelligence: Emotional Competence Framework includes 25 personal and social competencies (Goleman, 1998): http://www.eiconsortium.org/pdf/emotional_competence_framework.pdf

- National League for Nursing, essential nursing education curricular competencies: http://www.nln.org

- Oregon Consortium of Nursing Education, competency-based curriculum: http://ocne.org/index.html

- Quality and Safety Education for Nurses (QSEN), instructional videos with reflective questions, teaching strategies, and annotated bibliography: www.qsen.org

- SBAR: A Shared Structure for Effective Team Communication: An Implementation Toolkit, 2nd Edition: http://www.uhn.ca/TorontoRehab/Education/SBAR/Documents/SBAR_Toolkit.pdf

- TeamSTEPPS, a free interdisciplinary multimedia curriculum for teaching teamwork available from the Agency for Healthcare Research and Quality: http://teamstepps.ahrq.gov

- Watson Caring Science Center Webinars: www.nursing.ucdenver.edu/caringscience

- Watson Caring Science Institute: https://www.watsoncaringscience.org/

Part II: Reflection and Mindful Practice

- American Mindfulness Research Association: https://goamra.org/

- The Association for Contemplative Mind in Higher Education: http://www.acmhe.org

- Association for Mindfulness in Education: http://www.mindfuleducation.org/

- Center for Contemplative Mind in Society: http://www.contemplative-mind.org/

- Center for Healthy Minds: https://centerhealthyminds.org/

- Contemplative Studies: http://home.sandiego.edu/~komjathy/Homepage_of_Louis_Komjathy/Contemplative_Studies.html

- Mindful Meditation Audio: http://marc.ucla.edu/body.cfm?id=22

- Mindfulness and the Brain, Wisdom 2.0 Conference:

- Mindfulness at the Center (resource section): http://www.mindfulnessatthecenter.com/

Part III: Supporting Reflective Learning: In Didactic and Clinical Practice Contexts

- Evaluating Reflection: http://learningforsustainability.net/evaluation/

- Learning, Reflection, and Change: http://www.infed.org/thinkers/et-schon.htm

- Reflection for Learning: http://sites.google.com/site/reflection4learning/Home

- Reflective Practice: http://www.tandf.co.uk/journals/RP

- YouTube video introducing reflective writing: http://www.youtube.com/watch?v=0plCU9oyZlM&feature=related

- YouTube video on reflective teachers: http://www.youtube.com/watch?v=9HQlYNViOdA&feature=related

- Visual Thinking Strategies: http://vtshome.org/

Part IV: Deepening the Foundation of Professional Practice Through Reflection

- Appreciative Inquiry: http://appreciativeinquiry.case.edu

- Center for Courage & Renewal: http://www.couragerenewal.org/

- Conversation Café: www.conversationcafe.org

- Liberating Structures: http://www.liberatingstructures.com/

- YouTube video on critical reflection for deepening learning through experiences: http://www.youtube.com/watch?feature=endscreen&NR=1&v=Fn3vqg31po0

Part V: Future Directions in Reflective Practice

- Center for Spirituality and Healing, University of Minnesota: https://www.csh.umn.edu/

- eLearning module on Interprofessional Collaboration for Patient and Family Centered Care: https://tahsn.pathlore.net/tahsn/courseware/MSH/IPE/player.html

- Institute for Alternative Futures: http://www.altfutures.com/home

- Institute of the Future for the Phoenix Research Institute, identified six drivers and ten skills necessary for a 2020 workforce: http://cdn.the atlantic.com/static/front/docs/sponsored/phoenix/future_work_skills_2020.pdf

- Interdisciplinary Journal of Partnership Studies: http://pubs.lib.umn.edu/ijps/aimsandscope.html

- National Center for Healthcare Leadership: http://nchl.org/index.asp

- Plexus Institute Complex Change & Innovation: http://www.plexus institute.org/

Appendix B
QSEN Prelicensure Competencies

QSEN competencies for prelicensure students are listed in Table B.1. These are embedded in accreditation criteria for nursing curricula. QSEN competencies for graduate students are listed in Appendix C.

Cronenwett, L., Sherwood, G., Barnsteiner, J., Disch, J., Johnson, J., Mitchell, P., . . . Warren, J. (2007). Quality and safety education for nurses. Nursing Outlook, 55(3), 122–131.

TABLE B.1 Patient-Centered Care

Definition: Recognize the patient or designee as the source of control and full partner in providing compassionate and coordinated care based on respect for patient's preferences, values, and needs.

KNOWLEDGE	SKILLS	ATTITUDES
Integrate understanding of multiple dimensions of patient-centered care: • Patient/family/ community preferences, values • Coordination and integration of care	Elicit patient values, preferences, and expressed needs as part of clinical interview, implementation of care plan, and evaluation of care. Communicate patient values, preferences, and expressed needs to other members of healthcare team.	Value seeing healthcare situations "through patients' eyes." Respect and encourage individual expression of patient values, preferences, and expressed needs.

continues

TABLE B.1 (continued)

KNOWLEDGE	SKILLS	ATTITUDES
• Information, communication, and education • Physical comfort and emotional support • Involvement of family and friends • Transition and continuity Describe how diverse cultural, ethnic, and social backgrounds function as sources of patient, family, and community values.	Provide patient-centered care with sensitivity and respect for the diversity of the human experience.	Value the patient's expertise with own health and symptoms. Seek learning opportunities with patients who represent all aspects of human diversity. Recognize personally held attitudes about working with patients from different ethnic, cultural, and social backgrounds. Willingly support patient-centered care for individuals and groups whose values differ from own.
Demonstrate comprehensive understanding of the concepts of pain and suffering, including physiologic models of pain and comfort.	Assess presence and extent of pain and suffering. Assess levels of physical and emotional comfort. Elicit expectations of patient and family for relief of pain, discomfort, or suffering. Initiate effective treatments to relieve pain and suffering in light of patient values, preferences, and expressed needs.	Recognize personally held values and beliefs about the management of pain or suffering. Appreciate the role of the nurse in relief of all types and sources of pain or suffering. Recognize that patient expectations influence outcomes in management of pain or suffering.
Examine how the safety, quality, and cost-effectiveness of healthcare can be improved through the active involvement of patients and families.	Remove barriers to presence of families and other designated surrogates based on patient preferences. Assess level of patient's decisional conflict and provide access to resources.	Value active partnership with patients or designated surrogates in planning, implementation, and evaluation of care. Respect patient preferences for degree of active engagement in care process.

KNOWLEDGE	SKILLS	ATTITUDES
Examine common barriers to active involvement of patients in their own healthcare processes. Describe strategies to empower patients or families in all aspects of the healthcare process.	Engage patients or designated surrogates in active partnerships that promote health, safety and well-being, and self-care management.	Respect patient's right to access personal health records.
Explore ethical and legal implications of patient-centered care. Describe the limits and boundaries of therapeutic patient-centered care.	Recognize the boundaries of therapeutic relationships. Facilitate informed patient consent for care.	Acknowledge the tension that may exist between patient rights and the organizational responsibility for professional, ethical care. Appreciate shared decision-making with empowered patients and families, even when conflicts occur.
Discuss principles of effective communication. Describe basic principles of consensus-building and conflict resolution. Examine nursing roles in ensuring coordination, integration, and continuity of care.	Assess own level of communication skill in encounters with patients and families. Participate in building consensus or resolving conflict in the context of patient care. Communicate care provided and needed at each transition in care.	Value continuous improvement of own communication and conflict resolution skills.

TABLE B.2 Teamwork and Collaboration

Definition: Function effectively within nursing and interprofessional teams, fostering open communication, mutual respect, and shared decision-making to achieve quality patient care.

KNOWLEDGE	SKILLS	ATTITUDES
Describe own strengths, limitations, and values in functioning as a member of a team.	Demonstrate awareness of own strengths and limitations as a team member.	Acknowledge own potential to contribute to effective team functioning.

continues

TABLE B.2 (continued)

KNOWLEDGE	SKILLS	ATTITUDES
	Initiate plan for self-development as a team member.	Appreciate importance of intra- and interprofessional collaboration.
	Act with integrity, consistency, and respect for differing views.	
Describe scopes of practice and roles of healthcare team members.	Function competently within own scope of practice as a member of the healthcare team.	Value the perspectives and expertise of all health team members.
Describe strategies for identifying and managing overlaps in team member roles and accountabilities.	Assume role of team member or leader based on the situation.	Respect the centrality of the patient/family as core members of any healthcare team.
Recognize contributions of other individuals and groups in helping patient/family achieve health goals.	Initiate requests for help when appropriate to situation.	Respect the unique attributes that members bring to a team, including variations in professional orientations and accountabilities.
	Clarify roles and accountabilities under conditions of potential overlap in team member functioning.	
	Integrate the contributions of others who play a role in helping patient/family achieve health goals.	
Analyze differences in communication style preferences among patients and families, nurses, and other members of the health team.	Communicate with team members, adapting own style of communicating to needs of the team and situation.	Value teamwork and the relationships upon which it is based.
Describe impact of own communication style on others.	Demonstrate commitment to team goals.	Value different styles of communication used by patients, families, and healthcare providers.
Discuss effective strategies for communicating and resolving conflict.	Solicit input from other team members to improve individual, as well as team, performance.	Contribute to resolution of conflict and disagreement.
	Initiate actions to resolve conflict.	

KNOWLEDGE	SKILLS	ATTITUDES
Describe examples of the impact of team functioning on safety and quality of care. Explain how authority gradients influence teamwork and patient safety.	Follow communication practices that minimize risks associated with handoffs among providers and across transitions in care. Assert own position/perspective in discussions about patient care. Choose communication styles that diminish the risks associated with authority gradients among team members.	Appreciate the risks associated with handoffs among providers and across transitions in care.
Identify system barriers and facilitators of effective team functioning. Examine strategies for improving systems to support team functioning.	Participate in designing systems that support effective teamwork.	Value the influence of system solutions in achieving effective team functioning.

TABLE B.3 Evidence-Based Practice (EBP)

Definition: Integrates best current evidence with clinical expertise and patient/family preferences and values for delivery of optimal healthcare.

KNOWLEDGE	SKILLS	ATTITUDES
Demonstrate knowledge of basic scientific methods and processes. Describe EBP to include the components of research evidence, clinical expertise, and patient/family values.	Participate effectively in appropriate data collection and other research activities. Adhere to Institutional Review Board (IRB) guidelines. Base individualized care plan on patient values, clinical expertise, and evidence.	Appreciate strengths and weaknesses of scientific bases for practice. Value the need for ethical conduct of research and quality improvement. Value the concept of EBP as integral to determining best clinical practice.

continues

TABLE B.3 (continued)

KNOWLEDGE	SKILLS	ATTITUDES
Differentiate clinical opinion from research and evidence summaries.	Read original research and evidence reports related to area of practice.	Appreciate the importance of regularly reading relevant professional journals.
Describe reliable sources for locating evidence reports and clinical practice guidelines.	Locate evidence reports related to clinical practice topics and guidelines.	
Explain the role of evidence in determining best clinical practice. Describe how the strength and relevance of available evidence influences the choice of interventions in provision of patient-centered care.	Participate in structuring the work environment to facilitate integration of new evidence into standards of practice. Question rationale for routine approaches to care that result in less than desired outcomes or adverse events.	Value the need for continuous improvement in clinical practice based on new knowledge.
Discriminate between valid and invalid reasons for modifying evidence-based clinical practice based on clinical expertise or patient/family preferences.	Consult with clinical experts before deciding to deviate from evidence-based protocols.	Acknowledge own limitations in knowledge and clinical expertise before determining when to deviate from evidence-based best practices.

TABLE B.4 Quality Improvement (QI)

Definition: Use data to monitor the outcomes of care processes and use improvement methods to design and test changes to continuously improve the quality and safety of healthcare systems.

KNOWLEDGE	SKILLS	ATTITUDES
Describe strategies for learning about the outcomes of care in the setting in which one is engaged in clinical practice.	Seek information about outcomes of care for populations served in care setting. Seek information about quality improvement projects in the care setting.	Appreciate that continuous quality improvement is an essential part of the daily work of all health professionals.

KNOWLEDGE	SKILLS	ATTITUDES
Recognize that nursing and other health professions students are parts of systems of care and care processes that affect outcomes for patients and families. Give examples of the tension between professional autonomy and system functioning.	Use tools (such as flow charts, cause-effect diagrams) to make processes of care explicit. Participate in a root cause analysis of a sentinel event.	Value own and others' contributions to outcomes of care in local care settings.
Explain the importance of variation and measurement in assessing quality of care.	Use quality measures to understand performance. Use tools (such as control charts and run charts) that are helpful for understanding variation. Identify gaps between local and best practice.	Appreciate how unwanted variation affects care.
Describe approaches for changing processes of care.	Design a small test of change in daily work (using an experiential learning method such as Plan-Do-Study-Act). Practice aligning the aims, measures, and changes involved in improving care. Use measures to evaluate the effect of change.	Value measurement and its role in good patient care. Value local change (in individual practice or team practice on a unit) and its role in creating joy in work. Appreciate the value of what individuals and teams can do to improve care.

TABLE B.5 Safety

Definition: Minimizes risk of harm to patients and providers through both system effectiveness and individual performance.

KNOWLEDGE	SKILLS	ATTITUDES
Examine human factors and other basic safety design principles as well as commonly used unsafe practices (such as workarounds and dangerous abbreviations). Describe the benefits and limitations of selected safety-enhancing technologies (such as barcodes, Computer Provider Order Entry, medication pumps, and automatic alerts/alarms). Discuss effective strategies to reduce reliance on memory.	Demonstrate effective use of technology and standardized practices that support safety and quality. Demonstrate effective use of strategies to reduce risk of harm to self or others. Use appropriate strategies to reduce reliance on memory (such as forcing functions, checklists).	Value the contributions of standardization/reliability to safety. Appreciate the cognitive and physical limits of human performance.
Delineate general categories of errors and hazards in care. Describe factors that create a culture of safety (such as open communication strategies and organizational error reporting systems).	Communicate observations or concerns related to hazards and errors to patients, families, and the healthcare team. Use organizational error reporting systems for near miss and error reporting.	Value own role in preventing errors.
Describe processes used in understanding causes of error and allocation of responsibility and accountability (such as root cause analysis and failure mode effects analysis).	Participate appropriately in analyzing errors and designing system improvements. Engage in root cause analysis rather than blaming when errors or near misses occur.	Value vigilance and monitoring (even of own performance of care activities) by patients, families, and other members of the healthcare team.
Discuss potential and actual impact of national patient safety resources, initiatives, and regulations.	Use national patient safety resources for own professional development and to focus attention on safety in care settings.	Value relationship between national safety campaigns and implementation in local practices and practice settings.

TABLE B.6 Informatics

Definition: Use information and technology to communicate, manage knowledge, mitigate error, and support decision-making.

KNOWLEDGE	SKILLS	ATTITUDES
Explain why information and technology skills are essential for safe patient care.	Seek education about how information is managed in care settings before providing care. Apply technology and information management tools to support safe processes of care.	Appreciate the necessity for all health professionals to seek lifelong, continuous learning of information technology skills.
Identify essential information that must be available in a common database to support patient care. Contrast benefits and limitations of different communication technologies and their impact on safety and quality.	Navigate the electronic health record. Document and plan patient care in an electronic health record. Employ communication technologies to coordinate care for patients.	Value technologies that support clinical decision-making, error prevention, and care coordination. Protect confidentiality of protected health information in electronic health records.
Describe examples of how technology and information management are related to the quality and safety of patient care. Recognize the time, effort, and skill required for computers, databases, and other technologies to become reliable and effective tools for patient care.	Respond appropriately to clinical decision-making supports and alerts. Use information management tools to monitor outcomes of care processes. Use high-quality electronic sources of healthcare information.	Value nurses' involvement in the design, selection, implementation, and evaluation of information technologies to support patient care.

Appendix C
Graduate/Advanced Practice Nursing Competencies

Table C.1 lists the QSEN competencies developed for graduate nursing education. Reprinted with permission from Elsevier. Reprinted from Cronenwett, L., Sherwood, G., Pohl, J., Barnsteiner, J., Moore, S., Sullivan, D. T., … Warren, J. (2009). Quality and safety education for advanced nursing practice. Nursing *Outlook, 57*(6), 338–348.

TABLE C.1 Patient-Centered Care

Definition: Recognize the patient or designee as the source of control and full partner in providing compassionate and coordinated care based on respect for patient's preferences, values, and needs.

KNOWLEDGE	SKILLS	ATTITUDES
Analyze multiple dimensions of patient-centered care: • Patient/family/community preferences, values • Coordination and integration of care	Elicit patient values, preferences, and expressed needs as part of clinical interview, **diagnosis**, implementation of care plan, and evaluation of care.	Value seeing healthcare situations "through patients' eyes." Respect and encourage individual expression of patient values, preferences, and expressed needs.

continues

TABLE C.1 (continued)

KNOWLEDGE	SKILLS	ATTITUDES
• Information, communication, and education • Physical comfort and emotional support • Involvement of family and friends • Transition and continuity Analyze how diverse cultural, ethnic, spiritual, and social backgrounds function as sources of patient, family, and community values. Analyze social, political, economic, and historical dimensions of patient care processes and the implications for patient-centered care. Integrate knowledge of psychological, spiritual, social, developmental, and physiological models of pain and suffering. Analyze ethical and legal implications of patient-centered care. Describe the limits and boundaries of therapeutic patient-centered care.	Communicate patient values, preferences, and expressed needs to other members of healthcare team. Provide patient-centered care with sensitivity, empathy, and respect for the diversity of human experience. **Ensure that the systems within which you practice support patient-centered care for individuals and groups whose values differ from the majority or your own.** **Assess and treat pain and suffering in light of patient values, preferences, and expressed needs.** **Respect** the boundaries of therapeutic relationships. **Acknowledge the tension that might exist between patient preferences and organizational and professional responsibilities for ethical care.** Facilitate informed patient consent for care.	Value patients' expertise with their own health and symptoms. Honor learning opportunities with patients who represent all aspects of human diversity. **Seek to understand** your personally held attitudes about working with patients from different ethnic, cultural, and social backgrounds. Willingly support patient-centered care for individuals and groups whose values differ from your own. **Value cultural humility.** **Seek to understand your personally held values and beliefs about the management of pain or suffering.** **Value** shared decision-making with empowered patients and families, even when conflicts occur.
Analyze strategies that empower patients or families in all aspects of the healthcare process. **Analyze** features of physical facilities that support or pose barriers to patient-centered care.	Engage patients or designated surrogates in active partnerships **along the health illness continuum.** **Create or change organizational cultures so that patient and family preferences are assessed and supported.**	Respect patient preferences for degree of active engagement in care process. **Honor** active partnerships with patients or designated surrogates in planning, implementation, and evaluation of care.

KNOWLEDGE	SKILLS	ATTITUDES
Analyze reasons for common barriers to active involvement of patients and families in their own healthcare processes.	Assess the level of patients' decisional conflict and provide access to resources. **Eliminate** barriers to presence of families and other designated surrogates based on patient preferences.	Respect patients' rights to access personal health records. **Value system changes that support patient-centered care.**
Integrate principles of effective communication **with knowledge of quality and safety competencies.** **Analyze** principles of consensus-building and conflict resolution. **Analyze advanced practice nursing roles in assuring coordination, integration, and continuity of care.** **Describe process of reflective practice.**	**Continuously analyze and improve** own level of communication skill in encounters with patients, families, and teams. **Provide leadership in** building consensus or resolving conflict in the context of patient care. Communicate care provided and needed at each transition in care. **Incorporate reflective practices into own repertoire.**	Value continuous improvement of own communication and conflict resolution skills. **Value consensus.** Value the process of reflective practice.

TABLE C.2 Teamwork and Collaboration

Definition: Recognize the patient or designee as the source of control and full partner in providing compassionate and coordinated care based on respect for patient's preferences, values, and needs.

KNOWLEDGE	SKILLS	ATTITUDES
Analyze your own strengths, limitations, and values as a member of a team. **Analyze impact of your own advanced practice role and its contributions to team functioning.**	Demonstrate awareness of your own strengths and limitations as a team member. Continuously plan for improvement in use of self in effective team development and functioning. Act with integrity, consistency, and respect for differing views.	Acknowledge your own contributions to effective or **ineffective** team functioning.

continues

TABLE C.2 (continued)

KNOWLEDGE	SKILLS	ATTITUDES
Describe scopes of practice and roles of all healthcare team members. **Analyze** strategies for identifying and managing overlaps in team member roles and accountabilities. **Analyze strategies that influence the ability to initiate and sustain effective partnerships with members of nursing and interprofessional teams.** Analyze the impact of cultural diversity on team functioning.	Function competently within your own scope of practice as a member of the healthcare team. Assume the role of team member or leader based on the situation. **Guide the team in managing areas** of overlap in team member functioning. **Solicit input from other team members to improve individual as well as team performance.** **Empower** contributions of others who play a role in helping patients/families achieve health goals. **Initiate and sustain effective healthcare teams.** Communicate with team members, adapting your own style of communicating to the needs of the team and situation.	Respect the unique attributes that members bring to a team, including variation in professional orientations, competencies, and accountabilities. Respect the centrality of the patient/family as core members of any healthcare team. Appreciate importance of interprofessional collaboration. **Value collaboration with nurses and other members of the nursing team.**
Analyze differences in communication style preferences among patients and families, **advanced practice** nurses, and other members of the health team. **Describe the impact of your own communication style on others.**	**Communicate respect for team member competence in communication.** Initiate actions to resolve conflict.	Value different styles of communication.

KNOWLEDGE	SKILLS	ATTITUDES
Describe examples of the impact of team functioning on safety and quality of care. **Analyze** authority gradients and their influence on teamwork and patient safety.	Follow communication practices that minimize risks associated with handoffs among providers and across transitions in care. Choose communication styles that diminish the risks associated with authority gradients among team members. Assert your own position/ perspective **and supporting evidence** in discussions about patient care.	Appreciate the risks associated with handoffs among providers and across transitions in care. **Value the solutions obtained through systematic, interprofessional collaborative efforts.**
Identify system barriers and facilitators of effective team functioning. Examine strategies for improving systems to support team functioning.	**Lead** or participate in the design **and implementation** of systems that support effective teamwork. **Engage in state and national policy initiatives aimed at improving teamwork and collaboration.**	Value the influence of system solutions in achieving team functioning.

TABLE C.3 Evidence-Based Practice

Definition: Integrate best current evidence with clinical expertise and patient/family preferences and values for delivery of optimal healthcare.

KNOWLEDGE	SKILLS	ATTITUDES
Demonstrate knowledge of **health research** methods and processes. Describe evidence-based practice to include the components of research evidence, clinical expertise, and patient/family values.	**Use health research methods and processes, alone or in partnership with scientists, to generate new knowledge for practice.** Adhere to institutional review board (IRB) guidelines.	Appreciate strengths and weaknesses of scientific bases for practice. Value the need for ethical conduct of research and quality improvement. Value **all components of evidence-based practice.**

continues

TABLE C.3 (continued)

KNOWLEDGE	SKILLS	ATTITUDES
	Role-model clinical decision-making based on evidence, clinical expertise, and patient/family preferences and values.	
Identify efficient and effective search strategies to locate reliable sources of evidence.	Employ efficient and effective search strategies to answer focused clinical questions.	Value development of search skills for locating evidence for best practice.
Identify principles that comprise the critical appraisal of research evidence. Summarize current evidence regarding major diagnostic and treatment actions within the practice specialty. Determine evidence gaps within the practice specialty.	Critically appraise original research and evidence summaries related to area of practice. Exhibit contemporary knowledge of best evidence related to practice specialty. Promote research agenda for evidence that is needed in practice specialty. Initiate changes in approaches to care when new evidence warrants evaluation of other options for improving outcomes or decreasing adverse events.	Value knowing the evidence base for practice specialty. Value public policies that support evidence-based practice.
Analyze how the strength of available evidence influences the provision of care (assessment, diagnosis, treatment, and evaluation). Evaluate organizational cultures and structures that promote evidence-based practice.	Develop guidelines for clinical decision-making regarding departure from established protocols/standards of care. Participate in designing systems that support evidence-based practice.	Acknowledge your own limitations in knowledge and clinical expertise before determining when to deviate from evidence-based best practices. Value the need for continuous improvement in clinical practice based on new knowledge.

TABLE C.4 Monitoring Outcomes with Data

Definition: Use data to monitor the outcomes of care processes and use improvement methods to design and test changes to continuously improve the quality and safety of healthcare systems.

KNOWLEDGE	SKILLS	ATTITUDES
Describe strategies for improving outcomes of care in the setting in which you are engaged in clinical practice. Analyze the impact of context (such as access, cost, or team functioning) on improvement efforts.	Use a variety of sources of information to review outcomes of care and identify potential areas for improvement. Propose appropriate aims for quality improvement efforts. Assert leadership in shaping the dialogue about and providing leadership for the introduction of best practices.	Appreciate that continuous quality improvement is an essential part of the daily work of all health professionals.
Analyze ethical issues associated with quality improvement. Describe features of quality improvement projects that overlap sufficiently with research, thereby requiring IRB oversight.	Assure ethical oversight of quality improvement projects. Maintain confidentiality of any patient information used to determine outcomes of quality improvement efforts.	Value the need for ethical conduct of quality improvement.
Describe the benefits and limitations of quality improvement data sources and measurement and data analysis strategies.	Design and use databases as sources of information for improving patient care. Select and use relevant benchmarks.	Appreciate the importance of data that allows you to estimate the quality of local care.
Explain common causes of variation in outcomes of care in the practice specialty.	Select and use tools (such as control charts and run charts) that are helpful for understanding variation. Identify gaps between local and best practice.	Appreciate how unwanted variation affects outcomes of care processes.

continues

TABLE C.4 (continued)

KNOWLEDGE	SKILLS	ATTITUDES
Describe common quality measures in the practice specialty.	Use findings from root cause analyses to design and implement system improvements. Select and use quality measures to understand performance.	Value measurement and its role in good patient care.
Analyze the differences between micro-system and macro-system change. Understand principles of change management. Analyze the strengths and limitations of common quality improvement methods.	Use principles of change management to implement and evaluate care processes at the micro-system level. Design, implement, and evaluate tests of change in daily work (using an experiential learning method such as Plan-Do-Study-Act). Align the aims, measures, and changes involved in improving care. Use measures to evaluate the effect of change.	Appreciate the value of what individuals and teams can do to improve care. Value local systems improvement (in individual practice, team practice, on a unit, or in the macro-system) and its role in professional job satisfaction. Appreciate that all improvement is change but not all change is improvement.

TABLE C.5 Safety

Definition: Minimize risk of harm to patients and providers through both system effectiveness and individual performance.

KNOWLEDGE	SKILLS	ATTITUDES
Describe human factors and other basic safety design principles as well as commonly used unsafe practices (such as workarounds and dangerous abbreviations).	Participate as a team member to design, promote, and model effective use of technology and standardized practices that support safety and quality.	Value the contributions of standardization and reliability to safety. Appreciate the importance of being a safety mentor and role model.

KNOWLEDGE	SKILLS	ATTITUDES
Describe the benefits and limitations of selected safety-enhancing technologies (such as barcodes, Computer Provider Order Entry, and electronic prescribing). **Evaluate** effective strategies to reduce reliance on memory.	**Participate as a team member to design, promote, and model effective use** of strategies to reduce risk of harm to self and others. **Promote a practice culture conducive to highly reliable processes built on human factors research.** Use appropriate strategies to reduce reliance on memory (such as forcing functions, checklists).	Appreciate the cognitive and physical limits of human performance.
Delineate general categories of errors and hazards in care. **Identify best practices for organizational responses to error.** Describe factors that create a just culture and culture of safety. **Describe best practices that promote patient and provider safety in the practice specialty.**	Communicate observations or concerns related to hazards and errors to patients, families, and the healthcare team. Identify and correct system failures and hazards in care. **Design and implement micro-system changes in response to identified hazards and errors.** Engage in a systems focus rather than blaming individuals when errors or near misses occur. **Report errors and support members of the healthcare team to be forthcoming about errors and near misses.**	Value your own role in reporting and preventing errors. **Value systems approaches to improving patient safety in lieu of blaming individuals.** **Value the use of organizational error reporting systems.**
Describe processes used to analyze causes of error and allocation of responsibility and accountability (such as root cause analysis and failure mode effects analysis).	Participate appropriately in analyzing errors and designing, implementing, and evaluating system improvements.	Value vigilance and monitoring of care, including your own performance, by patients, families, and other members of the healthcare team.

continues

TABLE C.5 (continued)

KNOWLEDGE	SKILLS	ATTITUDES
Describe methods of identifying and preventing verbal, physical, and psychological harm to patients and staff.	Prevent escalation of conflict. Respond appropriately to aggressive behavior.	Value prevention of assaults and loss of dignity for patients, staff, and aggressor.
Analyze potential and actual impact of national patient safety resources, initiatives, and regulations.	Use national patient safety resources: • For your own professional development • To focus attention on safety in care settings • To design and implement improvements in practice	Value relationship between national patient safety campaigns and implementation in local practices and practice settings.

TABLE C.6 Informatics

Definition: Use information and technology to communicate, manage knowledge, mitigate error, and support decision-making.

KNOWLEDGE	SKILLS	ATTITUDES
Contrast benefits and limitations of common information technology strategies used in the delivery of patient care. Evaluate the strengths and weaknesses of information systems used in patient care.	Participate in the selection, design, implementation, and evaluation of information systems. Communicate the integral role of information technology in nurses' work. Model behaviors that support implementation and appropriate use of electronic health records. Assist team members to adopt information technology by piloting and evaluating proposed technologies.	Value the use of information and communication technologies in patient care.

KNOWLEDGE	SKILLS	ATTITUDES
Formulate **essential information that must be available in a common database to support patient care in the practice specialty.** Evaluate **benefits and limitations of different communication technologies and their impact on safety and quality.**	Promote access to patient care information for all professionals who provide care to patients. Serve as a resource for how to document nursing care at basic and advanced levels. Develop safeguards for protected health information. Champion communication technologies that support clinical decision-making, error prevention, care coordination, and protection of patient privacy.	**Appreciate the need for consensus and collaboration in developing systems to manage information for patient care.** **Value the confidentiality and security of all patient records.**
Describe and critique taxonomic and terminology systems used in national efforts to enhance interoperability of information systems and knowledge management systems.	Access and evaluate high quality electronic sources of healthcare information. Participate in the design of clinical decision-making supports and alerts. Search, retrieve, and manage data to make decisions using information and knowledge management systems. Anticipate unintended consequences of new technology.	**Value the importance of standardized terminologies in conducting searches for patient information.** **Appreciate the contribution of technological alert systems** **Appreciate** the time, effort, and skill required for computers, databases, and other technologies to become reliable and effective tools for patient care.

Index

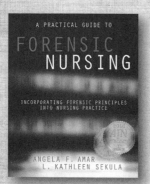
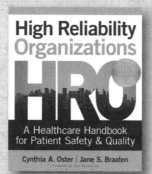
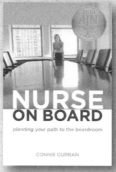
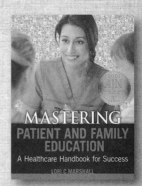
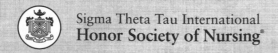
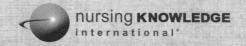

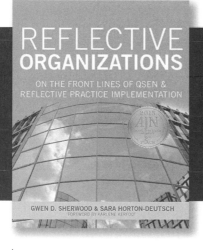

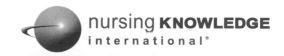

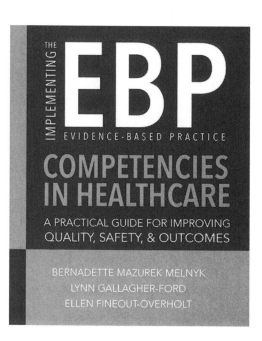
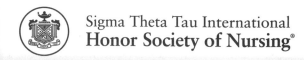
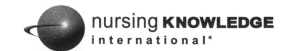

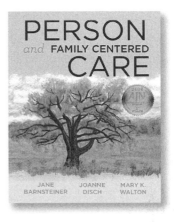
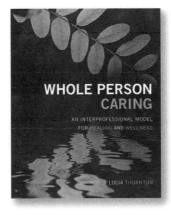
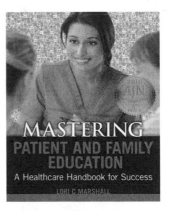
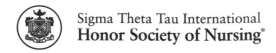
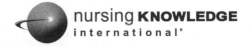

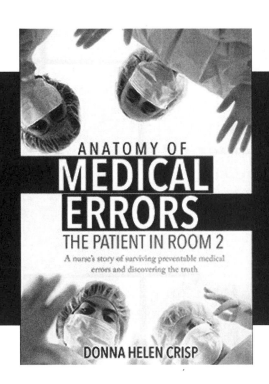

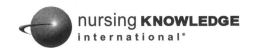